THE

Life Extension
REVOLUTION

Disease Prevention and Treatment, a comprehensive reference published by the Life Extension Foundation, contains more than 1,600 pages of up-to-the-minute research and treatment protocols. A searchable CD-ROM of the entire book is available free to anyone who has purchased *The Life Extension Revolution.* If the postage-paid response card is missing from your book, simply call 1-877-877-9705, and request the CD by mentioning code REV.

THE
Life Extension
REVOLUTION

THE NEW SCIENCE
OF GROWING OLDER
WITHOUT AGING

PHILIP LEE MILLER, M.D.
and the
LIFE EXTENSION FOUNDATION
with Monica Reinagel

A Lynn Sonberg Book
BANTAM BOOKS

The therapies described in this book are designed to be used with the assistance of an accredited anti-aging physician. Such a specialist is necessary to evaluate your status, fine-tune your dosages, watch for any side effects, and monitor your ongoing progress. The organizations listed in the appendix can refer you to members or board-certified anti-aging physicians in your area.

THE LIFE EXTENSION REVOLUTION
A Bantam Book / May 2005

Published by
Bantam Dell
A Division of Random House, Inc.
New York, New York

Book design by Sabrina Bowers

Bantam Books is a registered trademark of Random House, Inc.,
and the colophon is a trademark of Random House, Inc.

LIBRARY OF CONGRESS CATALOGING-IN-PUBLICATION DATA
Miller, Philip Lee.
The life extension revolution : the new science of growing older without aging /
Philip Lee Miller and the Life Extension Foundation with Monica Reinagel.
p.   cm.
"A Lynn Sonberg book."
Includes bibliographical references and index.
ISBN 0-553-80353-0
1. Longevity.   I. Reinagel, Monica.   II. Life Extension Foundation.   III. Title.
RA776.75.M54 2005
613.2—dc22   2005043086

Printed in the United States of America
Published simultaneously in Canada

www.bantamdell.com

10 9 8 7 6 5 4
BVG

To Maimonides, Paracelsus, Galileo, Semmelweiss, and Linus Pauling. We stand on the shoulders of the giants who, before us, had the courage to challenge entrenched ideas and beliefs. That is the true measure of human progress.

—P.M.

Contents

THE
Life Extension
REVOLUTION

Introduction

The Life Extension Vision

I DID NOT BEGIN MY career practicing anti-aging medicine—far from it. My specialty was emergency medicine and neurology. The patients I treated were in crisis, suffering from chest pains, difficulty breathing, loss of circulation, or in full-blown cardiac arrest. Even then, I knew that most of them were suffering from conditions that might have been avoided through a healthier lifestyle, nutrition, and preventive medicine. But in the emergency room, there's no time for that. There is just a never-ending flow of sick and dying people needing aggressive or even heroic measures to save their lives.

Burnout is common among emergency room doctors. After a while, it begins to feel like fighting a fire that continues to blaze out of control because no one has time to turn off the gas. After several years in emergency medicine, I was looking for a new direction. When I saw a notice for a conference being held by a new organization called the American Academy of Anti-Aging Medicine (known as the A⁴M), I immediately knew that this was my future, and the future of medicine as a whole.

I can remember the electricity and excitement that was in the air at that first meeting. Here was a group of outspoken doctors and scientists who were no longer willing to accept the conventional approach to medicine but had a much different vision—one in which common diseases are obsolete, eighty-year-olds are fit and healthy, and the outer limit of human life span is measured in centuries rather than decades. It was—and still is—a radical vision, but one that is fueled by stunning recent advances in our understanding of the mechanisms of aging, right down to the molecular level. You'll find these cutting-edge discoveries throughout the chapters—and the anti-aging program—that follows.

THE LIFE EXTENSION FOUNDATION

It was at that meeting that I met the organizers of the Life Extension Foundation (LEF), a group of researchers, writers, and advocates for anti-aging and life extension medicine. I was immediately impressed by their courage in challenging the conventional wisdom with provocative new ideas about health and medicine. LEF's track record for getting it right and getting it first is long and impressive:

➢ Since the early 1990s, antioxidants have been widely recognized as essential to maintaining health and preventing disease. But LEF first put forward the notion that antioxidant nutrients could stave off disease back in 1980, long before others in the medical community were paying attention to these important compounds.

➢ In 1981, LEF identified the importance of lowering homocysteine to prevent stroke and heart disease. Over ten years went by before mainstream researchers began to acknowledge the role of homocysteine in heart disease.

➢ In 1983, LEF published its conclusion that aspirin therapy could prevent heart attacks, a position that the American Heart Association didn't fully endorse until 1997.

➢ By the time mainstream medicine began looking into a little-known nutrient called coenzyme Q_{10}, LEF members had already been reaping the benefits of this miracle anti-aging nutrient for many years. In fact, LEF was the first to introduce CoQ_{10} in the United States, in 1983.

> LEF introduced its findings on lycopene in 1985, but it was well over a decade before the nutrient became widely recognized for its ability to prevent and slow the growth of certain types of cancer.

> In 1999, LEF took the controversial and highly contested position that leading estrogen replacement therapies might not provide protection against heart disease—a position that later was proven to be entirely correct.

Science has repeatedly ratified the many controversial positions LEF has advanced. Over the years, the foundation's careful, rigorous, and responsible approach has made it well regarded by even the most conventional of physicians.

The foundation has also been tireless and outspoken in its advocacy for the rights of doctors and patients to have access to the best information and most promising treatments. More than a decade ago, LEF helped to convince the FDA to fast-track approval for lifesaving experimental drugs. It has since sponsored bills that allow Americans to purchase prescription medications more cheaply, and fought against government opposition to legitimate alternative medicine therapies. LEF's commitment to freedom of information and access has led to landmark court decisions that protect these rights. I can think of no other organization that is so purposeful and articulate on this issue.

In addition to making important information more widely available, LEF has contributed greatly to our knowledge about disease and aging by supporting much-needed research through its nonprofit foundation. It has funded a wide variety of groundbreaking research, including an experimental antioxidant/drug cocktail that can protect the brain against severe oxygen deprivation, cutting-edge technology to preserve organs for transplant, and a project that will identify the genes that control aging and longevity. Now celebrating its twenty-fifth anniversary, LEF is the largest organization of its kind, dedicated to radically extending the healthy human life span by developing methods to control aging and disease.

FROM CRISIS TO TURNING POINT

It was also at the A⁴M conference that I met Dr. Julian Whitaker, one of the pioneers of preventive and nutritional medicine. As a result of that encounter, I spent a year at the Whitaker Wellness Institute, immersing myself in an entirely new approach to medicine—one that emphasized nutritional therapies for the treatment and prevention of disease. Whitaker was fond of saying, "We don't practice alternative medicine here. We practice good medicine." I've never forgotten those words.

Prior to my time at the Whitaker Institute, my own health had taken a sudden turn for the worse. A blood test revealed that I had developed a severe lipid imbalance. My cholesterol—which had always been ideal—was suddenly 280 and my triglycerides had skyrocketed to 650! Reflexively, I went to see an internist whom I had known when I practiced emergency medicine, and he recommended aggressive treatment with cholesterol-lowering drugs. But I realized that this was a chance to put the new principles I had been working with to the test. I had been "talking the talk"; now it was time to "walk the walk."

I put myself on a serious regimen of vitamins and antioxidants. I radically changed my diet and got serious about reducing stress. Against the advice of my conventionally minded colleague (and contrary to my own early training), I took no drugs. And it worked! Within five weeks, my cholesterol went from 280 to 160, and my triglycerides were down to 300. I stuck with it, and over the next year, I lost a total of 38 pounds, my cholesterol declined to 140, and my triglycerides went down to 98. And I felt so much better—younger, more energetic, fantastic!

From that point, there was no turning back. I was completely committed—personally *and* professionally—to a new way of practicing medicine. In 1996, I founded the Los Gatos Longevity Institute, a center devoted to providing comprehensive anti-aging medical care. Several years later, I was greatly honored when the Life Extension Foundation invited me to join its medical advisory board.

FROM REVOLUTION TO REALITY

My colleagues at LEF include some of world's leading scientists and anti-aging researchers, as well as hundreds of physicians who practice anti-aging medicine. In addition, LEF includes well over a hundred thousand members of every background and profession who are united by their desire to live longer and healthier lives. Every member of LEF has access to the most cutting-edge information and research on life-saving therapies and disease prevention protocols, in a forum that is constantly challenging, updating, and refining our understanding of these complex issues.

And now, for the first time, this phenomenal store of information is being shared with a wider audience. The anti-aging program offered in this book is the culmination of the very latest LEF research as well as my own years of clinical experience. These are the same therapies and protocols that have helped hundreds of my own patients and thousands of Life Extension Foundation members to grow older without aging. The program is also supported by hundreds of studies and clinical trials, including LEF-funded research on anti-aging and life extension. You'll find complete references to all of this research at the end of the book, organized by chapter and listed in the order in which studies are discussed in the text.

! Anti-aging medicine uses powerful tools—therapies that can rejuvenate and disease-proof your body. And like any power tools, these therapies must be used with care. The caution icons throughout the book highlight important warnings and safeguards that will help you use these protocols safely and effectively. You won't find miracle cures or hype here. Instead, you'll find a comprehensive, balanced, and responsible approach that will profoundly slow the rate at which your body is aging.

Throughout the following pages, you will also see text marked by a CD icon, indicating that additional information is available in LEF's *Disease Prevention and Treatment,* a comprehensive reference tool that includes over 1,600 pages of up-to-the-minute research and protocols. A searchable CD-ROM of the entire book is free to purchasers of this book. To request your free CD, simply return the card inserted into every copy or call the toll-free number on page ii. You'll also find updates to this invaluable material at www.lef.org.

The Life Extension Foundation has a compelling vision of the future as a time when we will no longer live in anxiety and fear of premature death and wasting illness. We will retire from one career at 65 and embark on a new course of education, or launch another full-time career. We will have the option of starting our families at the age of 50, with every expectation of seeing our grandchildren graduate from college. This vision is not simply a futuristic fantasy. The stark reality is that unless we can discover how to grow older without growing sicker and more disabled, we simply will not have the resources to care for our rapidly aging population. This is a challenge we *must* meet—and win.

To those who are not following anti-aging medicine closely, it may seem that we are no closer to making these dreams a reality than we were fifty years ago. But as LEF members know, we are in truth on the very brink of discoveries that could radically change the course of human history, thanks in large part to research supported and conducted by LEF itself. Within the last five years, thanks to advances in cellular, molecular, and even atomic medicine, we have made unprecedented progress in understanding the factors that drive disease and aging. Within the next ten to twenty years, much of the LEF vision will have become everyday reality.

That's why this book was written—and why it is more urgently needed than ever before. Your customized anti-aging and life extension program will give you a more youthful, energetic, and disease-proof body and mind. More importantly, it will help to ensure that you'll be there to take full advantage of all that the ever-expanding future holds.

PART I

EXTENDING THE PRIME OF LIFE

Extending the prime of life is about growing older without aging. Over the course of the twentieth century, the average life span for Americans almost doubled, to 76.5 years of age. Unfortunately, we have not done as good a job of slowing the degenerative processes that accompany aging. We now see a ballooning population of sick, elderly people, who face years of pain, disability, isolation, and infirmity.

The goal of anti-aging medicine is not just to extend your life span but to lengthen your healthy, functional life span. In this part of the program, we focus on the anti-aging strategies that will help you retain your physical vigor, mental clarity, and youthful appearance as you grow older.

CHAPTER 1

A New Role for Medicine

Every man desires to live long, but no man would be old.
—JONATHAN SWIFT

RIAN BECAME A PATIENT of mine about three years ago. He was 47 years old. He came to see me not because he was sick but because he wanted to feel better. Brian had built a successful software consulting firm and had worked hard to keep his business going while the high-tech industry went through difficult times. Now he was looking forward to enjoying the fruits of his labors. "I feel like the next twenty years should be the best of my entire life," he told me, "and I want to be in good health. No, in the best health possible."

By all conventional measures, Brian was in fairly good health already. Nonetheless, he felt that he was slowing down. He wasn't planning to retire for another ten years or so, but he was finding it harder and harder to stay focused and motivated at work. His sex life with his wife had tapered off. To add insult to injury, he noticed that his hair was getting thinner at about the same rate that his waistline was getting thicker. In short, Brian was experiencing physical and mental changes typical for someone his age.

Tina first consulted me at age 66, a little over a year ago. Like Brian, she wasn't sick but was sure she could feel better than she did. Tina is a gregarious, widely traveled woman who has always loved meeting new people and new challenges. She'd been looking forward to her retirement as a time when she'd be free for travel and adventure. But she'd noticed that she had begun to have trouble remembering details and names and felt more easily fatigued. "I hate feeling like a befuddled old woman," she said. "It's just not who I am!"

Widowed eight years before, Tina was still a warm and vibrant woman with a lot to offer. She was open to the possibility of meeting someone to enjoy her later years with. But she was becoming less confident about her appearance. She felt that she looked older than she was—and certainly older than she felt. Although everything Tina described was fairly normal for a 66-year-old, she was frustrated and upset by the changes she was noticing.

Both Brian and Tina wanted to know what anti-aging medicine could offer.

THE PROMISE OF ANTI-AGING MEDICINE

Twenty-five years ago, it probably wouldn't have occurred to someone in Brian or Tina's situation to seek help from a doctor. It would have been even harder to find a doctor who would have known what to do for them. Neither one of them was significantly overweight; neither smoked or drank to excess. Because they took reasonably good care of themselves, neither was suffering (yet) from heart disease, diabetes, or other conditions that might require treatment. By conventional standards, there was nothing wrong with them. They were in acceptable health . . . *for their age.*

By those standards, people such as Tina and Brian could do little besides wait for the aging process to unfold, and hope for the best. Along the way, doctors would assure them that aches and pains, failing body parts, and increasing weakness and frailty were simply a normal part of the aging process. As the diseases of aging (heart disease, arthritis, osteoporosis, diabetes, Alzheimer's disease, prostate cancer, etc.) set in, drugs would be prescribed to manage them.

Most people are accustomed to this style of medicine—and this rather hopeless view of the aging process. Anti-aging medicine, on the other hand, takes an entirely different approach. Whereas the focus of conventional medicine is on the diagnosis and treatment of disease, the goal of anti-aging medicine is to promote *optimal* health and wellness throughout every phase of the human life span. This visionary approach is built on four basic but radical principles:

> **Anti-aging medicine is *functional*.** By this, I mean that we are not just concerned with what might be going wrong in your body. Instead, we aim to improve and rejuvenate every function of the body—making the body stronger, healthier, and more youthful.

> **Anti-aging medicine is *preventive*.** Once full-blown disease has taken hold, even the best drugs and therapies sometimes offer only limited hope. Therefore, we take aggressive action to *prevent* the diseases of aging with nutritional and metabolic therapies.

> **Anti-aging medicine is *holistic*.** Too often, the conventional medical system sees patients as a collection of parts to be fixed by various specialists. As a result, many people continue to feel lousy despite the fact that they have an entire team of doctors working on them. By contrast, anti-aging medicine takes a holistic view of the body and of each person. Each aspect of your health is considered and treated in view of the whole person.

> **Anti-aging medicine is *integrative*.** Unfortunately, our medical community has been fractured into highly politicized camps, with a great deal of mistrust and even hostility between the conventional and alternative movements. There are some conventional doctors who insist that all herbal and nutritional remedies are snake oil, just as there are some alternative physicians who consider all pharmaceutical drugs to be poison. Of course, neither of these extreme statements is true, and this sort of dogmatic rigidity gets in the way of progress. Anti-aging medicine offers the distinct advantage of being truly *integrative* medicine. By remaining open-minded but science-based, we can combine the best and most effective therapies from conventional and alternative approaches.

It may indeed be normal for people to get weaker, slower, sicker, or more forgetful as they get older. But I want something better for my patients, and for you. No matter what your age or health status right now, my goal is for you to experience a state of exceptional wellness, and to maintain that healthier, more youthful state as you get older. That, in a nutshell, is the goal—and the promise—of anti-aging medicine.

DELIVERING ON THE PROMISE

With both Tina and Brian, I went through the same steps that you will be going through in this book, building a comprehensive anti-aging program that was personalized for their individual needs. First, we analyzed every aspect of their health, including hormone levels, nutrient status, organ function, body composition, stress levels, disease risk factors, mood, performance, and cognitive function. All of these factors are *biomarkers of aging.* They indicate the functional status of your cells and organs and reveal how quickly or slowly you are aging.

Based on this information, I developed programs for each of them. First, I coached them on diet and nutrition, exercise, stress reduction, and other lifestyle factors that are the foundation of an anti-aging program. (You'll find these discussed in detail in Part III.) Gradually, each of them implemented a customized program of anti-aging nutrients and hormonal supplements, based on the science and principles that we will be discussing in the next chapters. Over the course of weeks and months, as their cells, organs, and glands began to function better and better, both Brian and Tina began to notice big changes.

Six weeks after beginning his anti-aging program, Brian was already feeling on top of the world. He was fired up at work, instead of fighting off the Monday (and often Tuesday and Wednesday) blues. He'd lost about 8 pounds, although he had not been eating any less, and reported that things in the bedroom had taken off. "I feel like I did when I was a freshman in college," he said. Brian couldn't wait to continue with the next levels of the program. Three years later, he has met and exceeded every goal he set for himself.

If you met Brian today, you'd probably guess he was at least ten years younger than he is. Although his chronological age is now 50, I would judge his biological age, as measured by his hormone profiles, neurological function, heart health, immune status, organ function, and body composition, to be somewhere between 38 and 43, and holding. Seeing a patient experience this sort of metamorphosis is the reason I love practicing anti-aging medicine.

Tina also felt a huge surge in energy during the first few weeks of her anti-aging program. Over the next three months, she noted steady improvement in her memory and recall and general mental clarity. Instead of feeling her horizons narrowing, Tina felt that the world was once again her playground.

Not only did she feel better, but Tina also looked younger as a result of the anti-aging therapies she implemented. You could see the difference in her skin, the way she moved, and her attitude. Coming back from a trip, she told me that a man in the group who was ten years younger than she was had asked her for a date! "I never thought I'd see those days again," she said. A year later, Tina says she hates to think what her life would look like today if she hadn't taken action against aging.

Throughout this book you will meet more people like Tina and Brian, who not only feel and look years younger as a result of anti-aging therapies but have also pulled themselves back from the brink of serious disease, resolved lifelong health issues, and reduced or discontinued unnecessary or harmful medications.

No matter what your age or current health, anti-aging medicine offers you the same opportunity. With the program outlined in this book and the help of a qualified anti-aging medical professional, you can rejuvenate your body inside and out. You can vastly reduce your chances of disease and disability. You can enjoy the most vibrant health of your lifetime.

HOW AND WHY DO WE AGE?

The key to controlling the aging process lies in a better understanding of how and why we age the way we do. Only then can we take steps to slow or reverse that process. In just the past few years, we have gathered an enormous amount of new information about how our bodies age. This insight has already led to dramatic advances in effective anti-aging therapies, with the promise of more to come in the very near future.

Aging, we have learned, is not just a matter of mechanical wear and tear, cellular exhaustion, environmental toxins, or genetic programming. It is not simply hormonal, nor is it caused entirely by free radical damage, pathogens, or structural changes. And yet, all of these things play a role.

> **Cellular "programming."** To a certain extent, the decline in function and wellness we experience as we age is programmed by nature. The cells in your body are continually reproducing, replacing old and damaged cells with new ones. But every cell, even the ones that are newly formed, has an internal clock that remembers how old you are. That clock determines how that cell behaves, affecting how quickly the cell responds to messages from other cells and what quantities of hormones, enzymes, and other cellular chemicals are produced.

> **Biochemistry.** As cellular behavior changes with age, the resulting changes in biochemistry and hormone profiles have a sort of domino effect throughout the body. Your metabolism slows, and more fat is stored under the skin and around organs. The body breaks down muscle and connective tissue more quickly, while its rebuilding capacities slow down. The digestive system becomes less efficient at extracting nutrients from food. Cells and organs become less effective at detoxification functions. Nerve cells in the brain shrink and stiffen. The immune system becomes less vigilant against invading microbes or mutated cells.

> **Environmental influences.** The effects of changing biochemistry on your organs and tissues are compounded by factors from the external environment. Every day, our bodies are bombarded by ultraviolet radiation, assaulted by free radical molecules, and exposed to a multitude of bugs and germs as well as natural and man-made toxins. All of these interact with our genetic "program" to speed (or slow) the aging process.

> **Heredity.** In addition to the changes that are programmed to occur as we get older, we each also have a unique set of inherited genetic influences that affect how quickly or slowly we age, and may predispose us to certain diseases or conditions.

> **Lifestyle factors.** Our daily lifestyle habits, such as how much sleep we get, how much stress we are under, and what we eat or don't eat, also play a huge role in how our bodies cope with the internal and external factors that drive the aging process.

We'll be discussing all of these aspects in greater detail in the coming chapters. But even this brief outline shows that aging is a very complex process involving many factors. Figure 1.1 on the following page shows how these various factors interact with one another and flow down through multiple, overlapping layers of cause and effect. Notice that the typical symptoms and diseases of aging, seen at the very bottom of the diagram, are actually the culmination of a very long process that begins much earlier, long before we are old or even middle-aged.

THE AGING YOU CAN SEE IN THE MIRROR

Let's make this abstract discussion a bit more concrete by looking at a specific example of the aging process—one you can observe in the mirror. As we get older, the smooth, firm, and unlined skin we all have when we are young gradually becomes looser, less firm, and increasingly creased and wrinkled.

FIGURE 1.1. THE AGING PROCESS: AN OVERVIEW

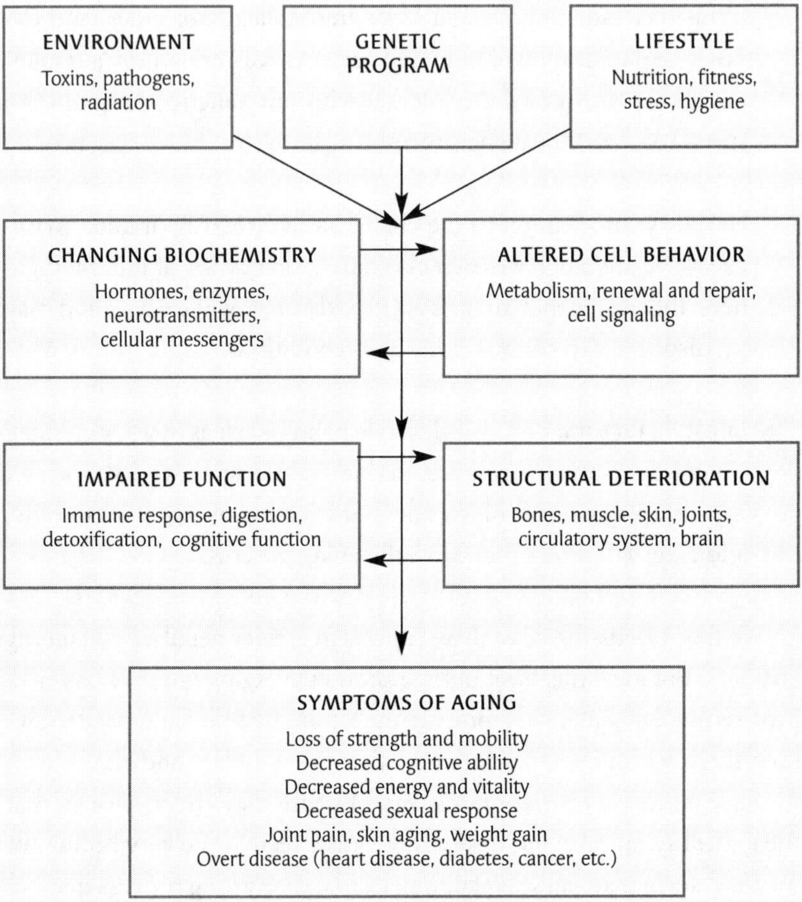

ENVIRONMENT Toxins, pathogens, radiation	GENETIC PROGRAM	LIFESTYLE Nutrition, fitness, stress, hygiene

CHANGING BIOCHEMISTRY Hormones, enzymes, neurotransmitters, cellular messengers	ALTERED CELL BEHAVIOR Metabolism, renewal and repair, cell signaling

IMPAIRED FUNCTION Immune response, digestion, detoxification, cognitive function	STRUCTURAL DETERIORATION Bones, muscle, skin, joints, circulatory system, brain

SYMPTOMS OF AGING
Loss of strength and mobility
Decreased cognitive ability
Decreased energy and vitality
Decreased sexual response
Joint pain, skin aging, weight gain
Overt disease (heart disease, diabetes, cancer, etc.)

Factors from the environment, our lifestyle habits, and our genetic programming all contribute to a cascade of cause and effect that ultimately produces symptoms of aging.

Like all aging, skin aging is the result of a combination of genetic and environmental factors. As we get older, changes in cellular behavior lead to changes in hormone levels that cause the skin to become thinner. The barrier function of the skin, which attracts and retains moisture in the skin, also becomes less effective, making the skin drier as well.

Underneath the skin is a flexible support structure made up of collagen fibers. But aging skin cells produce more collagenase, an enzyme that breaks down collagen. At the same time, the cells become less responsive to signals that tell them to increase production of fresh collagen. Because the skin is breaking down collagen faster than it is replacing it, the collagen layer underneath the skin begins to shrink and collapse. On the surface, the skin becomes loose and spongy and begins to fold in on itself, forming lines and wrinkles.

All of this is part of the genetic program for aging. The speed and timing of your particular aging program will be determined in part by heredity. But environmental factors greatly compound these genetically triggered changes in skin function. Ultraviolet radiation from the sun further stimulates the production of collagenase, the enzyme that breaks down collagen. It also creates enormous numbers of free radicals in the skin. That's where lifestyle issues (diet and nutrition) come into play. If there are sufficient antioxidant reserves in the body, excessive free radicals are largely neutralized. But if nutrition is poor and antioxidant levels are low, the free radicals can damage skin cell membranes, causing changes in pigmentation that show up as age spots or darkened patches of skin on the hands and face.

Of course, aging affects more than just the cosmetic appearance of skin. It also affects its health and function. Many people, for example, spend a lot of time outdoors in the sun when they are young. And yet skin cancer is relatively rare in younger people. But as we get older, skin cancer becomes more and more common. Why?

At any age, ultraviolet rays and free radicals can damage the DNA in skin cells, causing them to mutate and begin abnormal replication. This is the first step toward developing skin cancer. But in a youthful, healthy body, these mutated cells are destroyed by the immune system before they can cause a problem. As we get older, hormonal and cellular changes render the immune system less vigilant. As a result, mutated and malignant cells are more likely to survive and continue dividing, eventually forming cancerous growths.

Do you see how genetic, biochemical, environmental, and lifestyle

FIGURE 1.2. SKIN AGING: A SPECIFIC EXAMPLE

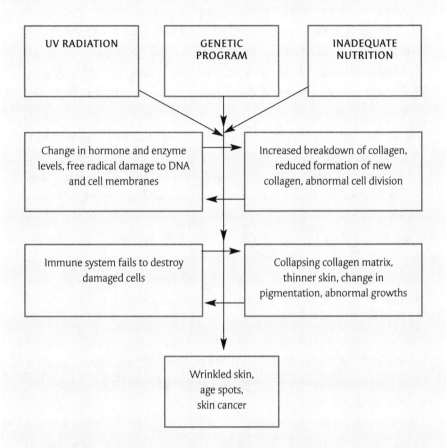

The same environmental, genetic, and lifestyle factors that contribute to the aging of our organs are responsible for the visible signs of aging in the skin.

factors interact to cause the changes in structure and function that we can observe in aging skin? These same factors are affecting every system, organ, and tissue of your body. Together, they produce the effect that we know as aging.

WHAT CAN BE DONE TO SLOW AGING?

The good news is that we can do a lot to reduce, correct, or compensate for the many biochemical and metabolic changes that occur as our bodies get older. At the genetic level, we are getting very close to isolating and identifying the precise parts of the genetic code that cause our cells to function differently as we age. This may eventually allow us to halt or reverse the genetically programmed changes that contribute to aging.

In the meantime, we can compensate for age-related hormonal declines with bioidentical hormone replacement protocols. This can help to prevent the changes in biochemistry, metabolism, and cell function that lead to poor health as we age.

Nutrient protocols can enhance immune surveillance, support organ function, improve detoxification, and improve cellular repair. Dietary and lifestyle changes support metabolism, detoxification, and disease resistance. On the environmental front, we can reduce our exposure to radiation, toxins, and pathogens. Each of these approaches is described in detail in the chapters that follow.

Any one of these steps will lead to a remarkable improvement in your health. In fact, you will come across many nutrients and therapies in the following pages that at one time or another were heralded as the silver bullet that would prevent all aging. As the field of anti-aging medicine has matured, we now know that as powerful and important as these discoveries have been, no one hormone or vitamin can prevent aging.

Just as there is a cascade effect in aging, with changes triggering further changes and effects compounded by other effects, anti-aging therapies likewise have cascading and compounding effects. The true power of anti-aging medicine is the integration of all of these tools into a comprehensive approach.

FIGURE 1.3. INTEGRATED ANTI-AGING PROGRAM

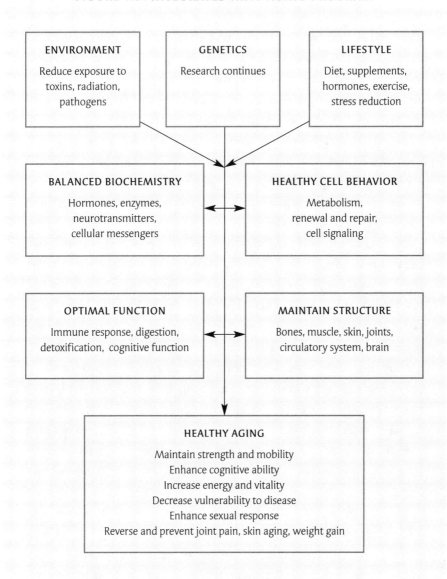

A comprehensive program, addressing all the different causes of aging, can positively affect the cascade, slowing the symptoms of aging and maximizing health as we get older.

THE FUTURE HAS ARRIVED

Anti-aging medicine is now the fastest-growing medical specialty in the United States. This reflects more than merely a change in attitude and philosophy. It reflects the enormous scientific advances that have been made in our understanding of the causes and treatments for aging.

It also recognizes the economic and social imperative we face as senior citizens become the largest sector of our society. With dwindling government resources and a crippled medical safety net, the pursuit of anti-aging therapies is a matter not of vanity but of survival.

It's no longer acceptable or responsible for doctors to dismiss a gradual deterioriation of function and wellness as "what happens when you get older." It's also not good enough to medicate symptoms as they arise, using pain relievers, antacids, arthritis drugs, and cholesterol medications. We must find a way to remain healthy, vital, and productive as we enjoy the longer life span that modernity has made possible.

The program you are about to embark upon will allow you to grow older *without becoming aged*. It will maximize your chances of not only a long life but a long and healthy life. Anti-aging medicine is more than just a medical specialty. It is the future of medicine and the future of humankind.

CHAPTER 2

Overcoming the Aging Effects of Stress

Every stress leaves an indelible scar, and the organism pays for its survival after a stressful situation by becoming a little older.
—HANS SELYE

I HAVE KNOWN PEOPLE—and perhaps you are one of them—who claim to thrive on stress. They feel that stress, challenge, and competition motivate them to perform better, to achieve and accomplish more. This makes perfect sense. Adrenaline and cortisol, the hormones that your body produces when you are excited or challenged (or angry or threatened), are specifically designed to help you function at a higher level, making you stronger, faster, and smarter.

While it is true that cortisol and adrenaline can have these very beneficial effects, your body is simply not designed to live on a steady diet of these hormones. Adrenaline works much like caffeine in the body, stimulating the sympathetic nervous system to create a hyperalert state. But in the same way that drinking too much coffee can leave you feeling weak and jittery, too much adrenaline is exhausting to the system.

The effects of excess cortisol are even more dangerous. Over time, too much cortisol in your system can harden your arteries, poison your brain cells, thin your bones, pad your waistline, and put your immune system to sleep. What's more, stress also burns up your supply of DHEA, a crucial anti-aging hormone. In fact, stress can quickly give you the hormone profile of someone twice your age.

Have you ever heard a story about someone's hair turning white as a result of a shock or trauma? New research shows that this old tale has a basis in fact. A fascinating study reported by the National Academy of Sciences in late 2004 showed that the biological impact of stress extends all the way to the genetic level, where it affects the part of our genes which, among other things, determine when our hair begins to turn gray.

Researchers at the University of California at San Francisco looked at the DNA of about five dozen women, some of whom were caring for children with severe disabilities. Not surprisingly, the mothers with disabled children felt that they were under heavy stress. And, in fact, the scientists found that the stress of caring for these children could actually be seen in the mothers' DNA—which resembled the DNA of much older women.

More common than the go-getters who thrive on stress are those who—like these mothers—feel mentally and physically exhausted by the stress in their lives. But I don't find that it's very helpful simply to advise people to reduce stress. Obviously, if they could see how to make their lives less stressful, they would have done so already. And even if they could somehow manage to schedule a vacation or make time for a yoga class, reversing the physiological damage caused by chronic stress may require more aggressive intervention.

Here's the point that many people don't understand about stress: It doesn't matter whether the stress is good or bad. It doesn't matter whether you win or lose. If you have a chronic imbalance of stress hormones (too much cortisol and too little DHEA), you are aging faster than you need to, and opening the door for diseases from heart disease to diabetes to depression. Even if you can't have—or don't want—a less stressful life, you need to buffer your body from the aging effects of stress hormones.

STRESSED FOR SUCCESS

Dr. Hans Selye, the brilliant physician who first identified and mapped out the stress response, acknowledged that stress was an unavoidable fact of life. After a lifetime of research on the health effects of stress,

Selye ultimately concluded that stress was absolutely necessary to our survival, and even desirable for its ability to enhance our performance. As he wrote in *The Stress of Life* (a highly readable—and highly recommended—treatise that remains as seminal today as it was when he wrote it five decades ago), "the complete absence of stress is death."

But as Selye and later stress researchers have shown, our individual response to stress is the critical factor that determines its impact on our health. (See also Robert Sapolsky's entertaining book *Why Zebras Don't Get Ulcers.*) Some personality types handle stress more successfully than others. Others (the so-called type A's) are at particular risk from stress-related disease. Herbert Benson, Jon Kabat-Zinn, and other relaxation researchers have shown that we can all learn to respond to stress more skillfully, using mind-body techniques to minimize the damage to our systems. Anti-aging medicine adds another powerful dimension by offering therapies that counteract the hormonal imbalances caused by stress.

Living on the Edge

Carrie is one of those people who seem to go from crisis to crisis. Carrie is smart and ambitious, but she tends to take on a little more than she can handle. She has so much going on all the time that things frequently seem to be on the verge of falling apart. When she first consulted me, she was once again going through a difficult time.

As the office manager for a busy marketing firm, Carrie had a lot of responsibility at work. She was also going to school at night to earn her MBA. The workload at school was overwhelming, and her boss was not sympathetic or understanding about the extra demands that her schoolwork was making on her time. To top it all off, she'd recently broken up with her live-in boyfriend and was sleeping on a friend's couch until she could move into a new apartment. But she couldn't seem to muster the energy to look for an apartment in addition to everything else she was juggling.

Not surprisingly, Carrie's stress level was very high. She was experiencing a variety of physical and emotional symptoms, including depression, panic attacks, and difficulty sleeping. The antidepressants that her doctor had prescribed didn't seem to be helping very much. When I questioned her a bit more, I learned that although the present circumstances were extreme, Carrie actually had been suffering from these kinds of stress-related symptoms for years. This suggested to me that Carrie might be at risk of more serious health problems, due to a chronic stress hormone imbalance.

Treating the Symptoms of Stress Just Masks the Problem

Doctors typically treat stress-related symptoms such as Carrie's with everything from sleeping aids and antidepressants to beta-blockers and antianxiety medications. Not only do these drugs carry serious side effects and risks of their own, but none of them addresses the hormonal impact of stress.

With my own patients, I aim to do more than relieve the symptoms of stress. I also want to bring the stress hormones back into a healthy balance. Interestingly, I find that the symptoms usually improve or disappear altogether in the process. Medications can be avoided or reduced. At the same time, risk factors can be reversed. The aging process can be slowed. This chapter will show you how to do exactly that.

How Well Are You Coping?

Some people are able to handle a lot of stress; others seem to unravel over relatively minor problems. Our individual tolerance for stress has a lot to do with genetics and personality type. Even those who do well under stressful conditions, however, may be suffering from the invisible effects of stress hormone imbalance. A blood test can give you and your physician a more precise picture of how well or how poorly your body is coping with stress.

To evaluate the impact of stress, I look at the levels of two important hormones. Cortisol is one of the "fight-or-flight" hormones produced by the adrenal glands in response to stress. People under stress have elevated levels of cortisol, which, as we have already seen, can be a serious health risk. The other hormone that I look at is dehydroepiandrosterone

(DHEA), which is also produced by the adrenals (as well as by the ovaries or testicles, in smaller amounts). Chronic stress tends to depress DHEA levels.

Often referred to as *the* anti-aging hormone, DHEA is the most abundant of all the steroid hormones. It is anabolic in nature, meaning that it promotes the renewal and replacement of tissues. For example, it stimulates the activity of osteoblasts (bone-building cells) and fibroblasts (skin-renewal cells), which translates into strong bones and youthful skin.

DHEA is highly active in the brain, increasing the levels of neurotransmitters that are crucial for both short- and long-term memory and learning. By promoting neurotransmitter production, DHEA appears to protect the brain against age-associated decline.

A robust immune response likewise depends on DHEA to boost the number of immune cells and increase their vigilance and activity. DHEA regulates immune function by modulating the release of interleukins, interferons, tumor necrosis factor, and other immune chemicals that can have a positive or negative effect on your health.

DHEA is also converted in the body to other steroid hormones, including testosterone and estrogen. Low levels of this master hormone can mean that levels of other important hormones become depressed as well. In this way, the effects of low DHEA cascade throughout the entire endocrine system, affecting the cardiovascular system, immune system, and metabolism.

In general, those patients who look and feel young for their age generally have higher DHEA levels than other people their age. People with low DHEA levels are more likely to suffer from heart disease, diabetes, cancer, and depression.

THE IDEAL BALANCE
BETWEEN DHEA AND CORTISOL

In a healthy, youthful body, DHEA is high and cortisol is low. If you look at the graph below, you can see that in a healthy person, the ratio between DHEA and cortisol is very high, with fifteen times the amount of DHEA as cortisol.

As we get older, we tend to produce less DHEA and, at the same time, more cortisol. Stress creates the same effect, only more dramatically. In a stressed or aging person, the ratio between DHEA and cortisol is much lower than in a youthful person, with perhaps only two or three times as much DHEA compared to cortisol. This is why I think of stress as the great aging accelerator. It mimics and exaggerates aging and disease processes.

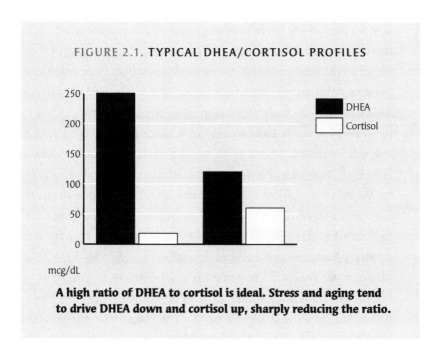

FIGURE 2.1. TYPICAL DHEA/CORTISOL PROFILES

mcg/dL

A high ratio of DHEA to cortisol is ideal. Stress and aging tend to drive DHEA down and cortisol up, sharply reducing the ratio.

Given what I saw and heard in my initial interview with Carrie, I wasn't surprised at the results of her blood work when they came back from the lab. She displayed the classic hormone profile of someone under extreme stress: very high levels of cortisol and extremely low levels of DHEA. Her DHEA/cortisol ratio was very low (only two times as much DHEA as cortisol). The stress Carrie was experiencing had altered her hormone profile and was literally aging her body, both inside and out.

THE DANGERS OF EXCESS CORTISOL

Many of the most common health problems that plague us as we get older—high blood pressure, weight gain, memory loss, lowered immune response—are driven in part by the effects of too much cortisol. When stress elevates your cortisol levels, it simply speeds the whole process up.

> ➤ **High Cortisol Promotes Heart Disease, Obesity, and Diabetes**
> One of the ways that cortisol helps you to respond to emergencies is by rapidly increasing your blood sugar. When cortisol rises, it signals your body to release sugar from the tissues where it is stored into the bloodstream. In response to the elevated blood sugar levels, your pancreas secretes insulin, which clears the sugar from your blood and into your cells, where it is used for energy. This provides the fuel that your muscles might need to leap out of harm's way or lift a child to safety. While a burst of blood sugar might be crucial to your survival in a life-or-death situation, chronically high blood sugar is not at all healthy.
>
> When your cortisol level is chronically elevated due to stress, it creates a devastating cycle of alternating high blood sugar and high insulin. After a while, your body can begin to lose its sensitivity to insulin and become less effective in regulating your blood sugar levels. This common phenomenon is known by a number of names, including insulin resistance syndrome, metabolic syndrome, and syndrome X. The dangerous progression from elevated cortisol to elevated blood sugar to insulin resistance is one of the chief ways that stress contributes to disease and even death.
>
> Insulin resistance is the first step toward some very serious health consequences. To compensate for the effects of insulin resistance, your pancreas secretes more and more insulin. Excessive insulin, or hyperinsulinemia, increases fat storage, leading to weight gain and obesity. It can also have a negative effect on your blood pressure, cholesterol, and triglycerides. It is, in itself, a major risk factor for heart disease. Hyperinsulinemia is also a precursor to

adult-onset (type 2) diabetes, in which the pancreas becomes unable to sustain insulin production.

Today's high-stress lifestyle and sugar-laden diet make this silent, invisible syndrome perhaps the most widespread and dangerous health concern of the modern era. We will be discussing how to avoid the effects of insulin resistance again in Parts II and III.

> **Cortisol Derails the Immune Response** Chronic, long-term stress—and the resulting high cortisol levels—can eventually start to degrade your immune response. You may become less able to fight off infections, especially viral infections. Stressed-out people are more susceptible to colds and flu.

When the immune response is impaired, viruses that may reside in your body in a dormant state, such as many herpes family viruses, also get the green light. This is why cold sores and shingles often flare up in stressful times. And for people with cancer, high cortisol levels can suppress the body's ability to fight the cancer, increasing the chances that the cancer will metastasize throughout the body.

> **Cortisol Impairs Neurological Function** Cortisol is also harmful to your brain cells. Studies have shown that elevated cortisol, caused by stress or aging, can impair your memory and your cognitive function. High cortisol ages the brain and damages the neural cells. The decline in cognitive function (memory, reaction time, problem solving, learning ability) that is commonly seen in older people appears to be at least partly the result of higher cortisol levels. By increasing cortisol, stress mimics and hastens the effects of aging on the brain.

DHEA: THE ANTIDOTE TO STRESS AND AGING

DHEA is your body's own natural antidote to the negative effects of cortisol. In fact, in a healthy body, a rise in cortisol will trigger a compensating rise in DHEA, which in addition to all its other benefits also acts to suppress cortisol production. In other words, the body has a check-and-balance system in place to protect you from the harmful effects of cortisol and to keep the ratio of DHEA to cortisol high.

If your body is continually overproducing cortisol, however, this delicate balancing act is disturbed. Eventually, elevated cortisol levels start to *suppress* the production of DHEA. The check-and-balance system stops working, and the DHEA/cortisol ratio can quickly spiral downward. When this happens, high cortisol begins to impair the cardiovascular, neurological, and endocrine systems. The immune system begins to flag. The body begins to age more quickly.

Replenishing DHEA Levels

In my first consultation with Carrie, I recommended that she try to get at least seven to eight hours of sleep a night, preferably going to bed and getting up at around the same time every day. Despite her fatigue, I also asked her to try to push herself to get in a brisk twenty-minute walk every evening before dinner.

I'm fully aware that it is very difficult to find the energy for even mild exercise when just getting through the day is a challenge. But it is a critical step in breaking the cycle of stress and fatigue. Regular exercise and good sleep habits both help to increase DHEA and reduce cortisol. Stress reduction and relaxation techniques such as meditation, yoga, and martial arts also positively affect stress hormone profiles. These and other lifestyle issues will be discussed in much more detail in Part III, as we build and implement your complete anti-aging and life extension program.

In addition, if your cortisol and DHEA levels are severely out of balance, whether from stress, aging, or both, DHEA replacement therapy is a powerful and necessary intervention. DHEA is one of those nutrients that was once promoted as a cure-all and fountain of youth. While it may have been somewhat oversold at first, there is no doubt that it is a very important and powerful agent in the fight against aging.

The benefits of DHEA therapy have been the subject of intense study at the Life Extension Foundation. While no one nutrient is the answer to every health problem, researchers around the world have documented a host of positive effects from DHEA supplementation.

> **DHEA protects against bone loss and osteoporosis.** A study conducted at Washington University in St. Louis, Missouri, found that DHEA supplementation increased bone mineral density in both men and women after just six months. In the words of the researchers, DHEA was able to "partially reverse age-related changes" in these elderly subjects. DHEA provides the building block for estrone, a form of estrogen that stimulates bone-building cells to create more bone tissue. A steep drop in estrogen after menopause is one of the chief reasons for the rapid loss of bone mass in women during the years immediately following menopause.

> **DHEA protects the skin against aging.** As we age, our skin cells produce more collagenase, a collagen-destroying enzyme. This enzyme breaks down the collagen beneath the skin, causing the skin to droop and crease. DHEA helps to maintain collagen levels in the skin, promoting smoother, younger-looking skin. French scientists studied the effects of DHEA replacement therapy in about three hundred men and women between the ages of 60 and 80 over the course of a year. One of the findings to come out of this well-known study (known as the DHEAge Study) was that DHEA supplementation greatly improved the color, tone, thickness, and hydration of the subjects' skin.

> **DHEA was shown to reduce body fat and increase lean body mass** in both the male and female subjects of the French DHEAge study. Other researchers have found that DHEA increases the metabolic rate, which helps decrease fat storage. DHEA also helps to protect against diabetes by regulating blood sugar.

> **DHEA has a powerful beneficial effect on mood.** Several studies have noted that DHEA supplementation can increase positive well-being and energy levels, especially in the elderly and in

postmenopausal women. DHEA directly affects the neuroreceptors in the brain that govern mood. German researchers report that DHEA significantly reduced feelings of anxiety and depression in women who had low DHEA levels due to adrenal dysfunction.

➢ **DHEA enhances sexual performance and satisfaction.** Placebo-controlled studies carried out at an impotence treatment center in Vienna, Austria, have shown DHEA to improve sexual function in men with erectile dysfunction. It has also been shown to increase libido and sexual responsiveness in women.

➢ **DHEA also reduces symptoms associated with menopause.** As a precursor to other hormones, including estrogen and testosterone, DHEA replacement can accomplish many of the same goals as traditional estrogen replacement therapy for postmenopausal women. Italian researchers recently documented that DHEA therapy helped significantly with mood and emotional symptoms common in postmenopausal women.

➢ **DHEA boosts immune function.** A number of studies have shown DHEA to completely restore the impaired immune function of aging or immune-impaired animals within a few days of administration. Studies on a group of elderly but otherwise healthy men showed dramatic increases in several areas of immune function, including T-cell activity, natural killer cell activity, B-cells, and monocytes.

➢ **DHEA protects against excessive cortisol.** Last but certainly not least, DHEA lowers elevated cortisol levels caused by stress and/or aging.

Seeing the Effects

Because her blood work showed that Carrie's DHEA levels were extremely low, it was not surprising that DHEA supplementation brought profound improvement in many of her symptoms. We started with a low dosage (10 mg per day) of pharmaceutical-grade DHEA, taken in the morning to avoid the chance that any stimulating effect might affect her sleep patterns. In addition, Carrie began a basic program of nutritional support, similar to the core nutrient regime outlined for you in Chapter 11.

Over a period of six weeks, we gradually increased her dosage to 30 mg per day. At this dosage, Carrie felt an enormous improvement in her sense of well-being. She felt more centered and better able to cope with stress of work and school. She found the energy to focus on finding a new apartment and began to get her life back on track. Her friends noticed the difference, saying she seemed much calmer and happier. Carrie, who was about to turn 40, also mentioned to me that she felt younger, "just like I did when I was in my teens." I, too, could see a difference in her appearance since her initial appointment.

All of these changes are exactly what I would expect to see when DHEA levels are restored to healthy levels. After a couple of weeks on the 30 mg per day dosage, we repeated her blood tests. Her DHEA levels were out of the basement and well into the optimal range. At the same time, the dangerously high cortisol levels had settled back down to healthy levels. The combined effect of these shifts produced a much improved ratio between DHEA and cortisol (approximately twenty-five times as much DHEA as cortisol).

Carrie's second blood test simply confirmed what Carrie herself had already felt and others could clearly see: her hormone levels were once again those of a healthy young woman. The transformation was evident in the relaxed and smiling patient across from me.

DHEA AS A TREATMENT FOR DEPRESSION

One of the biggest improvements Carrie experienced was a lifting of the cloud of depression that had persisted despite her long-term use of antidepressant medications. The connection between low DHEA levels and depression has not been widely recognized, but this is a pattern I see over and over again in my practice.

Doctors now write over thirty-five million prescriptions a year for drugs such as Prozac, Zoloft, and Effexor. These are the selective serotonin reuptake inhibitors (SSRIs), which are designed to relieve symptoms of depression by keeping more serotonin in the brain. But I believe the medical culture has overlooked stress as a major cause of depression, as well as the potential of DHEA to fight depression and other symptoms of stress.

Studies have found that women with the lowest DHEA levels are the most likely to be depressed, even when they are taking antidepressant drugs. Moreover, DHEA has been known to be an effective antidepressant for over fifty years. Studies in the 1950s showed that DHEA supplements increased energy, mood, and confidence and alleviated depression. Unlike pharmaceutical antidepressants, DHEA also offers a wide range of anti-aging and disease prevention benefits. When properly used, DHEA has no unpleasant side effects. By contrast, about a quarter of those who try SSRIs eventually stop taking them because the side effects (weight gain, sexual dysfunction, and others) are simply not worth it.

For some reason, this early research on DHEA was abandoned. Fortunately we are now seeing a revival of interest in DHEA as an antidepressant. Researchers at the National Institute of Mental Health found that DHEA alleviated depression in about 60 percent of subjects with chronic mild depression. That's a better response rate than SSRIs generally produce for this condition. What's more, the subjects reported improvement after only ten days. By contrast, SSRIs can take six to eight weeks to product an effect. Another study in San Francisco showed that DHEA was even able to help subjects who were already taking antidepressants but were still not getting relief from their depression.

In my own practice, I have been using DHEA to treat depression successfully for years. It has fewer side effects and far more potential benefits, and I have found it to be more effective than SSRIs in the vast majority of cases. Occasionally, as with Carrie, I find that using DHEA together with a lower dose of antidepressants yields the best results.

If you are one of the thirty-five million Americans taking antidepressants, you, like Carrie, may find that DHEA replacement therapy offers either an alternative or a valuable adjunct. Working with an anti-aging physician will help you find the best protocol.

BEYOND STRESSED: ADRENAL EXHAUSTION

Before we get into the details of your DHEA replacement protocol, I want to talk briefly about adrenal fatigue. This stress-related syndrome seems to be becoming more and more common among my patients. Adrenal fatigue is a more advanced stage of the stress response in which the adrenal glands simply run out of gas. After prolonged stress and prolonged overproduction of cortisol, the adrenals can become unable to produce very much cortisol at all.

With adrenal fatigue, the symptoms can be somewhat different than the classic symptoms of stress. In general, people with adrenal fatigue find themselves feeling overwhelmed and defeated by even minor challenges. Extreme fatigue, depression, and a lack of motivation (especially in the afternoon) are all typical. It is also common to experience periods of anxiety and to have trouble relaxing and falling asleep at night.

SIGNS OF ADRENAL EXHAUSTION

> Anxiety
> Depression
> Low blood pressure, light-headedness
> Sugar cravings
> Tendency to infection (such as colds or flu)
> Difficulty recovering from infection
> Crashing in the afternoon
> Difficulty falling asleep, even when tired
> Being overemotional or irritable at the first sign of stress or difficulty

How much stress does it take to exhaust the adrenal glands? This seems to be a highly individual equation. Some people can sustain high levels of stress for their entire lives and never reach this phase. Others reach adrenal exhaustion relatively quickly and never completely recover.

Willow came to see me after consulting a number of conventional and nonconventional doctors. A 41-year-old actress, Willow told me she'd been fatigued "all her life." In her late 20s, Willow had been diagnosed with depression. Although she said antidepressants had brought some improvement, she never felt really good—but she continued to take the drugs.

Willow also struggled with carbohydrate cravings, anxiety, and insomnia. If you compare her complaints to the box of symptoms of adrenal exhaustion above, you can see that she had classic symptoms of that syndrome. To be fair, these symptoms could also suggest a number of other medical problems. But in Willow's case, the lab work offered confirmation that her adrenals were at least part of her problem.

Diagnosing adrenal fatigue can be tricky. In many cases, blood tests will indicate low to normal cortisol levels. A doctor who was looking at only this one marker could easily miss the signs of adrenal fatigue. But very low DHEA in conjunction with low cortisol can be the tip-off that the body has gone beyond the initial phase of stress response and entered into adrenal fatigue.

As we'll discuss in more detail in Chapter 10, far too many physicians rely entirely on the reference ranges provided by laboratories when interpreting blood tests. Because they are based on what is "normal," as opposed to what is ideal, these ranges are frequently not sensitive enough to identify subtle problems that can lead to larger problems later on. The standard lab values also fail to consider the relationships between the different hormones, which is often the most important part of the story.

Willow's cortisol level was, in fact, on the low end of the normal range. But in her case, the low cortisol level was suspicious. She'd told me that she was feeling a lot of stress in her professional life as well as her personal life. Given what I knew about her circumstances, I would have expected her cortisol to be somewhat elevated, reflecting the stress she was experiencing.

In addition, her DHEA levels were quite low, which was further indication that her hormonal reserve had been severely depleted by stress. Although a standard lab might have interpreted Willow's blood work to be completely normal, the whole picture—her hormone levels, her symptoms, and what was going on in her life—all added up to adrenal fatigue.

Whenever adrenal fatigue is suspected, it's important to have your doctor rule out the possibility of Addison's disease, a rare condition in which the adrenals stop functioning. In the vast majority of cases, however, adrenal fatigue can be treated with adrenal extracts or small amounts of cortisone to support and stimulate adrenal function. In addition, DHEA replacement therapy is usually needed.

In Willow's case, I prescribed very low doses of hydrocortisone to compensate for her underproducing adrenals. Patients are often alarmed when I suggest an extended course of cortisone therapy. Most people believe that it is dangerous to take cortisone or any steroid for a long period of time. However, I am talking about a *very low* dose, just a fraction of the dose that would be prescribed for other types of conditions. Supplying this very small amount of medical cortisone (10–20 mg a day) allows the adrenal glands to rest and recover their normal function. With medical supervision, this very low dose can safely be used as long as necessary and then tapered off. In addition, I prescribed DHEA replacement therapy to help raise Willow's DHEA levels.

Willow felt tremendous improvement from the combination of DHEA replacement and hydrocortisone. She was able to break free of the twenty-year cycle of depression and fatigue that had followed her throughout her adult life. With these long-standing issues finally showing improvement, Willow was then motivated to embark on a more ambitious and comprehensive anti-aging protocol, such as the one we'll be customizing for you in Part III of the book.

For more information on the treatment of adrenal fatigue, consult the LEF Disease Prevention and Treatment database under the heading "Adrenal Disease."

Using DHEA Safely

The reason DHEA is so powerfully effective is that it is a highly active substance in the body. As such, it needs to be used judiciously. Using hormone therapies such as DHEA, as well as the hormone replacement protocols we'll discuss in the next chapter, is much like driving a race car. A race car will definitely get you from point A to point B very quickly. But it takes a lot of skill and training to handle a race car without getting hurt.

! The use of any hormone therapy, including DHEA, should be done with the assistance of a trained anti-aging specialist who can evaluate your hormone status, fine-tune your dosage, watch for any side effects, and monitor your ongoing progress. The appendix lists some resources for finding accredited anti-aging physicians. The Life Extension Foundation also offers guidance, assistance, and resources to its members.

WHO NEEDS DHEA REPLACEMENT THERAPY?

Carrie didn't need a blood test to tell her she was stressed. It was obvious to both of us that stress was a major problem in her life. Mitchell, on the other hand, *did* need a blood test to realize the extent to which his health was being compromised by stress hormones.

Mitchell is a 60-year-old executive with a well-known telecommunications company. He's accustomed to the high-stress environment of big business and corporate politics. Mitchell's only complaint was that he was beginning to lose enthusiasm for the fight. Not yet ready to retire, he nonetheless found himself less interested and motivated by what he was doing, in a way that was beginning to diminish his effectiveness. Although there didn't seem to be anything wrong with his health, Mitchell's wife (who was a patient of mine) finally convinced him to schedule an appointment with me for a general evaluation.

Even though Mitchell wouldn't have said that stress was a problem for him, his blood work told another story. Mitchell's DHEA/cortisol ratio was only 3.4. High cortisol levels were setting him up for some serious medical consequences, while dwindling DHEA levels were literally draining the vitality out of him. As with Carrie and Willow, I started Mitchell on a program of DHEA replacement therapy to bring his levels up and improve his DHEA/cortisol ratio. Not only did his hormone profile quickly improve, but he experienced a profound upswing in his mood, energy, and general enthusiasm for life. Mitchell also reported a renewed sexual drive and vigor that he had assumed was a thing of the past.

Determining Your DHEA Levels

To find out your own DHEA status, you can have your hormone levels measured by either saliva test or blood test. Although the saliva tests offer some advantages in convenience, the methodology and interpretation of this kind of testing have not yet been well established or standardized. I prefer a blood test that measures the levels of DHEA-S (a metabolite of DHEA) in your blood. (See also the discussion of testing methods in Chapter 10.)

The following chart shows typical DHEA ranges for men and women of various ages. As you see, DHEA levels begin to drop off after age 30 and can be almost negligible after the age of 60, paralleling the general decline in our health and vitality as we age. Stress accelerates the natural decline of DHEA levels and the aging process.

Normal vs. Optimal DHEA Levels (mcg/dL)			
Sex	*Age*	*Normal*	*Optimal*
Male	18–30	125–619	250–450
	31–50	59–452	
	51–60	20–413	
	61–83	10–285	
Female	19–30	29–781	150–350
	31–50	12–379	
	Postmenopause	10–260	

You can also see that what is "typical" or "normal" is not necessarily optimal. A laboratory or physician who is not trained as an anti-aging specialist may believe that DHEA values in the normal range are acceptable. However, the conventional medical community also believes that aging and disease are both normal and acceptable. As you will see throughout this book, my colleagues at the Life Extension Foundation and I practice medicine from a completely different perspective. Our goal is not "normal" aging. Our goal is optimal health and longevity.

Anyone with less than optimal DHEA levels—whether due to aging or to stress—will likely benefit from DHEA replacement therapy. Over the last two decades, the Life Extension Foundation has analyzed thousands of blood tests and has determined that most people over the age of 40 can benefit from DHEA supplementation.

The Goal of DHEA Therapy

DHEA levels may be low due to the suppressive effects of ongoing stress or to the dropoff in our natural production of DHEA as we age. Whatever the reason, the goal of DHEA replacement therapy is to restore DHEA levels to youthful or optimal ranges.

DHEA can be administered in a gel that is rubbed into the skin, in a liquid suspension that is placed under the tongue, or by oral supplements, which is the form I prefer. DHEA is considered to be a nutritional supplement, not a drug, and this means that you can buy it without prescription in health food stores, in pharmacies, by mail order, and even in large grocery stores. But it is important to select a supplement from a reputable manufacturer, one that uses a pharmaceutical grade of DHEA. This helps to ensure the purity and consistent dosage of the supplement. Your medical advisor will be able to recommend a good brand.

Dosage Guidelines

Most of the studies on DHEA supplementation in women have used the same dosages as are typically used for men, 50 mg per day or higher. But women often need less DHEA than men do in order to get good results.

Because DHEA is a precursor to the sex hormones, it can be converted to both estrogen and testosterone in the body. For women, a small boost in testosterone can bring about a very positive increase in energy levels, libido, and overall sense of well-being. But you want to be careful not to overdo it.

Too much DHEA can sometimes lead to some undesirable (but not serious) side effects in women, such as increased sweating, oilier skin or acne, or hair growth. These effects are generally not seen in dosages below 50 mg per day, but if they do occur, they are easily reversed when the dosage is reduced.

I find it works best to start conservatively. Some women are exquisitely sensitive to even a small amount of DHEA, and for them, 10 mg per day, or even 5 mg per day, is plenty. Others will need a larger dose before they achieve the desired effects. The goal is to find the lowest dose that will be effective. I generally start with 10 mg per day and increase the dosage by 10 mg at a time (to a maximum of 50 mg per day) until the ideal level is attained. You should allow two to four weeks to evaluate the effectiveness of each level before increasing the dosage.

Because men have higher testosterone levels to start out with, they don't seem to be as sensitive to DHEA, and the dosage guidelines are fairly straightforward. Most men will do very well on a replacement dosage of 50 mg per day. If needed, the daily dosage can be increased by 10 mg increments to a maximum safe dosage of 100 mg per day.

Because DHEA can be energizing, it is best taken in the morning so that it doesn't have too stimulating an effect when you are trying to sleep. Some people prefer to take DHEA in two or three smaller doses throughout the day. If you want to do this, make sure to take your last dose of the day before 6 p.m.

Monitoring Your Progress

How you feel is one valuable guideline that your doctor will use to determine the proper dose of DHEA. If you have not experienced a notable improvement in energy and mood, you may need to increase the dosage (up to the recommended maximum dosage) in order to feel the benefits. If you begin to feel overly stimulated, restless, or unpleasantly

Dosage Guidelines for DHEA

If you are:	Male	Female
Start with:	50 mg/day	10 mg/day
Increase as needed by increments of:	5–10 mg/day	5–10 mg/day
To a maximum of:	100 mg/day	50 mg/day

aggressive or are experiencing any other side effects, that would be an indication to decrease your dose.

When it comes to hormone replacement, the dosage that is both safe and effective can vary greatly from individual to individual. In addition to evaluating how you feel, your doctor will probably want to retest your blood levels of DHEA-S after six to eight weeks of supplementation, or after any significant change in your dosage.

A stress hormone profile, which tests both cortisol and DHEA, will give the most accurate picture of your progress. Increasing your DHEA levels will likely also cause elevated cortisol levels to decline somewhat, so even a small improvement in DHEA can have a very positive effect on your DHEA/cortisol ratio.

To calculate your DHEA/cortisol ratio, first be sure that both are being reported in the same unit of measurement. (For most labs, this will be mcg/dL.) Then divide your DHEA value by your cortisol value. For example, if your DHEA level is 210 and your cortisol is 14, you would divide 210 by 14. The result is your DHEA/cortisol ratio. In this case, $210 \div 14$ equals a ratio of 15.

If the result is somewhere between 15 and 25, you are in the target range. If your result is lower than 15 *or* your DHEA level is lower than 150 mcg/dL, you would most likely benefit from increasing the amount of DHEA you are taking. If your result is higher than 25 *and* your DHEA levels are higher than 350 (for women) or 450 (for men), your doctor will probably reduce the amount of DHEA you are taking.

Please remember that every person's medical situation is different. These guidelines are not a substitute for professional and ongoing medical advice.

Fine-tuning DHEA Dosages	
Indications to increase DHEA dosage	*Indications to decrease DHEA dosage*
DHEA/cortisol ratio lower than 15	DHEA levels higher than 450 mcg/dL (men) or 350 mcg/dL (women)
DHEA level lower than 150 mcg/dL	Restlessness, aggression, overstimulation
No improvement in mood, energy	Oily skin or acne, increased hair growth (in women)

WHO SHOULD NOT TAKE DHEA

With proper monitoring and medical guidance, DHEA replacement therapy is a very safe and extraordinarily effective anti-aging therapy for most people. However, the use of DHEA by people with certain types of cancer is an area of potential concern. In general, we have seen that DHEA enhances immune function, including the body's ability to fight cancer. In the laboratory, DHEA has also been shown to inhibit the growth of breast and prostate cancer cells and to protect against the formation of cancerous lesions. This suggests that maintaining optimal DHEA levels as we age may be important in preventing cancer. In fact, one study found that those with the highest DHEA levels have a slightly lower risk of colon cancer.

However, there is some concern that DHEA supplementation may fuel the growth of preexisting prostate cancer. Prostate cancer is fueled by a form of testosterone, and DHEA can be converted to testosterone in the body, although it is hotly debated whether or not the form of testosterone that is enhanced by DHEA is the type that promotes the growth of cancer. The research to date on this question is inconclusive, and we will need more information to fully understand all the mechanisms at work. Until we do, it is best to err on the side of caution.

! Men with prostate cancer are advised not to use DHEA supplementation, or to use it only under the close supervision of their cancer specialists. Men taking DHEA should also have annual screenings to monitor any change in prostate-specific antigen (PSA), a marker for prostate cancer. This basic cancer screening is recommended for all men over the age of fifty, whether or not they are taking DHEA.

There has also been concern over the effect of DHEA supplementation on cholesterol levels in women. Some research suggested that DHEA might cause a decrease in HDL (the "good" kind of cholesterol) in women. The effect was not significant enough to be a major concern, nor has it been seen consistently in other studies. In fact, the ability of DHEA to protect against heart disease by preventing oxidation of LDL (the "bad" cholesterol) appears much more significant.

However, it serves as yet another reminder that anyone using any type of hormone replacement therapy should be working with a medical advisor who will be monitoring any and all developments in your health status.

You can find more information in the LEF Disease Prevention and Treatment database under the headings "DHEA Replacement Therapy" and "Prostate Cancer." To follow the research on DHEA as it unfolds, log on to the LEF Web site (www.lef.org) for the most current research findings and recommendations on DHEA and cancer protocols.

BEYOND DHEA REPLACEMENT

As we've seen in this chapter, stress hormone imbalance is one of the most common (and preventable) causes of accelerated aging and disease. Restoring a balance between cortisol and DHEA is the first important step in creating a more youthful hormone profile. The next chapter takes us further into the heart of anti-aging medicine, with a more comprehensive approach to hormone replacement. Until we crack the genetic code of aging (more about that in Part IV), hormone replacement therapy may be the closest thing we have to a true fountain of youth.

CHAPTER 3

Tuning the Sex Hormones

None are so old as those who have outlived enthusiasm.
—HENRY DAVID THOREAU

WORKING WITH HORMONES IS one of the things I enjoy most about practicing medicine, because the effects can be almost magical. Of course, successful anti-aging requires more than just hormone modulation. The right diet, supplements, exercise, stress reduction, and disease prevention are all critical to achieving your goal of a long and healthy life. But few things have as immediate and profound an impact on quality of life as restoring hormones to optimal levels.

For my patients, especially those in their 40s, 50s, and 60s, the difference can be nothing short of life changing. Within a few weeks of beginning hormone therapy, patients typically report that their entire outlook has changed. They have a renewed sense of enthusiasm, physical vitality, and well-being. And the benefits of hormone modulation, which include a more youthful skin and physique, improved mental function, and increased resistance to disease, continue to accrue with time.

Hormone modulation has been practiced in different forms by both conventional and alternative physicians for decades, with varying degrees of success and safety. Through years of clinical experience and research, I've arrived at a unique method for keeping all of the various hormones in balance as individual levels are optimized with hormone supplements. This balancing act is, I believe, the key to safe and effective hormone modulation.

HORMONAL ATROPHY LEADS TO AGING

The reason hormone modulation plays such a central role in anti-aging medicine is that hormonal decline is a primary factor in the aging process. Hormones are the chemical messengers that control virtually every biological process in the body. They tell your cells what proteins to manufacture and your organs which functions to perform. When hormone levels decline, less information is transmitted, and the body functions less effectively. Research compiled by the Life Extension Foundation clearly shows that declining hormone levels are a potent risk factor for disease, aging, and death.

In the last chapter, for example, we saw that the production of DHEA by the adrenal glands peaks in the mid-20s and then begins a slow decline. The same is true with other glands, including the thyroid and pituitary. Although hormone production begins to taper off during our 20s, the effects are often not felt until we reach our 40s or 50s, when hormone levels have declined to the point that our function is noticeably affected.

Just as we reach midlife, another hormonal shift takes place. The production of sex hormones (estrogen, progesterone, and testosterone) begins to decline. For women, the hormonal changes that lead up to and follow menopause are fairly dramatic. Men also experience a decline in sex hormone production known as andropause. Andropause has only recently been recognized as medically significant. Both menopause and andropause contribute to symptoms of aging and the susceptibility to disease.

One of the most powerful things we can do to slow biological aging is to compensate for these age-related changes in hormone production. The goal of hormone modulation is never to achieve unnaturally high levels of any hormone, but always to replicate the optimal levels and ratios of youth. By restoring hormone profiles to youthful levels, you literally create a younger body. A more youthful appearance, improved function, and increased resistance to disease follow naturally.

Sex hormones are, in particular, the "joie de vivre" hormones. Supporting the levels of these hormones with natural supplements leads to enhanced confidence, mood, and body image, as well as increased sexual interest, ability, and satisfaction. Some of my patients say that their marriages have benefited dramatically from their hormone replacement regimens.

HORMONE MODULATION FOR MORE YOUTHFUL BODIES

For decades, women routinely have been given estrogen to compensate for the decline in the production of this hormone after menopause. With the recent collapse of medical claims for conventional hormone replacement therapy (HRT), this practice is now changing. As we will discuss in more detail later in this chapter, the Women's Health Initiative study on hormone replacement vividly demonstrated the dangers of artificial hormone regimens. Unfortunately, we are now in danger of turning our backs on a therapy that can be highly beneficial when properly used.

In addition to underestimating the risks of artificial hormones, conventional medicine also has taken a strangely narrow and lopsided approach to hormone replacement. Although women were given estrogen to supplement their declining hormone levels, men were not offered testosterone to compensate for the corresponding decline in their hormone production. Furthermore, conventional medicine virtually ignored age-related declines in other hormones such as thyroid or DHEA.

Anti-aging physicians, by contrast, take a more comprehensive and consistent approach to hormone replacement. We typically evaluate and correct the levels of many different hormones, including DHEA and the sex hormones (testosterone, estrogen, and progesterone) as well as thyroid and growth hormone.

The conventional medical community remains skeptical of—even hostile to—the anti-aging approach to hormone modulation. Experts representing the mainstream routinely insist that the use of hormones for anti-aging purposes is "unnatural" and "unsafe," although they present no evidence for either claim.

This is ironic, to say the least, because the widely accepted practice of estrogen replacement was itself the original anti-aging hormone therapy. Estrogen replacement therapy really took off following the publication in 1966 of a book entitled *Feminine Forever*, by gynecologist John Wilson. In his best-selling book, Wilson promoted estrogen primarily as a way to forestall the physical changes (i.e., aging) that follow the onset of menopause. Only years later did the medical community attach medical benefits to estrogen therapy, such as protection against heart disease and osteoporosis. (The latest research appears to show that the heart-protective effects are, in fact, nonexistent.)

Today, HRT is recommended primarily as a way to delay osteoporosis and relieve menopausal discomforts such as hot flashes, mood disorders, and vaginal dryness, without much emphasis on its anti-aging effects. But whether or not the conventional medical community wants to admit it, the fact remains that estrogen therapy has anti-aging effects on women.

Wilson once claimed that the rejuvenating benefits of estrogen were so apparent that he could tell at a distance of twenty paces whether a woman was taking estrogen or not. But why stop with estrogen? The same is true with other hormones as well. Restoring healthy hormone levels promotes health and slows aging.

ARE HORMONES SAFE?

Not only does the conventional medical community largely ignore the benefits of hormone modulation, many are vehemently opposed to anti-aging hormone therapies on the grounds that hormones are dangerous. There seems to be a double standard at work here. As we will discuss in a moment, the safety—and even effectiveness—of "approved" hormone regimens, such as HRT for menopausal women (or even birth control pills for younger women), has now been refuted by the Women's Health Initiative study. Over the years, far more deaths have been caused or contributed to by HRT than by any other anti-aging hormone therapy.

Sadly, many athletes and bodybuilders have also been harmed by the illicit misuse of hormones in an effort to gain a competitive advantage. Some of this abuse was overseen by unscrupulous or uninformed medical professionals, but this is not the way that hormone therapy is practiced or promoted by the anti-aging community.

Clearly, hormones are powerful substances, and their actions and interactions in the body are highly complex. As such, they should be used with care, and always under the guidance of a qualified anti-aging specialist. But as we will explore in detail in this chapter, hormone replacement is *safe and highly beneficial,* providing that certain criteria are met.

Hormones should be administered in a way that most closely mimics the body's natural, optimal function:

> ➢ Supplemental hormones should be as similar as possible to the hormones produced in our own bodies.
> ➢ Dosages should be individually customized, using lab tests, symptoms, and experienced clinical judgment as a guide, and reevaluated regularly.
> ➢ Utmost care must be taken to maintain a natural and optimal balance between the various hormones in the body.

These guidelines are what separate anti-aging hormone modulation from the incomplete, unnatural, and often dangerous way that hormone replacement is practiced by conventional medicine.

Unfortunately, the majority of conventionally trained physicians are, in fact, not trained in the proper and effective use of hormone modulation as an anti-aging therapy. To complicate things, hormones are not regulated in a logical way by the FDA. Some hormones require a doctor's prescription, but others are available over the counter or on the Internet. It may even be tempting to take matters into your own hands. In order to emphasize what a bad and dangerous idea this is, let me add a fourth guideline to the ones listed above.

> ➢ Hormone therapies (including "natural" and nonprescription prepa-
>   rations such as progesterone cream or DHEA) should always be
>   administered and supervised by a qualified anti-aging specialist.

Now that we've established our guidelines, let's look at the specifics
of hormone modulation. We begin with the sex hormones, with protocols for men and women. As you will see, testosterone is not just a
"male" hormone, any more than progesterone or estrogen are "female"
hormones. Both protocols involve the same hormones (estrogen, testosterone, and progesterone) but, obviously, in different ranges and proportions.

If you are primarily interested in male hormone protocols, you can
skip to the second half of this chapter, where that discussion begins.
However, both men and women will benefit from reading through the
entire chapter, as much of the information in each protocol applies to
both sexes.

Our discussion of hormone modulation extends into the next chapter, which begins with a look at thyroid function and concludes with a
discussion of human growth hormone.

I.
WORKING WITH THE
FEMALE HORMONE SYSTEM

In my practice, I use the term *bioidentical hormone replacement therapy*
(BHRT) to distinguish the way anti-aging specialists administer hormones from the conventional HRT administered by the medical mainstream. As you will see, the differences are critical.

Female hormone modulation focuses largely on three hormones
(estrogen, progesterone, and testosterone) and has two primary goals.
The first goal is to compensate for age-related decline in natural hormone production, such as the decline in estrogen production at menopause. The second is to maintain an optimal balance between the various
hormones.

There is no standard prescription for BHRT. It is highly individual and flexible, based on each woman's changing hormonal status.

> ➢ Corinne at 36 was still producing plenty of estrogen but needed a small amount of natural progesterone to bring her hormone profiles into balance and eliminate premenstrual symptoms.

> ➢ Nora, a very youthful 50-year-old, had not yet gone through menopause but was beginning to notice the effects of declining estrogen levels. Her BHRT regimen included a small dose of natural estrogen plus a tiny amount of testosterone. The estrogen helped to keep her skin and other tissues youthful and enhance mental clarity. The testosterone helped to boost her mood, energy, and sex drive.

> ➢ Juanita, 48, suffered from hot flashes and insomnia caused by the surges and dips in her estrogen levels as she approached menopause. Juanita got relief from a nondrug regimen that included foods and supplements rich in phytoestrogens. These gentle, plant-based estrogens worked to smooth out the highs and lows in her estrogen levels and relieve the symptoms she was experiencing.

> ➢ At 66, Tina had been in menopause for fifteen years. Her low estrogen and progesterone levels contributed to bone loss and left her vulnerable to osteoporosis. Tina also complained that she was becoming increasingly forgetful. Her BHRT regimen included a balanced dose of natural estrogen and progesterone to rejuvenate her skin, increase her bone density, and help improve her memory. A small dose of testosterone greatly increased her physical stamina and overall drive. Testosterone is also a potent bone-building hormone.

These few examples from my own practice illustrate the many different ways BHRT can be used to promote greater health and well-being at any age. I want to stress again that the secret of successful hormone modulation lies not just in enhancing the levels of hormones in the body but in optimizing the balance between them.

WHAT PROGESTERONE CAN DO FOR YOU

Progesterone is a balancing hormone that works in a dynamic relationship with estrogen to regulate the menstrual cycle and the health of the reproductive organs. When women reach their 30s and 40s, it is very common to see a situation in which the balance of these two hormones is shifted too heavily toward estrogen. This excess of estrogen is commonly known as estrogen dominance.

The reasons for estrogen dominance syndrome are complex. Some research shows that many of the agricultural chemicals that have been widely used over the last decades have estrogenic effects on both men's and women's bodies, leading to estrogen overload. Eating habits are also to blame. Most women do not get enough dietary fiber, for example, which helps to absorb and excrete excess estrogen. The modern epidemic of obesity is another culprit, as fat cells also produce and store estrogen.

Estrogen dominance is often to blame for many symptoms experienced by women in this age group. These include premenstrual syndrome (PMS), night sweats, and depression. A small amount of natural progesterone can help to rebalance these hormones and relieve these symptoms.

In addition to relieving PMS symptoms, progesterone provides important benefits for breast and bone health as well. It helps to preserve bone density in women of all ages by stimulating bone-building cells (osteoclasts) and increasing the rate of new bone formation.

Studies have also shown that progesterone prevents excessive proliferation of both normal and cancerous breast cells. In trials conducted by Dr. Helene Leonetti at Bethlehem Obstetrics Clinic in Pennsylvania, progesterone therapy reduced fibrous (benign) breast lumps.

In addition, statistical analysis suggests that women with higher progesterone levels have a reduced risk of breast cancer. And among women who are diagnosed with breast cancer, a number of studies indicates that those with higher progesterone levels at the time of surgery have up to double the long-term survival rate as those with lower levels.

Renowned progesterone researcher Dr. John Lee has also noted that brain cells need progesterone to function well. It appears to act in the brain in a number of ways, by promoting energy production in brain cells and by protecting against nerve cell damage and brain aging. Progesterone therapy has also been shown to relieve depression in women.

The evidence clearly suggests that progesterone therapy has multiple benefits for women's health, both before and after menopause. Sadly, these benefits are almost completely overlooked in conventional practice. Most gynecologists believe that the only role of progesterone is to prevent endometrial cancer in women taking estrogen, either as hormone replacement or as birth control. There is a widespread misconception that women who have had a hysterectomy can be given estrogen replacement without progesterone because there is no longer any danger of endometrial cancer once the uterus has been removed. This ignores the many valuable benefits of progesterone.

Natural Progesterone Only, Please

The form of "progesterone" used in conventional contraceptives and HRT drugs is actually not progesterone at all, but a synthetic hormone called progestin. To many conventional physicians, progestins and progesterone are the same thing. Nothing could be farther from the truth.

Progestins are chemically different from the progesterone manufactured in the body and do not have the same benefits as natural progesterone. They also have significant risks, which include birth defects, breast cancer, blood clots, fluid retention, acne, rashes, weight gain, and depression. Most of the unpleasant side effects that cause women to stop taking HRT or birth control pills are caused by the progestins.

Natural progesterone, on the other hand, can be derived from sources such as soy and wild yam. These plants contain plant hormones, which are extracted and then chemically converted into hormones that are identical to human progesterone.

Once converted, natural progesterone can be mixed into a cream and delivered transdermally (through the skin). One argument for this method is that absorption through the skin allows the hormone to bypass the liver, which can break down much of the hormone before it reaches the target tissues.

While progesterone creams are extremely popular (in part because of their availability over the counter), I prefer an oral form of progesterone that has been micronized (broken down into tiny particles) and suspended in oil. This allows steady, gradual absorption of progesterone from the intestinal tract. I find the oral form of progesterone to be more potent in raising progesterone levels. This can be helpful in cases where the effects of progesterone cream are too subtle to relieve symptoms. The dosing for the oral form is also far more precise than the progesterone creams, which are simply measured out by the patient with a small spoon. In my experience, women tend to get a more accurate dose with the oral form and therefore have more predictable results.

Because it is more potent, the oral form also requires more scrupulous monitoring of blood levels to ensure that levels do not get too high and that the balance between progesterone and estrogen is maintained.

What Is the Ideal Progesterone Level?

Progesterone levels vary greatly depending on age and phase of the menstrual cycle. With the testing method that I use, progesterone levels for a nonpregnant woman can range anywhere from 2,000 to 14,000 pg/mL (picograms per milliliter). The range is so large that it, alone, is not very helpful.

In addition, there is so much variability between various testing methods and laboratories that there is no way to specify a single range that would apply to all the different ways to test progesterone. In Chapter 10, we'll discuss these issues in more detail, including guidelines on how to understand the results of your own medical tests.

However, the relationship between progesterone and estrogen is more significant and more meaningful than the individual levels of either hormone. Regardless of all the other variables, I have found that the ideal ratio between between progesterone and estrogen remains fairly constant. In my female patients, I like to see between ten and twenty times as much progesterone as estrogen. If the ratio of progesterone to estrogen is below 10, natural progesterone is often the solution.

This was the case with Corinne, a 36-year-old who suffered from severe premenstrual syndrome. Her natural estrogen levels were on the high side but not unhealthy. However, her progesterone levels were quite low, with only about four times as much progesterone as estrogen. Corinne's case is typical of the estrogen dominance syndrome described earlier.

A moderate dose of oral natural progesterone micronized in oil brought her progesterone levels up, which in turn brought the hormones into a much more favorable balance (twenty times as much progesterone as estrogen). Her premenstrual symptoms have almost disappeared.

When using the oral, micronized form of progesterone, I begin most women with 25 mg per day and increase to 50 mg per day if needed. In addition to blood tests, I monitor improvements in mood, clarity of thought, sleep quality, decrease in anxiety, and overall sense of well-being. Occasionally, I might prescribe 100 mg per day, or even 150 mg in rare cases.

How to Use Natural Progesterone Creams

Natural progesterone creams are available without a prescription. Unfortunately, there are a proliferation of "wild yam" and "natural progesterone" products available in health food stores. Some of these products do not contain any usable progesterone whatsoever. (Remember that the plant hormones found in soy and yams must be converted into the progesterone recognized by the body.) When selecting an over-the-counter product, check the label to be sure that it specifies a standardized amount of pharmaceutical-grade progesterone.

Natural progesterone creams can also be prescribed by your physician. Physician-dispensed preparations typically contain 20 to 30 mg per $\frac{1}{4}$ teaspoon, whereas over-the-counter products may contain only 10 to 20 mg per $\frac{1}{4}$ teaspoon. (A dose of $\frac{1}{4}$ teaspoon is about the size of a pea.)

Natural progesterone cream is extremely safe. There is little possibility of toxicity or overdose. A small minority of women may experience menstrual irregularities (breakthrough bleeding, skipped periods, cramping) or emotional symptoms such as depression from excessive doses of progesterone. A very small percentage of women react poorly to even small doses of progesterone, but any unpleasant symptoms are quickly resolved when dosages are adjusted downward or discontinued.

APPLICATION GUIDELINES FOR PROGESTERONE CREAM

These guidelines are for a progesterone cream providing 30 mg progesterone per $1/4$ teaspoon. Adjust as necessary if using a different concentration. Women using any progesterone preparation should be monitored by a qualified anti-aging physician.

Premenopausal women: $1/8$ to $1/4$ teaspoon per day during the second half of the menstrual cycle (beginning fifteen days after the beginning of your period and continuing to the first day of your next period)

Postmenopausal women: $1/8$ to $1/4$ teaspoon daily

Women with osteoporosis: $1/8$ to $1/4$ teaspoon twice a day

The cream should be rubbed into areas where the skin is soft and relatively thin, such as on the inner arm, thighs, stomach, or breasts. Avoid applying the cream to the same area day after day. If needed, the dosage can be safely increased under the supervision of a physician.

A trained anti-aging specialist will consider your age, hormone status and balance, and symptoms in determining how much progesterone (if any) is right for you, and whether natural estrogen therapy is also needed.

ESTROGEN KEEPS YOU YOUNG

Estrogen is, of course, a feminizing hormone. But its effects extend beyond the reproductive system. Produced in the ovaries (and in small amounts in the male testes), estrogen travels throughout the body to tissues that have estrogen receptors and promote youthful cell behavior. The female reproductive organs and genital tissues are extremely rich in estrogen receptors, as are breast tissue and skin. Brain cells also have estrogen receptors. Mood, memory, and cognitive activity are all supported by estrogenic activity in the brain.

As women enter their 40s, the ovaries begin to atrophy, and estrogen levels start to decline. Eventually, the ovaries fail entirely, estrogen levels bottom out, and menstruation ceases (menopause). The exact timing and pace of this transition is highly individual.

Some women experience a gradual decline in estrogen over the course of ten or fifteen years; some go through a briefer but more intense transition. For many, the decline is characterized by surges, sputters, and dips that leave them riding a hormonal roller coaster. Menopause itself can occur anytime between the late 30s and late 50s, although the average age is 51 years.

As estrogen levels drop, many women experience unpleasant symptoms such as hot flashes and insomnia. These symptoms occur as the body attempts to adjust to lower estrogen levels. These so-called menopausal miseries can actually be characterized as withdrawal symptoms.

If estrogen levels drop suddenly (as with surgical menopause) or fluctuate wildly, estrogen withdrawal symptoms can be more severe. Interestingly, Western women tend to have more severe estrogen withdrawal symptoms than their Japanese counterparts. Possible reasons for this are explored below in our discussion of phytoestrogens.

The good news is that as the body gradually gets used to having less estrogen, the withdrawal symptoms fade. The bad news is that low estrogen levels also have long-term effects on health. Estrogen deficiency results in vaginal dryness, atrophy of the sexual organs, loss of skin tone, depression, forgetfulness, and loss of bone density. Unlike hot flashes, the effects of estrogen deficiency do not improve with time and may get worse. Of particular concern is the accelerated bone loss that follows menopause.

EFFECTS OF ESTROGEN DEFICIENCY

> Loss of skin firmness and elasticity
> Dry skin and mucous membranes (including eyes, nasal passages, vagina)
> Genital atrophy and reduced sex drive
> Memory loss
> Reduced feeling of well-being
> Accelerated bone loss
> Hair loss

The symptoms of estrogen withdrawal as well as the consequences of estrogen deficiency can be avoided by replacing lost estrogen with hormone therapy. But as with any hormone therapy, it is very important that the body's natural balance be respected and maintained. This is where conventional HRT has gone wrong.

Estriol: The Forgotten Estrogen

The female body actually produces three different types of estrogen: estrone (E1), estradiol (E2), and estriol (E3). E1 and E2 are the stronger, more biologically active forms, while E3 is a relatively weak estrogen. Perhaps for this reason, mainstream medicine has largely ignored estriol and focused on estrone and estradiol. This has proved to be a critical mistake.

Because of their tendency to promote cell division, estrone and estradiol can both promote cancer growth. Estriol, on the other hand, acts as a natural cancer preventive, blocking cell proliferation and protecting against cancer in the breast and other estrogen-rich tissues.

In fact, estriol is widely used in Europe as a therapy to prevent cancer and as the first choice for estrogen replacement therapy. In the

United States, however, the most widely prescribed estrogen replacement drugs (Premarin, EstraDerm, Estrace) do not provide any cancer-protective estriol. Instead they contain only synthetic (or "conjugated") forms of estrone and estradiol. In the forty years since these drugs have been in wide use, the incidence of breast cancer in the United States has increased from one in thirty women to one in eight women.

HRT and Breast Cancer

In 2002, the Women's Health Initiative, a long-term study of the effects of hormone replacement therapy involving over 161,000 women, was abruptly halted when it was found that HRT was causing a significant increase in breast cancer rates. This study was not the first evidence of a connection between these drugs and breast cancer—there were other large-scale studies published in 1995 and 1997 that found essentially the same thing. But these earlier studies did not receive the same publicity as the 2002 finding. (This is, by the way, a very telling example of how the major media rather abitrarily determine which medical findings merit our attention.)

In any case, the 2002 study was front-page news, and I suspect that the phones in every gynecologist's office rang off the hook that week. Although the truth is that heart disease kills far more women than breast cancer, most women are far more anxious about breast cancer than they are about heart disease. Millions of women taking Premarin and Provera were panicked to learn that the hormones they had been prescribed might be increasing their chance of this dread disease.

Over the following two years, the bad news from the Women's Health Initiative (WHI) continued to emerge. Researchers found that the most common HRT regimen (Premarin plus Provera, sometimes called PremPro) also increases a woman's risk of heart disease, heart attack, and stroke. A smaller arm of the study, using estrogen (Premarin) without progestin, found that artificial estrogen alone, while not as dangerous as the Premarin/Provera combination, also increased the risk of stroke.

The researchers themselves were so convinced that the benefits of

Premarin and Provera were not worth the risks that they suspended the study early for ethical reasons, to allow subjects to discontinue therapy. As a result of the WHI debacle, many women and their doctors are now frightened about hormone replacement therapy in general. Many women are forgoing the profound benefits of hormone replacement out of fear of side effects and risks.

In the media coverage of this story, an important point got missed. The WHI study did not prove that hormone replacement therapy is unhealthy and risky. It found specifically that HRT using *Premarin and Provera* is unhealthy and risky. I couldn't agree more. These drugs violate all of the criteria for safe and effective hormone therapy. They use hormones that are foreign to the body and wreak havoc with the body's hormonal balance.

Premarin is an artificially conjugated estrogen that is derived from the urine of pregnant horses—thus the name: *Pre*(gnant)*mar*(e's)(ur)*in*(e). As you might imagine, horse estrogen is many times stronger than human estrogen. Premarin is primarily the dangerous estrone form, without the balancing estriol form of estrogen. In my opinion, it has no place in the human body. Provera, although it is considered to be "progesterone," is not progesterone at all but the artifical hormone progestin.

While I'm no fan of these drugs, I also think that the facts of the study were misrepresented in a sensational way that caused a lot of unnecessary anxiety for the millions of women who had been prescribed these drugs for HRT.

In the WHI study, the risk of breast cancer for those taking Premarin and Provera was shown to be 34 percent higher than for those who took placebo drugs. That does not mean that women who take these drugs have a 34 percent chance of getting breast cancer. In this study, woman taking HRT had less than a 2 percent incidence of breast cancer. Among those taking the drugs, 1.9 percent were diagnosed with breast cancer, compared with 1.5 percent of those who took a placebo.

By taking Premarin and Provera, the women in this study increased their *actual* risk of breast cancer by only 0.4 percent (four-tenths of 1 percent). Stated another way, the use of HRT was responsible for 4 additional cases of breast cancer per 1,000 women. Had the newspapers (or the researchers) reported it in that way, I doubt whether women would have been as upset as they were. This study is a prime example of the way that medical statistics can be manipulated for effect.

Nor were misleading statistics the only problem with the way this study was represented in the media. In addition to glossing over the critical difference between the artificial hormones used in this study and other more natural forms of HRT, many of the media reports failed to mention that this same study found that HRT resulted in a *decreased* incidence of colorectal cancer, hip fractures, vertebral fractures, and osteoporosis.

To summarize, here are the actual facts about hormone replacement that got lost in the media frenzy over the now infamous WHI study.

1. HRT offers many important anti-aging benefits.

2. Premarin and Provera contain hormones that are dangerous and foreign to the human body, and their use is associated with health risks.

3. These risks can be minimized and the benefits maximized when HRT is administered in a way that is natural, balanced, and individualized.

A Safer Estrogen Therapy

A much safer approach to estrogen replacement therapy (and the one favored by anti-aging physicians) is to provide a balance of estriol and estradiol or estrone. This approach mimics the body's own production. Often estriol alone can alleviate any symptoms of estrogen deficiency.

A large study conducted in Germany, for example, found that 92 percent of women using estriol got relief from hot flashes (with hot flashes completely eliminated for 71 percent). The researchers also documented improvement or elimination of depression in 57 percent of the subjects, and reversal of genital shrinkage or atrophy in 92 percent. The women also had fewer migraine headaches and improved skin quality. None of the women experienced any increase or worsening of their symptoms, and the estriol therapy was free of undesired side effects.

While it is extremely safe and well tolerated, estriol is not as biologically active as estrone or estradiol. For some women, estriol alone is not enough to prevent menopausal symptoms. When stronger estrogens (estradiol or estrone) are required in order to get sufficient relief of symptoms, including estriol in the mix helps to protect against any cancer-promoting effects.

The natural estrogens we use are derived from soybeans, not horse urine, and are chemically identical to the hormone produced in the body. With natural, balanced estrogen therapy we can provide all the rejuvenating and protective benefits of estrogen without the side effects and risks associated with synthetic and unbalanced hormones.

BENEFITS OF NATURAL ESTROGEN

> ➤ Alleviation of menopausal symptoms
> ➤ Alleviation of depression
> ➤ Improved skin firmness and elasticity
> ➤ Enhanced moistness of vaginal tissues and mucous membranes
> ➤ Reduced genital atrophy, enhanced sex drive
> ➤ Improved memory and neurological function
> ➤ Reduced bone loss and fewer bone fractures
> ➤ Protection against Alzheimer's disease
> ➤ Reduced risk of colon cancer

What Is a Healthy Estrogen Level?

As with progesterone, estrogen levels vary depending on age and whether a woman has gone through menopause or where she is in her menstrual cycle, as well as what testing methods are used. In my own practice, I prefer blood tests to other methods such as saliva or urine testing, but there can be dramatic differences in the way different labs process the blood tests.

With the blood test I use, for example, healthy estrogen levels can range from 180 to 200 pg/mL (picograms per milliliter) for women in their 30s and 40s. For women in their later 40s, 50s, and 60s, I consider estrogen levels from 60 to 120 pg/mL to be ideal. (Without estrogen replacement, estrogen levels commonly drop well below 10 pg/mL following menopause.)

Because the balance between the different estrogens is also important, I also use very sensitive tests that can measure the individual levels of estradiol and estrone. (I have not yet found a test that is sensitive enough to reliably measure estriol.) As a guideline, I like to see estradiol as 40 percent or more of the total estrogen. That translates into an estrogen/estradiol ratio of 2.5 or lower.

Target Estrogen and Progesterone Ranges
(Values may vary with different labs, but
ratios will remain roughly constant)

	Progesterone	Estrogen	Total estrogen/ estradiol ratio	Progesterone/ total estrogen ratio
Women under 50	2,000–14,000 pg/mL	180–200 pg/mL	2.5 or lower	10–20
Women over 50	2,000–8,000 pg/mL	60–120 pg/mL	2.5 or lower	10–20

MINIMAL INTERVENTION
FOR MAXIMAL BENEFIT

Hormone modulation is, quite literally, a balancing act. The goal is to achieve optimal hormone ratios as well as optimal hormone levels. Lab tests provide important clues about what hormones may be deficient or out of balance. Equally important, especially in determining the correct dosages, is how the patient actually feels before and after a regimen is instituted.

I use a "start low and go slow" approach. Dosages are gradually increased only as needed to achieve ideal hormone levels and maximum well-being and relief from symptoms.

Physicians have several options when working with natural hormones. Bi-Est and Tri-Est are two popular medications that combine estriol with estrone and/or estradiol, closely mimicking a woman's natural hormone production. Both Bi-Est and Tri-Est use bioidentical estrogens derived from soybeans. (Unlike natural progesterone, a physician's prescription is required for estrogen.)

Compounding pharmacists can also custom-blend a hormone preparation according to a physician's instructions, including any or all of the different estrogen forms as well as progesterone and even testosterone in the exact amounts needed. These can be prepared as oral medications or creams (or vaginal suppositories) for transdermal application.

With conventional HRT, a woman's estrogen levels frequently get pushed much higher than necessary due to strong synthetic estrogens. She is then given high doses of progestin to prevent problems from too much estrogen. When we use natural, bioidentical hormones and pay close attention to maintaining a natural balance of the different estrogens and progesterone, I find we can usually get great results with smaller doses than are used in conventional regimens.

Hormone Modulation in Early Menopause

Nora is a successful advertising executive who works in films, an industry that places enormous emphasis and value on youthfulness. Nora came to me seeking an aggressive anti-aging program. Her goal was to reverse her biological age by at least ten years.

At 50, Nora was actually navigating through the premenopausal years with relative ease. She was experiencing only occasional menopausal symptoms such as hot flashes, but she was concerned about other signs of aging. Nora described an increasing "spaciness" or brain fog that is a typical symptom of declining estrogen levels. She also noticed that her skin had gotten thinner and dryer and looked dull and aged.

Nora's blood tests indicated that her estrogen levels were normal, although on the low side of the range for her age. But her symptoms suggested she might feel better with a slightly higher estrogen level. I prescribed a low dose of estradiol plus estriol as part of her anti-aging regimen. As Nora's estrogen levels rebounded, she noticed a big improvement in her mental clarity and general sense of well-being. Nora's husband was the first to notice the rejuvenating effects of estrogen on her complexion. After several months, her skin had a noticeable glow and had a tauter, more toned appearance.

Nora's natural progesterone levels were already good. Once we brought her estrogen levels up, the balance between estrogen and progesterone was right in the target range (ten to twenty times as much progesterone as estrogen), so we did not add progesterone to her regimen at that time.

Hormone Modulation in Later Menopause

Tina, whom you met in Chapter 1, was 66 and had gone through menopause in her early 50s. For her, the transitional "menopausal miseries" were long since past, but she was clearly suffering from the effects of long-term estrogen deficiency.

Tina was headed toward full-blown osteoporosis, having lost a considerable amount of bone density following menopause. As you might recall, she was also bothered by forgetfulness and memory lapses, which made her nervous about traveling alone. Tina also worried that these symptoms might be early signs of Alzheimer's. A consultation with a neurologist was able to allay Tina's anxiety about Alzheimer's, but the doctor offered no solutions, telling her that forgetfulness was "normal for her age."

As we have already discussed, however, estrogen deficiency can lead to reduced neurological function, particularly the symptoms that Tina described. Her blood tests confirmed that her estrogen was quite low (27 pg/mL), as was her progesterone (400 pg/mL). This gave Tina a progesterone/estrogen ratio of 15, well within the target range, but in this case the fact that both hormones were significantly suboptimal was more critical.

I began Tina on a BHRT regimen that consisted of a low dose of natural estrogens (estradiol plus estriol) as well as a very low dose of natural progesterone. In a few months, Tina's estrogen levels had climbed to a healthy 63 pg/mL, but her progesterone remained low. At this point her progesterone/estrogen ratio was actually lower than when we started. It had gone from 15 to a very low 4.8. This did not, however, indicate that Tina's hormone profiles were getting worse. It was merely an interim step toward the ultimate goal.

I include this detail in order to illustrate that each of the guidelines that I've provided regarding levels and ratios must be considered as part of a bigger picture. (And the estrogen/progesterone picture is itself only one part of the larger picture of all the hormone systems.) For some patients, the optimal solution may even lie outside of these guidelines. This can be determined only by a trained anti-aging specialist.

In Tina's case, we fine-tuned her regimen by increasing the progesterone dosage a bit. Within a couple of months, her progesterone levels were also on the rise, and her progesterone/estrogen ratio was 13, once again in the target range.

The following chart shows the progression of Tina's case. Notice that during the initial stages of hormone modulation, the different values may move in and out of target ranges as the body adjusts and we fine-tune the regimen. Ultimately, however, we reach a state of alignment in which all the values approach the ideal.

Progression of Hormone Therapy (Tina)					
Lab Values	Baseline	Rx	After 3 months	Rx	After 5 months
Estrogen	27 (very low)	Low dose	63 (ideal)	No change	85 (ideal)
Progesterone	400 (very low)	Low dose	300 (very low)	Increase dose	1,100 (improved)
Progesterone/ Estrogen Ratio	15 (on target)		4.8 (below target)		13 (on target)

Equally important, Tina felt the effects of the higher estrogen levels. She was delighted to feel a noticeable improvement in the mental fuzziness that had been so distressing to her. She felt more confident, more in control of the details of her life. The estrogen, along with other bone-preserving supplements that are discussed in greater detail in Chapter 10, also appeared to slow the rate of bone loss that had posed perhaps the greatest threat to Tina's future health and independence.

DRUGS TO PREVENT OSTEOPOROSIS

Traditional HRT regimens have largely fallen from favor because of the increased risks of heart attack, stroke, and breast cancer demonstrated by the Women's Health Initiative study. But one of the chief benefits of estrogen replacement has been the prevention of bone loss following menopause. With so many women now opting *not* to use hormone replacement, doctors have begun to overprescribe drugs such as Fosamax to prevent osteoporosis in women not taking estrogen after menopause.

Drugs such as these are valuable therapies for women at extreme risk for, or already suffering from, osteoporosis. The drugs are also helpful in preventing bone loss in women who cannot take estrogen, such as those with or at risk of breast cancer. However, I consider these drugs to be inappropriate for routine preventive use, especially when there are natural alternatives. A significant percentage of women suffer side effects from the drugs, such as mild to severe nausea, reflux, or damage to the esophagus.

Bioidentical hormone replacement therapy allows women to enjoy the anti-aging benefits of hormone replacement—including the preservation of bone density—without the health risks that accompany the synthetic hormone regimens, or the side effects of the anti-osteoporosis drugs. In Part III we will also be discussing nutrients that support healthy bones, along with dietary factors and the importance of weight-bearing exercise.

NATURAL ALTERNATIVES TO ESTROGEN

For some women, even natural estrogen therapy is not an option, either because of personal preference or because of other medical considerations. Juanita, for example, had a family history of breast cancer. Because some forms of breast cancer are fed by estrogen, even natural estrogen therapy was thought to be a risk for Juanita.

Nonetheless, Juanita was suffering from estrogen withdrawal. Ferocious hot flashes made it almost impossible to get through the day without embarrassment. Her sleep was disturbed almost every night by night sweats and bouts of insomnia. Whether as a result of estrogen withdrawal or as a secondary effect of sleep deprivation, Juanita felt like an emotional wreck and was struggling with depression and anxiety.

Many women who choose not to use hormone replacement therapy turn instead to plants and herbs that contain phytoestrogens. These are plant hormones that are so similar to human estrogen that they can plug into the estrogen receptors in our cells. Phytoestrogens are very weak in comparison to human estrogens, which are a thousand to ten thousand times stronger. Nonetheless, phytoestrogens can stimulate those empty estrogen receptors enough to relieve the symptoms of estrogen withdrawal. For many women, phytoestrogens offer an effective, nonhormonal option for the relief of typical symptoms of early menopause.

Hormone-Modulating Herbs

Black cohosh has long been recognized by traditional cultures for its ability to ease symptoms of menopause, and modern chemical analysis reveals that it is rich in phytoestrogenic compounds. A standardized extract of black cohosh is a standard pharmaceutical treatment for menopausal symptoms in Europe and Australia. Clinical studies show that it is highly effective in reducing symptoms of estrogen "withdrawal" without side effects.

Licorice root extract has likewise been prized for centuries in traditional Chinese medicine for its multiple health benefits. Studies have shown that the phytoestrogens in licorice root are safe and effective in preventing menopausal symptoms.

Dong quai is another Chinese tonic for female health, although it is not directly estrogenic. Rather, it is believed to promote progesterone production, which can help to balance excessive estrogen levels.

There are many herbal formulations specifically for menopause, which contain a combination of hormone-modulating herbs. Because manufacturing methods vary greatly and affect the potency of the product, it is important to look for formulations that specify standardized plant extracts.

Typical Herbal Women's Health Formula
(taken 1 or 2 times per day)

Black cohosh (standardized potency)	20 mg
Licorice root extract (standardized potency)	10 mg
Dong quai (standardized potency)	10 mg

This type of formula can be used alone or in combination with low-dose BHRT to relieve hot flashes, vaginal dryness, and other symptoms of estrogen withdrawal. Whether you are using phytoestrogens, BHRT, or both, it is often helpful to use a low-dose natural progesterone cream (discussed on page 57) at the same time, to help to maintain estrogen/progesterone balance.

The Story on Soy

Another plant rich in phytoestrogens is the soy plant. Soy compounds called isoflavones are heavily promoted to women as a "natural" way to prevent hot flashes and to prevent bone loss and heart disease due to estrogen loss. In addition, they are now being advanced as a way to prevent hormone-related cancers such as breast and prostate cancer.

There is little doubt that soy isoflavones are effective in relieving menopausal symptoms. Several studies have found isoflavones to be nearly as effective or as effective as pharmaceutical estrogens, although far safer than synthetic estrogens. As little as 50 mg per day of soy isoflavones can also increase bone mass as well as lower your cholesterol and triglycerides.

Researchers are also very interested in soy as a possible way to prevent cancer. Asian cultures, which traditionally consume a lot of soy, have a far lower incidence of hormone-related cancers such as breast and prostate cancer than do Westerners, who traditionally eat less soy. The thought is that the weak estrogens in soy help to prevent hormone-related cancers in both men and women by blocking the action of other, stronger estrogens that can promote cancer growth.

However, an epidemiological observation such as this can never control for all the variables. It is also true that Asians eat far less red meat and saturated fats than Americans do, and drink large amounts of green tea. Both of these factors are known to decrease cancer risk. Obviously, it is impossible to say what part soy consumption plays in the incidence of cancer in Asia, based only on such observations.

Researchers have isolated several compounds in soy that appear to be anticancer agents, and controlled trials are beginning to test the hypothesis that adding soy isoflavones to the Western diet may protect us from cancer. I don't mean to imply that soy does not have health benefits, only that its value may have been somewhat oversold.

My chief concern is that people have begun to take large doses of soy isoflavones to prevent (and even to treat) cancer, based on this still evolving research. Women have assumed that if a little soy is good for menopausal symptoms, a lot of soy will be better. Although much research remains to be done on soy's ability to fight cancer, many seem to think that there is no harm in loading up on soy in the event that the research proves the theory to be correct.

There are those in the anti-aging community who will disagree with me, but I am not in favor of the consumption of large amounts of soy. First of all, many of its benefits (such as its ability to prevent cancer) have yet to be proven definitively. Others (such as its highly complex hormonal interactions) are still poorly understood. At best, it is but one part of a total approach to hormonal balance and disease prevention. In excess, soy (like just about everything else) can create certain problems.

I have seen a lot of health-conscious people seriously overdoing it with soy.

Soy is frequently promoted as a "healthier" source of protein, and as you will see in Chapter 12, when we discuss diet in more detail, adequate protein consumption is crucial for maintaining healthy tissues. As a source of protein, soy has certain advantages over meat. It is high in fiber and contains no saturated fat. It is, however, difficult to digest and can cause gas and constipation.

More importantly, there are other sources of protein, such as whey and egg, that are far more bioavailable and valuable to the body. For this reason, I recommend whey-based protein, not soy, as a primary source of protein supplementation.

Excessive amounts of soy also can suppress the function of the thyroid gland, especially in those prone to low thyroid function. As we will discuss in Chapter 4, proper thyroid function is essential to staying youthful as you grow older. Undermining your thyroid function by overdoing it with soy is really robbing Peter to pay Paul. Or, to take a different analogy, bodybuilders who build their biceps while ignoring the triceps muscles on the back of the arm eventually find themselves unable to straighten their arms. By the same token, for anti-aging to be effective, the body's systems must remain in balance with one another.

As with everything, moderation is the golden rule. If you enjoy soy foods such as tofu, tempeh, edamame, and soy nuts, these foods offer valuable nutrients and can be a healthy part of a varied diet. I recommend keeping your intake of soy foods to one or two servings a day.

Although I don't personally recommend soy (isoflavone) supplements, protein powders, or drinks, I do have patients who use them as a way to cover all the nutritional bases. Again, research and good sense suggests a healthy intake to be around 100 mg of isoflavones (or 25 grams of soy protein) per day. Many women find soy isoflavone supplements to be helpful in modulating symptoms of menopause, and promising research continues on their cancer-fighting and disease preventing properties. I think the evidence will ultimately reveal isoflavones to be an important *component* of an integrated program of nutrients. To that end, I support the moderate use of soy and isoflavones.

The Limitations of Phytoestrogens

In terms of hormone modulation, phytoestrogens, including soy, are of most value in relieving symptoms of early menopause. In my experience, however, they are not strong enough to provide the same sort of long-term anti-aging effects as bioidentical hormone replacement therapy. In my practice, I frequently see women who were able to make it through the transition into menopause without hormone replacement therapy by using phytoestrogens to ease the symptoms of estrogen withdrawal.

As they begin to get into their 50s and 60s, however, they begin to find that the herbs aren't enough to forestall the aging effects of hormonal decline. They are delighted to learn that bioidentical hormone replacement offers a safe and effective alternative to dangerous artificial hormones. And unlike conventional HRT, which is now recommended for only short periods of time due to the risks, the anti-aging and disease-preventing benefits of BHRT continue to accrue for as long as youthful hormone profiles are maintained.

TESTOSTERONE THERAPY FOR WOMEN

Most people are under the impression that women's bodies produce only tiny, insignificant amounts of testosterone. So you might be surprised to learn that women have far more testosterone in their blood than they do estrogen. Testosterone, in both men and women, is an energizing hormone. It is a natural antidepressant and is largely responsible for sexual drive and function in both men and women. It also helps maintain lean muscle mass.

Of course, in sufficient quantities, testosterone is also masculinizing. Accordingly, the level of testosterone in the male body is twenty to eighty times higher than in the female body.

In both men and women, most of the testosterone in circulation is tightly bound to protein and not biologically active. Only a small percentage (between 0.5 and 2.0 percent) of the total testosterone is free testosterone, and that is the amount that matters. Even these small amounts of free testosterone in a woman's body have an important effect on her health and well-being.

For women, I find that when free testosterone slips below a certain level (below about 1.2 pg/mL), depression, fatigue, and loss of libido are common. A slight rise in testosterone can bring profound benefits in the form of an elevated mood and reinvigorated sense of sexuality. And, of course, it is not just the testosterone level itself but the ratio of testosterone to other hormones that matters. As a rough guideline, I find that most women feel best when they have two to five times as much total testosterone as estrogen.

Target Hormone Ranges and Ratios for Women			
Estrogen	*Total testosterone*	*Free testosterone*	*Testosterone/ estrogen ratio*
180–200 pg/mL (under 50) 60–120 pg/mL (over 50)	120–900 pg/mL	1.2–3.0 pg/mL	2–5

Nudging Testosterone Levels Higher

At the beginning of her anti-aging program, Nora's blood tests indicated that her free testosterone levels were a bit low. But I did not immediately recommend testosterone therapy to her. First I wanted to see if her testosterone levels would respond to other, less direct stimulation.

You may recall that DHEA is converted in the body to other hormones, primarily testosterone. In women, particularly, supplementation with DHEA can bring about a mild increase in testosterone levels.

Like most people over 40, Nora's DHEA was indeed suboptimal, and I prescribed 50 mg per day of DHEA as part of her initial protocol. Even after her DHEA levels had been brought up to optimal levels, however, Nora's testosterone levels remained quite low. About six months into her anti-aging program, I suggested that Nora try a very low dose of testosterone, in the form of a prescription cream that is rubbed into the skin. This did the trick, nudging Nora's testosterone higher and giving her anti-aging protocol a noticeable boost in terms of her general sense of well-being.

As I mentioned earlier, Nora began her program with the goal of reversing her biological age by ten years. Over the course of the first year, Nora was indeed transformed by the benefits of a complete anti-aging program. She has lost 30 pounds, her skin has a tauter and more toned appearance, and her muscle strength and definition have improved. She's feeling more energetic, more vigorous, and more enthusiastic about her life, her work, and her marriage.

Although Nora did not mention a reduced libido as one of her concerns, she did mention that the hormone regimen had had a very noticeable effect on her sexual response. She was surprised and delighted when impulses that had been quiet for some time began to stir again. A big part of Nora's renewed sexual desire had to do with the greater ease she felt with her body. As she and her husband rekindled their physical romance, she also felt that her body was sexually more responsive than it had been in years.

Nora's program included much more than hormone modulation. It's hard to say for sure which elements of her program produced which specific changes. But from what we know about hormones and how they act in the body, it is clear that the hormone replacement part of her program deserves much of the credit for the transformation Nora has experienced. In particular, I would say that the natural estrogens and low-dose testosterone were largely responsible for Nora's enhanced sex drive, the more youthful appearance of her skin, and the improvement in the "brain fog" that plagues many menopausal women.

SUCCESSFUL HORMONE MODULATION

Although hormone modulation is obviously complex, the path to successful hormone modulation is fairly simple. Here are the basic steps that will help you maximize the benefits of hormone modulation:

1. First, you will need a qualified anti-aging specialist to guide your hormone replacement program.

2. Your symptoms, lab tests, and health history will help your anti-aging specialist pinpoint which hormones, if any, may be needed.

3. If hormone therapy is needed, "start low and go slow," using only natural and bioidentical hormones in the lowest amounts needed to restore optimal levels and balance.

4. Finally, remember that everything changes. Hormone levels are dynamic and are changing throughout our lives. If your protocol includes hormone modulation, I recommend that your hormone levels be retested annually. Periodic adjustments in your regimen may be necessary to keep things in balance.

For additional information, consult the section "Female Hormone Replacement Therapy" in the LEF Disease Prevention and Treatment database. See also Part III, which explains how to implement hormone testing and replacement into your complete anti-aging program.

II.
MALE HORMONE MODULATION

For men, sex hormone modulation is primarily a matter of supporting declining testosterone levels. But contrary to popular misconceptions, testosterone therapy is not just for bodybuilders and would-be Casanovas. It is for any man who wants to protect the health of his heart, bones, and brain. And yes, it also serves to enhance sexual function and maintain a more youthful physique.

As men approach middle age, levels of testosterone in the body typically begin to decline, and this is intimately connected to the physical, sexual, and cognitive changes that men experience as they get older. In my own practice, most of the men I see over the age of 45 or so are suffering from multiple symptoms due to declining testosterone.

A comprehensive research review of over two hundred published studies, compiled by the Life Extension Foundation, clearly shows that low testosterone levels due to aging are a prime risk factor for disease, disability, and even death. More to the point, low testosterone levels can be corrected with natural hormone supplements.

Yet men, and their doctors, are nervous about testosterone. The idea of hormone replacement for men is a relatively new one and, as such, it is not well-understood or widely accepted in conventional circles. First, there is some confusion about the dangers associated with anabolic steroid drugs. These synthetic forms of testosterone have been used irresponsibly by athletes and bodybuilders to artificially enhance their strength and performance. The use of natural testosterone in anti-aging protocols bears absolutely no resemblance to this dangerous practice.

Second, there is a widespread fear that raising testosterone levels may cause prostate disease. In fact, the evidence shows that prostate disease increases precisely as natural testosterone levels decline in the aging male and that the incidence of prostate dysfunction is at its lowest at the time when lifetime testosterone exposure is peaking.

I firmly believe that maintaining healthy testosterone levels is one of the most important things you can to do protect the health of your prostate. The newest research suggests that low testosterone *in combination with increasing estrogen* may be the true culprit in prostate dysfunction. Once again, the real story is in the balance between the various hormones. This is the key to safe and effective hormone therapy—a notion that is almost completely overlooked in conventional endocrinology.

As in the protocol for female hormones, my approach to male hormone modulation is not to push hormone levels higher blindly, but rather to mimic the body's own youthful equilibrium. With careful hormone modulation, men in their 40s, 50s, 60s, and beyond can maintain a hormonal environment that is similar to the peak physical environment of the youthful body. The anti-aging results are spectacular.

TESTOSTERONE'S ROLE IN SLOWING AGING

Testosterone levels have a big impact on neurological function and mood, particularly on one's sense of confidence, enthusiasm, and drive. The feeling that you can "take on the world" is a testosterone-driven feeling. Accordingly, the loss of testosterone in middle age can leave men feeling as if their life force is draining out of them. Low levels of testosterone have been correlated with depression in men.

Physically, testosterone fuels muscle growth and repair. Higher testosterone levels result in a higher percentage of lean muscle tissue, which is why men generally have less body fat and more muscle tissue than women who are equally fit. For men, the loss of muscle mass and strength and increased abdominal fat in middle age are telltale signs of declining testosterone.

Testosterone also protects the heart muscle from damage and helps prevent heart disease by keeping cholesterol and blood pressure down. The typical age-related decline in testosterone closely parallels the increase in heart disease as men get older, and testosterone therapy has been shown to improve heart conditions such as angina and to increase blood flow to the heart.

And, of course, the desire for sex, as well as sexual sensation and performance, is promoted by the stimulation of testosterone receptor sites in nerves, blood vessels, and the genitals. Declining testosterone levels are frequently behind a loss of libido (for both men and women) in midlife. Low testosterone can lead to atrophy of the male genitals, an effect that can be reversed if testosterone levels are increased.

Estrogen Dominance in Men

At the same time as testosterone production is fading in men, there is a tendency for estrogen levels to increase. In the preceding section on female hormone modulation, we talked about estrogen dominance syndrome, in which the balance between estrogen and progesterone tips too heavily toward estrogen.

In men, the same syndrome can occur, when the level of estrogen is too high compared with the levels of testosterone and progesterone. This comes as a shock to many of my male patients. We tend to think of estrogen as a "female" hormone and testosterone as a "male" hormone, forgetting that women's ovaries produce small amounts of testosterone, just as men's gonads produce small amounts of estrogen.

Estrogen imbalance in men is not only possible, it is common. In fact, men over the age of 50 frequently have estrogen levels that are even higher than those of women the same age. Too much estrogen in the male body can increase the risk of heart attack and stroke and lead to inflammation of the prostate (benign prostatic hyperplasia, or BPH). To make matters worse, excess estrogen can also suppress testosterone production in the testes.

As with women, estrogen dominance can be fueled by obesity, as fat cells in both men and women can produce and store estrogen. Estrogenic chemicals in the environment (such as those in commonly used pesticides) can also create estrogen imbalance in men. In fact, many researchers link these chemicals to the rising rates of infertility and impotence in American men.

There is one final complication that can increase estrogen levels in men. One of the particular qualities of steroid hormones (which includes the sex hormones as well as DHEA and cortisol) is that they can be converted into other steroid hormones in the body.

We've already seen that DHEA, for example, can be converted into testosterone and estrogen, depending on your sex. Testosterone is also converted into estrogen in both men and women (although estrogen cannot be converted back into testosterone). The conversion of testosterone to estrogen requires an enzyme called aromatase, thus the process is technically referred to as *aromatization*.

Excessive aromatization of testosterone is often a problem for men. Sometimes the problem is not that the testes are not producing enough testosterone, but that too much of that testosterone is being aromatized into estrogen. Paradoxically, as testosterone levels sink in the male body, the aromatization of testosterone into estrogen *increases,* which further lowers testosterone.

What Is an Ideal Testosterone Level?

Please remember that the ideal values for testosterone and all the other hormones vary greatly according to what testing methodology and laboratory process is used to measure the hormones. In Chapter 10, we'll discuss medical testing and interpretation in more detail. For purposes of illustration in this chapter, I am using the values that correspond to the lab that I personally use.

I use two different blood tests to measure the amounts of both total and free testosterone (in both men and women). For men, the optimal range for total testosterone is between 6,000 and 9,000 pg/mL. This is the level that you typically see in young, healthy men. Up to 99.7 percent of the total testosterone in circulation at any given time is bound up with proteins and is not in an active form. The amount of free, or available, testosterone should ideally be around 25 to 35 pg/mL.

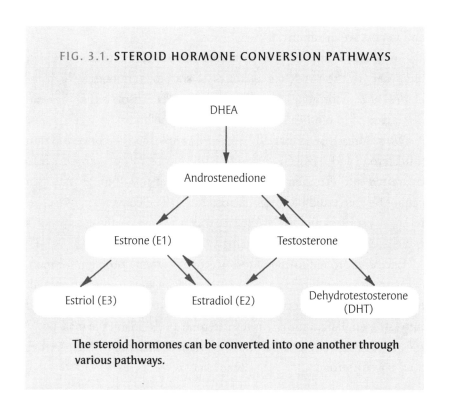

FIG. 3.1. STEROID HORMONE CONVERSION PATHWAYS

The steroid hormones can be converted into one another through various pathways.

In the chart below, Hormone Levels for Men, note the difference between normal ranges provided by the laboratory and my target levels for optimal health and function. The laboratory reference ranges reflect the levels found in the majority of a healthy test population. I have found, however, that men feel and function much better when testosterone levels are in the upper part of the normal range. Ideally, estrogen levels in men should be on the lower side of the normal range. As with women, I measure total estrogen levels as well as the individual types of estrogens, such as estradiol and estrone. (If you skipped the section on women's hormones, please refer back to the first half of this chapter for more information on the various types of estrogen.)

As with all hormones, the ratios between the various hormones are just as important as the individual hormone levels. These ratios are not standardized by any laboratory but instead have been developed through years of clinical experience. In observing how my male patients respond to hormone therapy and correlating that with lab results and other medical tests, clear patterns have emerged.

Hormone Levels for Men

Hormone	Lab Reference	Target
Testosterone (total)	2,700–9,700 pg/mL	6,000–9,000 pg/mL
Testosterone (free)	18–40 pg/mL	25–35 pg/mL
Estrogen	40–115 pg/mL	Less than 100 pg/mL
Estradiol (E2)	21–50 pg/mL	20–40 pg/mL

Men who are at their physical and mental peak generally have about 80 to 120 times as much total testosterone as estrogen. Another very sensitive and accurate measurement for male hormone balance is the ratio of estradiol (E2) to free testosterone, which should ideally be less than 1. For the great majority of men over the age of 40, these ratios can only be achieved with the help of bioidentical hormone replacement.

Target Hormone Ratios for Men	
Testosterone/estrogen	80–120
Estradiol/free testosterone	Less than 1

Laboratory testing offers invaluable insight into how the body is functioning. But hormone modulation can never be reduced to a paint-by-the-numbers project. Over the years, I have developed these target levels and ratios based on my clinical experience with scores of patients. But some of my most successful patients fall outside of these guidelines.

How you feel as a result of your therapy—what we call the "clinical picture"—is just as significant a piece of information as what your lab results say. Unfortunately, many conventional endocrinologists have all but forgotten this. I've had patients describe office visits in which the doctor never looked up from the lab report to see the patient sitting four feet away, and never asked a single question about how the patient was feeling.

Because each human body is wonderfully unique, the practice of hormone modulation—and medicine in general—must be a creative collaboration between doctor and patient, using the tools that science provides as well as the powers of observation, intuition, and insight that no test tube or petri dish can ever replace.

A Typical Scenario

In Chapter 1, I described my patient Brian as a typical example of how many people experience the aging process. While there was nothing medically wrong with Brian, he could clearly see that he was experiencing a gradual physical and mental decline. At 47 years old, Brian was 25 pounds heavier than he had been in graduate school, with most of it collecting around his waist. He was burned out at work, dragging himself through each day without enthusiasm. There was also increasing strain in his marriage because of his loss of interest in sex.

When we began working together, Brian's hormone pattern was quite typical for a middle-aged man. In the chart at the top of page 83,

Brian: 47-Year-Old Male

Hormone	Baseline	Optimal
Testosterone (total)	5,760 pg/mL	6,000–9,000 pg/mL
Testosterone (free)	16 pg/mL	25–35 pg/mL
Estrogen	145 pg/mL	Less than 100 pg/mL
Estradiol (E2)	21 pg/mL	20–40 pg/mL
Testosterone/ estrogen ratio	40	80–120
Estradiol/free testosterone ratio	1.3	Less than 1.0

you can see that low testosterone and high estrogen levels led to hormone ratios that were far from ideal.

The next chart shows the lab values for another patient of mine who first consulted me at age 66. Mark's hormone profile was also typical of an aging male. In fact, it gives a sense of how things might have contin-

Mark: 66-Year-Old Male

Hormone	Baseline	Optimal
Testosterone (total)	4,640 pg/mL	6,000–9,000 pg/mL
Testosterone (free)	19 pg/mL	25–35 pg/mL
Estrogen	170 pg/mL	Less than 100 pg/mL
Estradiol (E2)	16 pg/mL	20–40 pg/mL
Testosterone/ estrogen ratio	27	80–120
Estradiol/free testosterone ratio	0.8	Less than 1.0

ued for Brian had he not begun a program of hormone modulation. As testosterone and progesterone slowly sink lower and estrogen continues to climb, the imbalance between the hormones gets more and more extreme.

Mark was moderately overweight and was concerned about his rising high blood pressure and cholesterol. He was feeling old and tired, and lately he had begun to experience difficulty getting and maintaining an erection. All of this was very consistent with the hormonal imbalance revealed by his lab work.

I have worked with both Brian and Mark over a period of years, implementing and then maintaining a comprehensive anti-aging program with each of them. In addition to the nutritional and lifestyle protocols that we'll talk about in detail in Part III, their programs also included hormone replacement regimens, fine-tuned to their individual needs. As you can see from their initial values above, both Brian and Mark were suffering from low testosterone, exacerbated by high estrogen levels.

The obvious solution for testosterone deficiency would be to administer supplemental testosterone, much the way we used supplemental estrogen to raise the levels of estrogen in aging women. But in the case of testosterone, it turns out that the obvious solution is not the right solution.

The Testosterone Mistake

When the dangers of testosterone deficiency were first realized, researchers did experiment with testosterone replacement therapy as a possible treatment. However, the research failed to produce consistent benefits. Testosterone therapy did not reliably increase the amount of testosterone or free testosterone in the subjects.

Despite this, many doctors who are not specifically trained in antiaging medicine give in to pressure from male patients who believe that testosterone will make them more "virile," and prescribe testosterone patches or pills. And now, with the availability of prescription drugs from unreputable Internet vendors, men are able to obtain and use testosterone with no medical supervision whatsoever, vastly increasing the potential for harm.

! Hormone therapy is serious business that should be monitored by a *qualified* anti-aging physician. The abuse of testosterone is a perfect illustration of why this is so important. Unless it is correctly administered, testosterone replacement may be useless or can drive the testosterone/estrogen ratios even lower. In an effort to get the desired effect, men may be tempted to increase their dosage, even to harmful levels. Unfortunately, this will not help.

Previously, I mentioned that estrogen dominance syndrome in men can be driven in part by the aromatization of testosterone into estrogen. The aromatization issue has, in fact, turned out to be the key to successful male hormone modulation.

What the researchers studying testosterone replacement did not realize (because they were not measuring estrogen levels) was that for some men, most of the testosterone they were administering was being aromatized into estrogen. While researchers hoped to increase testosterone levels, the therapy produced the opposite effect of increasing estrogen levels and increasing hormonal imbalance, especially in older subjects.

THE PROBLEM WITH "ANDRO"

Androstenedione, commonly referred to as "andro," is a precursor hormone that is converted in the body to testosterone. Because it is available over the counter (whereas testosterone requires a prescription), andro has become popular as a do-it-yourself testosterone-boosting supplement.

Androstenedione, however, is also subject to aromatization into estrogen. (See Figure 3.1 on page 80.) There is no reliable way of controlling how much will be converted into testosterone and how much will be aromatized into estrogen. If testosterone levels are already low, this may increase the likelihood that aromatization will prevail.

A study published in the *Journal of the American Medical Association* showed that androstenedione actually increased estrogen levels in the subjects but failed to increase testosterone levels, strength, or muscle mass. Androstenedione is not recommended as a way to increase testosterone in men.

The Key to Successful Testosterone Therapy

In order to get the benefits of testosterone therapy, we need to take an extra step to block the conversion of testosterone into estrogen. This can be done with aromatase inhibitors, which are sometimes referred to as "estrogen-blocking" drugs. Arimidex and Aromasin are two such drugs. Originally developed to suppress estrogen levels in women with estrogen-dependent cancers, aromatase inhibitors can be used in much smaller dosages to block the conversion of testosterone to estrogen in men.

When testosterone therapy is administered together with Arimidex, testosterone goes up but estrogen stays low. When the ratio of testosterone to estrogen is increased, it makes a big difference in the way the body functions and feels.

In Brian's case, I recommended 50 mg of testosterone a day, in the form of gel that he rubbed into the thin skin on his inner arm in the morning. In addition, Brian took a very low daily dose of the prescription estrogen-blocking drug Arimidex.

Within three months, Brian's testosterone level increased dramatically to 10,950 pg/mL and his estrogen decreased to 123 pg/mL. If you compare this with the target ranges on page 83, you can see that both Brian's testosterone and estrogen levels were slightly higher than the target range. However, the testosterone/estrogen ratio was an ideal 89. Moreover, the ratio of estradiol to free testosterone had improved from 1.30 to 0.3. And best of all, Brian felt like a million bucks. Success!

The effects of Brian's anti-aging protocol on his quality of life were profound. Brian reported a vast improvement in energy, enthusiasm, and overall lust for life. He was working out regularly again and felt his body was responding to exercise better than it had in years. Perhaps most dramatic of all was the improvement in his sex drive, which he described as "like being back in college."

Progression of Hormone Therapy (Brian)			
Lab Values	Baseline	Rx	After 3 months
Testosterone	5,760 pg/mL (low)	Testosterone gel (50 mg)	10,950 pg/mL (slightly high)
Estrogen	145 pg/mL (high)	Arimidex	123 pg/mL (better, but still slightly high)
Testosterone/ estrogen ratio	39 (low)		89 (ideal)
Estradiol/ free testosterone	1.3 (high)		0.3 (ideal)

For Mark, I recommended a moderate dose of testosterone (100 mg per day), in the form of lozenges that are dissolved under the tongue. I also prescribed a low dose of Arimidex to prevent the aromatization of testosterone and to keep his estrogen levels down.

Two months later, Mark's estrogen levels were down to 104 pg/mL and his testosterone up to 10,960 pg/mL, for an ideal testosterone/estrogen ratio of 105. At this point I noticed that Mark's free testosterone levels were a bit high at 47, but his ratios were good and he felt great.

When hormone therapy is first initiated, it can take a few months for the body to adjust and balance itself. If you are testing your hormone levels frequently, you may see your levels changing somewhat erratically during that initial period. Furthermore, hormones are by nature constantly in flux. In addition to looking at the lab values, I am also looking at the bigger picture and the larger trends.

In Mark's case, we decided not to make any changes in his dosages but to test again after another month. The next month, his free testosterone had settled down to an ideal 33 pg/mL.

Like Brian, Mark felt a very noticeable improvement in his energy and mood from the higher testosterone levels. Much to his delight, he also found that his sexual performance improved. I was also very pleased to see improvement in many of his cardiac functions, including lower

Progression of Hormone Therapy (Mark)

Lab Values	Baseline	Rx	After 2 months	After 3 months
Testosterone	4,640 pg/mL (low)	Testosterone lozenges (100 mg)	10,960 pg/mL (slightly high)	8,230 pg/mL (ideal)
Testosterone (free)	19 pg/mL (low)		47 pg/mL (high)	33 pg/mL (ideal)
Estrogen	170 pg/mL	Arimidex	104 pg/mL (much better, but still slightly high)	102 pg/mL
Testosterone/ estrogen ratio	27 (low)		105 (ideal)	80 (ideal)

blood pressure and improved blood flow to and from the heart. While hormone modulation was just one aspect of Mark's program, these improvements are all consistent with the proven effects of higher testosterone levels.

The Importance of Natural Testosterone

In its natural form, testosterone cannot be absorbed when taken orally as a pill. The FDA has approved a synthetic methylated form of testosterone that can be taken as a pill, but I do not recommend this form. In high doses, methylated testosterone can be oncogenic (cancer-promoting) and can cause liver toxicity.

As with any hormone therapy, only natural, bioidentical hormones should be used, and only under the supervision of an anti-aging medical professional. Natural, bioidentical testosterone is available in various forms, including patches, creams, gels, and sublingual tablets or lozenges. All testosterone products require a prescription, and routine blood testing to monitor levels is essential.

IF TESTOSTERONE MAKES YOU "TESTY"

In most individuals, testosterone has very beneficial effects on mood, acting as a natural antidepressant and energizer. Less commonly, testosterone use can lead to irritability or unpleasant feelings of aggression. This is usually an indication that the dosage is too high and should be reduced.

HORMONES AND PROSTATE HEALTH

Sooner or later, most men over 40 (and some even younger) will experience prostate difficulties. The prostate is a doughnut-shaped gland that encircles the urethra. In middle age, this gland is prone to enlargement, a condition known as benign prostatic hyperplasia. This enlargement of the prostate can interfere with the flow of urine, leading to frequent and sometimes painful urination. And although BPH is by definition a benign condition, men with chronic BPH have an increased risk of prostate cancer later in life.

While the benefits of testosterone therapy can be life-changing, there is a widespread belief that testosterone replacement therapy may increase the risk of benign prostatic hyperplasia or prostate cancer. For this reason, many men think they have to live with the symptoms of testosterone deficiency.

Enlargement of the prostate is caused by excessive proliferation of the cells in the prostate. While many doctors believe that excess testosterone aggravates BPH, numerous studies show that high testosterone levels are in fact not a risk factor for BPH. In fact, the latest research suggests that it may actually be high *estrogen* levels that cause excessive proliferation of the prostate cells, in much the same way that estrogen can promote proliferation of cells in the breast.

Young men, who have the highest testosterone levels, rarely suffer from enlarged prostates. As men get older and testosterone levels drop, there is a greater tendency for testosterone to be aromatized into estrogen. There is also a greater incidence of BPH. Hormone modulation to support healthy testosterone levels may itself help slow down the aromatization process. The addition of aromatase inhibitors ensures that estrogen levels are kept in check, with benefits for prostate health.

Testosterone and Prostate Cancer

Prostate cancer is a more serious, but still related, concern. Benign growth of the prostate gland can eventually lead to malignant growth, or prostate cancer. Prostate cancer is extremely common, affecting one out of every eight men in their lifetimes. While prostate cancer can often be successfully treated, the treatments frequently cause permanent incontinence or impotence. One in every twenty-eight men will die of prostate cancer.

Most researchers now agree with my long-held belief that high testosterone is not itself a risk factor for prostate cancer. However, it is true that if prostate cancer is present, testosterone (or more accurately, the testosterone metabolite DHT) can fuel its growth.

For this reason, there is controversy over whether testosterone therapy should be used for anyone with established prostate cancer. While many anti-aging specialists prefer not to use testosterone replacement in the presence of prostate cancer, testosterone is actually being used in Europe as a treatment for prostate cancer. This is an issue that requires further research.

! Before beginning testosterone therapy, it is important to be screened for existing prostate cancer. This is usually done by measuring the prostate-specific antigen (PSA), in addition to a digital rectal exam. Contrary to popular notions, PSA is not a marker of prostate cancer but is instead a marker of prostate inflammation, or BPH. The correlation between PSA readings and prostate cancer is not exact, but PSA readings do provide a helpful (if incomplete) indication of prostate health.

If you were to have early prostate cancer, so early that it could not yet be detected by standard screening, testosterone therapy would most likely trigger an increase in your PSA readings. It's important to understand that the testosterone would not have caused prostate cancer in this case. It would merely have brought it to light sooner than it might otherwise have been. As with any cancer, early detection always improves the chances of successful treatment.

Because men with long-standing BPH have an increased likelihood of developing prostate cancer, those with moderate to severe BPH have a difficult decision regarding the benefits versus risks of testosterone therapy. The drug Proscar (finasteride) prevents the conversion of testosterone into DHT, much the way that aromatase inhibitors block the conversion of testosterone into estrogen. Because it is DHT (and not testosterone) that can fuel prostate growth, the combination of testosterone with Proscar may offer the health benefits of testosterone therapy while adding further protection against prostate cancer for those at increased risk.

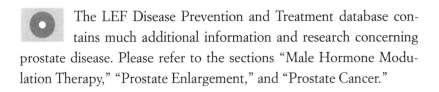 The LEF Disease Prevention and Treatment database contains much additional information and research concerning prostate disease. Please refer to the sections "Male Hormone Modulation Therapy," "Prostate Enlargement," and "Prostate Cancer."

Nutrients for Prostate Health

Because prostate disease is a concern for every man, I recommend a nutrient protocol to protect prostate health for all male patients, whether or not hormones are part of their anti-aging program. Taking these herbs as a preventive measure will help to promote healthy prostate function throughout life. Prostate health formulas containing these herbs are readily available at health food stores, drugstores, and groceries, by mail order, and over the Internet. As with any herbal formulation, look for a product that specifies pharmaceutical-grade standardized extracts for the active ingredients.

Nettle extract, or *Urtica dioica,* has been the pharmaceutical treatment of choice in Germany for over a decade. Studies have shown that it can reduce BPH symptoms by 86 percent after three months of use. Nettle extract appears to work by preventing the binding of testosterone proteins to prostate cell membranes.

Pygeum extract also has a successful record in the treatment and prevention of prostate difficulties. By blocking DHT from attaching to prostate cell receptor sites, it inhibits the proliferation of prostate cells. Pygeum is also anti-inflammatory, which can significantly reduce the size of an enlarged prostate.

Lycopene is an antioxidant nutrient found in tomatoes and to a lesser extent in watermelon and pink grapefruit. Studies have indicated that men who regularly consume lycopene have lower rates of prostate cancer.

Zinc is critical to sexual function and prostate health and is frequently found in men's health formulas. However, a recent study showed that too much zinc (more than 100 mg per day) can double your rate of prostate cancer.

! Total zinc intake (from all supplements, including any multivitamin or mineral formula) should not exceed 50 mg per day. Be sure to balance zinc by taking it along with its natural mineral partner, copper.

Selenium levels have been specifically linked to prostate cancer incidence (low levels increase your risk). Because selenium levels tend to decline with age, supplementation is increasingly important as you get older.

Nutritional Protocol for Prostate Health	
Nettle extract (standardized potency)	120–250 mg/day
Pygeum (standardized potency)	50–100 mg/day
Lycopene (standardized extract)	10–20 mg/day
Zinc	30–50 mg/day
Selenium	200 mcg/day

Saw Palmetto: Special Considerations

Saw palmetto is one of the most popular natural remedies to relieve symptoms of BPH. This herbal extract works by the same mechanism as the prescription drug Proscar, blocking the conversion of testosterone to DHT by inhibiting the enzyme needed for the conversion. Saw palmetto has been shown to be highly effective in reducing enlargement of the prostate and in relieving urinary symptoms. Saw palmetto extract also inhibits the growth of prostate cancer cells.

While it is very effective in relieving symptoms of BPH, I do not recommend long-term use of saw palmetto as a preventive therapy. As we have seen, the increase in estrogen levels that is common in older men helps to fuel prostate inflammation and cell proliferation.

My own clinical experience has led me to suspect that while saw palmetto blocks the conversion of testosterone into DHT, it may also increase the aromatization of testosterone into estrogen. This second action would obviously be at cross purposes with our goals for both anti-aging and prostate health.

This is an area that has not been widely studied and needs further research. Until these questions have more definitive answers, I think it is wise to limit the use of saw palmetto, using it as needed to relieve symptoms but not as an ongoing therapy. When I do use saw palmetto, I couple it with aromatase inhibitors to prevent an unintentional boost in estrogen.

Natural Progesterone Therapy for Men

As I pointed out in the previous section on women's hormone modulation, conventional medicine gravely underestimates the benefits of progesterone for women's health. However, the importance of progesterone for men's health has been overlooked completely.

Progesterone plays an important role in prostate health. In much the same way as it protects against proliferation of cells in the female breast, progesterone may protect against proliferation of cells in the prostate. It is a potent inhibitor of DHT (dehydrotestosterone), which is the metabolite of testosterone that fuels prostate growth and prostate cancer.

Progesterone also helps to prevent bone loss in men, as it does in women. Unfortunately, public health campaigns on the dangers of osteoporosis sometimes create the impression that osteoporosis is a woman's health issue. As a result, men are less likely to take action to prevent bone loss. Although it tends to strike later in life, osteoporosis is just as debilitating for older men as it is in postmenopausal women. By age 65, men are losing bone mass as fast as women their age. By age 75, osteoporosis is as common in men as it is in women. In fact, spinal and hip fractures due to osteoporosis are a major cause of disability and death in older men.

Progesterone therapy for men remains a somewhat controversial issue. Progesterone researcher Dr. John Lee reports anecdotal evidence that men using progesterone cream have seen a decrease in their PSA (a marker for prostate dysfunction). Given progesterone's known ability to inhibit DHT, this is logical. Unfortunately, progesterone replacement for men is an area that has not yet been well researched, but it deserves greater attention.

In my opinion, the biochemical evidence more than supports the use of low-dose progesterone therapy for men when it is needed to correct hormone levels and ratios. Maintaining healthy progesterone levels promotes prostate health and sexual function, and helps to prevent bone loss.

The reference ranges for progesterone in men are generally quite low. For example, the laboratory I use considers a progesterone level between 300 and 1,000 pg/mL to be normal for a middle-aged man. By these standards, my patients Brian and Mark were both in the normal range with progesterone levels of 800 and 400, respectively. (As in women, progesterone levels in men tend to get lower and lower with age.)

From my clinical experience, however, I have found that men with higher progesterone levels are healthier and more youthful. My target for men is between 1,500 and 2,500 pg/mL, although I frequently see even higher levels in patients who are using anti-aging therapies. I rarely observe problems due to high progesterone.

Your ideal progesterone level is also determined by your estrogen level. If your estrogen level is on the high side, more progesterone is needed to balance the effects. When estrogen is low, progesterone may also be a bit lower. For men, I aim for a ratio of fifteen to twenty-five times as much progesterone as estrogen.

Target Progesterone Levels and Ratios for Men	
Progesterone	1,500–2,500 pg/mL
Progesterone/ estrogen ratio	15–20

My experience has been that it takes only a very mild stimulus to lift progesterone levels in men. Therefore, I administer progesterone therapy with a very light touch. Progesterone cream can be purchased over the counter, but as described in the previous section, it is important to be sure that the cream contains a standardized concentration of pharmaceutical-grade natural progesterone.

For men with low progesterone levels, I recommend 25 mg ($\frac{1}{4}$ teaspoon) of progesterone cream rubbed into the inner arm or thigh before bedtime. While testosterone is stimulating and is best administered in the morning, progesterone has a natural sedative effect. When applied before bed, it can help to promote more restful sleep.

Because progesterone helps to balance excessive estrogen in men, progesterone therapy frequently has the welcome effect of boosting libido and sexual performance in men.

Pregnenolone: The Progesterone Stimulator

Another way to gently boost low progesterone is with the hormone pregnenolone. This precursor hormone can be converted into progesterone in the body. In Brian's case, 20 mg per day of pregnenolone brought his low progesterone up to target levels, which in turn also corrected his progesterone/estrogen ratios.

Pregnenolone is also available over the counter as a dietary

Progression of Hormone Therapy (Brian)			
Lab Values	*Baseline*	*Rx*	*After 6 months*
Progesterone	800 pg/mL (low)	20 mg pregnenolone	2,100 pg/mL (ideal)
Progesterone/ estrogen ratio	5.52 (very low)		23 (ideal)

supplement, but men taking either progesterone or pregnenolone should continue to seek guidance from a medical professional to monitor hormone levels on an ongoing basis. Although I have never seen adverse effects from excessively high progesterone levels, you want to be sure that the hormone levels are balanced.

I often find that low progesterone production corrects itself, making ongoing supplementation unnecessary. As the body is rejuvenated through a general anti-aging program and other hormones are brought into alignment, it seems to boost the body's natural hormone production. This was the case with Mark. Although I did not prescribe progesterone or pregnenolone therapy for Mark, his progesterone levels went up on their own as his anti-aging program was implemented. As his estrogen levels also dropped, the progesterone/estrogen ratio was brought into balance.

SUMMING IT UP

To maintain your health, strength, and vigor as you age, you need to support healthy, youthful hormone levels. Although I have tried to give you a detailed understanding of the issues involved with the various sex hormones, I hope I have also convinced you that hormone modulation is not a do-it-yourself proposition.

To get really great results from hormone modulation, you need to work with someone who understands the complexities of testing, hormone balance, and interaction. With expert guidance, hormones are one of the most powerful tools we have to rejuvenate and reinvigorate the body as it ages.

Here are the basic steps to follow in order to begin enjoying the benefits of hormone modulation:

1. First, an anti-aging specialist will evaluate your hormone levels and health status, including prostate health.

2. Using lab tests as well as your symptoms as a guide, your doctor will recommend natural, bioidentical hormones as needed to bring hormone levels and ratios into healthy, youthful ranges.

3. Always protect your prostate with nutrients that promote prostate health.

4. Finally, annual hormone testing is critical to monitor levels and maintain hormone balance. (Prostate cancer screening should be repeated every four to six weeks for the first six months of testosterone therapy to rule out undetected prostate cancer.)

As I stated in the beginning of this chapter, hormone modulation plays a central role in countering the effects of biological aging. But hormone therapy extends far beyond the sex hormones. In Chapter 4, we'll look at the critical role of the thyroid in maintaining a youthful metabolism. Then we'll delve into the power and promise of human growth hormone. In Part III, you'll see how all of these therapies fit into your complete anti-aging program.

CHAPTER 4

Tapping the Power of Thyroid and Growth Hormone

The biggest human temptation is to settle for too little.
—THOMAS MERTON

IN THE LAST CHAPTER, we saw the dramatic difference that hormone replacement made for my 50-year-old patient Nora, an advertising executive in the film industry. Nora's hormone profiles were typical for someone her age, reflecting the age-related decline in the production of many hormones. To compensate for this, I developed a hormone replacement regimen for Nora that included DHEA, estrogen, and small amounts of testosterone. As you may recall, Nora was delighted with the improvement in her mental clarity, mood, skin tone, and libido—all benefits of more youthful hormone profiles.

But anti-aging hormone modulation does not stop with the steroid hormones that we discussed in Chapters 2 and 3. This chapter details two other hormone systems that are central to my approach to anti-aging medicine. The first of these is the thyroid, an area that is very familiar to (but largely misunderstood by) conventional endocrinologists. The second is the more mysterious and powerful human growth hormone. Both thyroid and growth hormone are fundamental to maintaining a youthful, healthy body as you grow older.

I.
THYROID: THE METABOLIC ACTIVATOR

Nora was quite surprised when I suggested that low thyroid function was contributing to her symptoms of fatigue, constipation, and unexplained weight gain. Just a year before she consulted me for an anti-aging program, Nora's family doctor had tested her thyroid function as part of a general medical workup. Her blood test results were within the normal range, and the doctor informed Nora that her thyroid was fine.

In anti-aging medicine, of course, we're not interested in normal. Our goal is optimal function, optimal health, and optimal well-being. And as we've seen before, there is usually a big difference between normal and optimal.

Many people with supposedly normal thyroid function are actually suffering from symptoms of *suboptimal* thyroid function. When thyroid function is suboptimal, it often results in weight gain or difficulty losing weight, constipation, insomnia, and fatigue. You may be more susceptible to colds and infections. Cold hands and feet, sleepiness, and dry or flaky skin are other telltale signs of low thyroid function.

By contrast, when the thyroid is working well, you literally have energy to burn. A vigorous, youthful metabolism means more physical and mental energy to power you through the day and more restful sleep at night. The skin has a youthful glow. Excess weight drops off naturally. And your immune system is empowered to protect you against the diseases of aging.

Many of my patients—including those who have been told that their thyroid function is normal—are stunned at the difference they feel when suboptimal thyroid function is brought up to ideal, youthful levels.

For Nora, addressing her undiagnosed low thyroid function helped to end a long-standing battle with her weight, which had been creeping up by a pound or three a year for the past decade. With a moderate amount of thyroid hormone added to her hormone replacement regimen, Nora was delighted to see her weight begin to go down, to a total loss of about 30 pounds over the course of the following year. As you will see, there are many other important reasons to optimize thyroid function as well, such as protecting against heart disease and slowing the aging process.

WHAT YOUR THYROID DOES FOR YOU

The thyroid gland, located in your neck, secretes hormones that regulate your energy metabolism, controlling how much energy is stored in the form of fat and how much is actually released into the cells for use by the body. The thyroid helps to regulate your body temperature, your sleep rhythms, and your digestive function, and it is crucial to the immune system's ability to fight off infections and even cancer cells. It is also critical to cognitive functions and mood.

Symptoms of Low Thyroid Function

- Depression—both physical and mental
- Clouded thinking—loss of cognitive edge
- Fatigue
- Feeling cold
- Dry, flaky skin
- Poor digestion with frequent "bloated" feeling
- Constipation
- Low resistance to infection (such as colds and flu)
- Weight gain or difficulty losing weight
- Difficulty conceiving and/or miscarriages
- Heavy or prolonged menstrual bleeding that is not effectively controlled by appropriate estrogen/progesterone therapy

HIDDEN HORMONE DEFICIENCIES

There are a handful of diseases that can affect thyroid function, including cancer, benign growths, and autoimmune conditions such as Hashimoto's disease or Graves' disease. Any of these can cause your thyroid to produce too much hormone (hyperthyroidism) or too little (hypothyroidism). These diseases are relatively rare. If you were to suffer from one of them, it would most likely be quickly recognized and treated by a conventional endocrinologist.

While thyroid *disease* may be rare, thyroid *dysfunction* is rampant—especially as people get older. Thyroid function gradually slows down as we age. With decreased thyroid function come a host of symptoms that we have come to associate with aging, such as poor digestion, fatigue, constipation, weight gain, reduced immune function, and so on. This may all be a normal part of the aging process—but it does not have to be this way! With proper treatment, these typical symptoms of aging can be avoided or greatly reduced.

Despite the fact that low thyroid function is both common and easily treated, it usually goes undiagnosed and untreated. The American Association of Clinical Endocrinologists (AACE) estimates one out of every five women and one out of ten men over the age of 60 suffer from an underactive thyroid gland. In fact, I believe that the number of people who can benefit from thyroid support is far higher than the AACE acknowledges. Once again, there is a critical distinction between what conventional medicine accepts as normal and what anti-aging medicine views as optimal.

How Thyroid Function Is Measured

The thyroid takes its orders from the pituitary gland (and the hypothalamus), which are constantly monitoring the amount of thyroid hormone (thyroxine) that is circulating in the blood.

When the level of thyroxine gets low, the pituitary gland releases thyroid stimulating hormone, or TSH. As the name suggests, TSH signals the thyroid to produce more thyroxine. As the amount of thyroxine in the blood increases, the production of TSH is suppressed. This in turn slows the production of thyroxine. This feedback loop between the pituitary and thyroid works to keep the level of thyroid hormone relatively constant.

We can use TSH levels as one measure of thyroid function, but the relationship is an inverse one. In other words, *high* TSH levels may indicate *low* thyroid function and vice versa. When TSH levels are high, it means that the pituitary is signaling for more thyroid hormone. This suggests that the thyroid is underactive and is not producing enough thyroid hormone for the body's needs. On the other hand, if TSH is very low, it suggests that an overactive thyroid might be secreting too much thyroid hormone, which would suppress the level of TSH.

When TSH is neither too high nor too low, it indicates that the body has just enough thyroid hormone. The critical issue here is how you define what is "too high" or "too low." Once again, the anti-aging approach is somewhat more particular than the conventional approach. Where TSH levels anywhere from 0.2 to 5.5 may be considered normal by conventional endocrinologists, the optimal range is between 1.0 and 2.0.

Unrecognized Health Hazards

When I tested her blood, Nora's TSH level was 2.41, well within the normal reference range. However, researchers have shown that people with TSH levels higher than 2.0 are at a higher risk of future thyroid problems. In other words, slightly elevated TSH levels are likely to continue to climb.

! If your TSH levels are above 4.0 (still well within the "normal" range), *you are at increased risk of heart disease.* This is serious business.

We hear a lot about heart disease, both from the government as well as from the pharmaceutical companies selling cholesterol and other heart disease drugs on television. It is, as we all know, the number one killer in America. You would think that the link between TSH levels and heart disease would be taken more seriously by the conventional medical world. This connection alone should be more than enough reason to update the reference ranges for TSH.

Despite all the evidence to the contrary, however, unless your TSH is over 5.5, a conventional doctor will most likely tell you that your thyroid is just fine. Most of my patients, however, do not consider premature aging and an increased risk of heart disease to be fine, especially when there is something they can do to reduce the risk.

Evaluating Thyroid Function

TSH (mU/L)	Conventional approach	Anti-aging paradigm	TSH (mU/L)
Over 5.5	Underactive thyroid	Increased risk of heart disease	Over 4.0
0.2–5.5	"Normal"	Increased risk of future thyroid deficiency	2.0–4.0
		Optimal thyroid function	1.0–2.0
		Overactive thyroid	Less than 1.0
Less than 0.2	Overactive thyroid		

Research has shown, for example, that treatment with thyroid hormone may lower high cholesterol levels. In my opinion, no one should be prescribed cholesterol-lowering drugs until steps have been taken to bring the body into optimal hormonal and nutritional balance. (We will be discussing the pros and cons of cholesterol drugs and their alternatives in more detail in Part II.) Many times, treating a thyroid deficiency will bring cholesterol down naturally.

! If you have heart disease (or are at risk), and your thyroid function has not been checked recently, request a blood test to rule out low thyroid function. If your TSH level is over 4.0, ask your doctor to consider treatment.

ANTI-AGING BENEFITS OF THYROID REPLACEMENT

Once identified, low thyroid function can be easily corrected by augmenting the body's own production with bioidentical thyroid hormones.

As part of Nora's hormone augmentation program, I prescribed a low dose (37 mcg per day) of thyroxine. If you follow alternative medicine, you may be familiar with the position that Armour dessicated thyroid, which is derived from porcine thyroid tissue, is a more "natural" form of thyroid hormone. As you will see below, I use Armour in patients whose bodies cannot properly convert thyroxine into the active form of the hormone. But for many patients, the thyroxine form works as well or better.

When we retested her blood several months later, her TSH had settled to 1.7. More importantly, Nora noticed an enormous change in the way she felt. She reported a dramatic increase in energy, to the extent that she had stopped drinking coffee in the morning because she no longer needed the caffeine to wake her up. If you are someone who can't get both eyes open until you've had your first cup of coffee, you will appreciate the magnitude of the change Nora felt.

As I have mentioned, Nora also lost quite a bit of weight over the course of the first year we worked together—30 pounds altogether. This was not the result of dieting. Although Nora did make some changes in her diet similar to the ones that I've outlined for you in Chapter 11, she did not try to restrict her intake of food or calories. Her weight loss was primarily the result of a more youthful metabolism. Although many things in the anti-aging program contribute to this effect, optimizing thyroid function is a chief factor.

Undertreatment Is Also a Major Problem

As we have seen, low thyroid function often goes undiagnosed, and many suffer unnecessarily from symptoms that could be easily resolved. But equally shocking is the number of people who continue to suffer from low thyroid symptoms, *even though they have been diagnosed and are receiving treatment.*

A group of researchers in Colorado measured thyroid hormone levels in over twenty-five thousand people. In that very diverse group, about one in ten had abnormally high levels of TSH (and in this study, TSH levels had to be higher than 5.2 in order to be considered too high). One of the most striking things about their findings, however, was that *40 percent of people who were already taking thyroid medications still had abnormally high TSH levels.*

In other words, *almost half* of those who were diagnosed with low thyroid function were not receiving adequate treatment for their condition. And once again, that number (40 percent) only includes those whose TSH levels were higher than 5.2. Had these researchers used the guidelines for optimal thyroid function as their criteria, the numbers would have been even higher.

This was precisely the situation with my patient Willow, who, as you may recall from Chapter 2, was suffering from adrenal exhaustion. When I started treating Willow, she had been taking thyroid medication for years. Nonetheless, she continued to experience symptoms of thyroid insufficiency.

Like many people who are diagnosed with an underactive thyroid, Willow had been given a standardized dose of Synthroid (thyroxine). In her case, this was clearly not enough to completely correct the problem. Her continuing symptoms were a signal that the issue required more attention. Sadly, far too many endocrinologists are guilty of treating their patients strictly by the numbers. If the blood tests are normal, they consider the problem solved, regardless of how the patient feels. At this point, many patients are told that any remaining symptoms must be in their heads, as the laboratory reports "prove" that the problem has been solved.

DON'T SETTLE FOR TREATMENT
BY THE NUMBERS

It's true that a blood test can provide your doctor with valuable information about what's happening from a biochemical point of view. However, no lab test is more important or significant than your own evaluation of how you feel. Your lab results might be perfect. But if you don't feel fantastic, your doctor should continue to look for solutions.

In fact, Willow's blood tests confirmed that despite the thyroid hormone she was taking, her thyroid profile was not optimal—although it was within the range generally accepted as normal. As part of her total hormone rebalancing program, which included DHEA therapy and cortisol to support her adrenal glands, I also made some adjustments in her thyroid medication.

A slight increase in her thyroxine prescription, from 50 mcg per day to 75 mcg per day, made all the difference. After decades of ineffective treatment for an underactive thyroid, Willow finally got to experience what it feels like to be operating under optimal thyroid function. This underscores the importance of paying attention to how you feel, regardless of what the tests indicate. The treatment of the thyroid should always involve experienced clinical judgment, with the help of complete, thorough, and up-to-date lab testing.

Willow's case also illustrates the importance of looking at the hormones in relationship to one another and not in isolation. In Willow's case, both thyroid and adrenal function were low—a fairly common phenomenon. She had been treated for thyroid problems for years, without getting relief. I suspect that her untreated adrenal exhaustion was one of the reasons that Willow's thyroid symptoms had not completely responded to treatment.

WHEN THYROID TREATMENT DOESN'T WORK

Whenever thyroid problems are suspected or treated, it is important to monitor adrenal function as well. Attempting to treat low thyroid levels without supporting the adrenals can deplete the adrenal glands. At the same time, if your adrenals are weak, symptoms of low thyroid may persist even after your thyroid levels have been restored.

❗ If you have been treated for low thyroid function but continue to have a lot of the same symptoms, adrenal exhaustion may be a hidden factor. Treating low adrenal function (discussed in Chapter 2) can bring about a dramatic improvement in persistent thyroid problems.

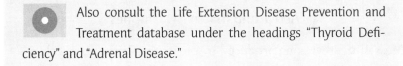

Also consult the Life Extension Disease Prevention and Treatment database under the headings "Thyroid Deficiency" and "Adrenal Disease."

Recognizing and treating the adrenal exhaustion *in conjunction with* her thyroid problem finally brought Willow some relief from her long-standing fatigue, anxiety, and depression. Stabilizing her mood and energy levels then gave her a foundation upon which to build a more ambitious anti-aging program.

Low Thyroid Function Is Not Just a Problem for Women

The conventional wisdom is that thyroid problems are relatively un-common in men. Therefore, men are rarely screened for thyroid defi-ciency. This is a serious error. In my practice, I find that men are just as likely to suffer from suboptimal thyroid function as women. Many of these men start out with TSH levels that indicate an increased risk of heart disease. And yet most of them would be overlooked by conven-tional doctors using "normal" reference ranges for thyroid function.

Finn was a 50-year-old man who came to me for an anti-aging pro-gram after attending a lecture that I gave at a local college. Something in my talk (which was on changing attitudes toward aging and health) struck a chord with Finn. Perhaps it had something to do with the mile-stone birthday he'd just celebrated, but Finn realized that his health and general vitality were slipping away from him. He decided that he wanted to take action against aging.

As part of his initial workup, I tested Finn's thyroid function and found that his TSH was slightly elevated at 2.67. But TSH, which is ac-tually produced by the pituitary gland, is only one part of the picture: it measures the body's *need* for thyroid hormone. To get a complete picture of how the thyroid itself is working, I also look at the level of thyroxine in the blood. (Unfortunately, doctors are frequently forced to evaluate thyroid function based solely on TSH levels because of limitations placed on them by insurance companies.)

Active and Inactive Hormones

Most of the thyroxine produced by the thyroid is in a form called T4, because each molecule of hormone contains four atoms of iodine. Before T4 can be used in the tissues of the body, however, it has to be converted into a form containing only three atoms of iodine, called T3. Both T4 and T3 can be measured with blood tests.

In order to get the most complete and accurate picture of thyroid function, I measure T4 and T3 along with TSH. The TSH reading tells me whether the tissues of the body are getting enough thyroid hormone. The level of T4 tells me whether or not the thyroid is able to produce adequate amounts of hormone. The level of T3 tells me whether the T4 form is being converted properly into the biologically more potent T3 form. When the thyroid is working well, all three of these hormones will usually be in the optimal ranges shown below. (Note: a complete thyroid workup will also include other tests, such as reverse T3 and thyroid antibodies.)

Similar to testosterone, much of the T4 and T3 in circulation is tightly bound to protein molecules, with a smaller amount of each hormone circulating in an unbound (or free) format. Tests that measure only the amount of free T3 and free T4 give a more accurate idea of how much hormone is available to the tissues. Although I prefer to test for free hormones, reference ranges and optimal values for both total and free T3 and T4 are shown on page 109.

Fine-Tuning the Program

In Finn's case, his free T4 was 1.2, just within the target range, but his free T3 levels were on the low side at 2.70. I suspected that Finn's problem was twofold. First, his thyroid was slowing down with age, producing less thyroid hormone. Complicating this was the fact that Finn's body was having trouble converting the inactive form of T4 to the active T3 form. It's quite possible that Finn may have suffered from low-grade thyroid deficiency for most of his life, due to an inability to convert T4 into T3 efficiently.

As long as the conversion from T4 to T3 is taking place, low thyroid function can be treated successfully with T4 (Synthroid or Levoxyl) alone. But when I suspect problems with the conversion, I use another form of thyroid hormone that supplies both T4 and T3 (Armour desiccated thryoid). I prescribed a low dose of Armour thyroid (¼ grain per day) for Finn. Over the next six months, we watched his T3 levels come up nicely, but the TSH remained a bit high.

Thyroid Hormones		
Hormone	*Normal reference range*	*Optimal values*
TSH (mU/L)	0.2–5.5	1.0–2.0
Free T3 (pg/mL)	2.60–4.80	2.80–3.20
Free T4 (ng/dL)	0.70–1.53	1.2–1.4
Total T3 (ng/dL)	60–181	120–124
Total T4 (mcg/dL)	4.5–12.0	7.5–8.1

With hormone modulation, I frequently work with patients intensively over the course of a year or more, making small adjustments in their regimen, in order to find just the right balance. Over time, and with some experimentation, we arrived at a somewhat unusual but effective formula for Finn. In the end, it was a combination of Armour (T3 and T4) and Levoxyl (T4) that succeeded in bringing his thyroid profile into optimal balance. To Finn, it felt like waking up. The constant feeling of sleepiness that had dogged him throughout his life was gone. "I feel like someone just replaced my batteries!" he told me.

How to Get the Right Kind of Treatment

Thyroid hormone is available only with a doctor's prescription. But as you have seen, low thyroid function is often overlooked and undertreated by conventional doctors. You can and should ask to see the results of any laboratory tests your doctor orders, and discuss them with your doctor. (See also Chapter 10 on medical testing.) A qualified anti-aging physician will evaluate and treat the thyroid with optimal, youthful function as a goal, and in the context of a complete anti-aging protocol. (The appendix lists resources for locating anti-aging medical professionals.)

Progression of Treament (Finn)					
Hormone	Baseline	Rx	After 4 months	Rx	After 1 year
TSH	2.67 mU/L (high)	$^1/_4$ grain Armour	3.7 mU/L (high)	$^1/_4$ grain Armour plus 25 mcg Levoxyl (T4)	1.55 mU/L (ideal)
Free T4	1.2 ng/dL (ideal)		1.2 ng/dL (ideal)		1.2 pg/mL (ideal)
Free T3	2.70 pg/mL (low)		3.60 pg/mL (ideal)		3.00 pg/mL (ideal)

Optimizing thyroid function was only one aspect of Finn's anti-aging program. Like most men over 40, Finn also had low levels of DHEA and testosterone, which we treated with the protocols described in Chapters 2 and 3. As he saw his health and his body change in response to his anti-aging program, Finn became more and more enthusiastic about anti-aging therapies. He decided to take his program to the next level: the addition of human growth hormone.

Personally, I consider growth hormone therapy to be the gold standard in anti-aging hormone therapies. However, there is a lot to consider before deciding whether this powerful therapy is for you.

II.
GROWTH HORMONE:
THE ULTIMATE ANTI-AGING HORMONE

The remarkable growth and development of our bodies, from tiny babies to full-size adults, is orchestrated largely by human growth hormone, or HGH. Growth hormone is responsible for the astonishing growth spurts of childhood, in which a pair of shoes or pants can be outgrown in a matter of weeks. The remarkable healing powers of children, in which wounds seem to disappear overnight, is also a feature of growth hormone activity.

As we reach adulthood and our physical maturation is complete, the role of HGH downshifts to one of repair and regeneration (or rejuvenation). If tissues or organs are damaged by trauma or disease, growth hormone works to regenerate them. Growth hormone also works throughout life to maintain bone strength, muscle tone, brain function, and the integrity of the hair and skin.

As with other hormones, the body's production of growth hormone diminishes with age. By the age of 60, levels of growth hormone are commonly one-quarter of their youthful levels. The loss of growth hormone, along with other hormonal declines, leads to symptoms we associate with aging:

- Thinning, sagging, and wrinkled skin
- Thinning bones (osteopenia or osteoporosis)
- Loss of muscle strength
- Accumulation of fat tissue
- Decreasing heart function
- Failure of the immune system
- Thinning hair
- Loss of sexual function and desire
- Decreased stamina and vigor

Perhaps more powerfully than with any other hormone system we have discussed so far, supplementing the body's waning production of growth hormone with bioidentical replacement hormones can reduce and even reverse the changes normally associated with the aging process. Growth hormone replacement therapy enhances the effects that we have already seen with testosterone and estrogen therapy: more youthful skin, increased lean muscle mass, and increased mental and physical vitality. But with the addition of growth hormone, the changes are even more dramatic and profound.

In 1990, the *New England Journal of Medicine* published a study that put growth hormone therapy and anti-aging medicine in the headlines. The now famous Rudman study documented the amazing results of growth hormone therapy in a pilot study of twenty-one men between the ages of 61 and 81. In six months of therapy, the subjects experienced some very dramatic and positive changes in their bodies. Measurements showed an increase in lean muscle tissue (+8.8 percent), a decrease in fat deposits (−14.4 percent), an increase in skin thickness (+7.1 percent), and an increase in lumbar bone density (+1.6 percent). A control group that received no therapy had no significant changes in any measures. As Rudman and his colleagues summed it up, the six months of growth hormone therapy resulted in changes equivalent to the reversal of ten to twenty years of biological aging.

The Rudman study unleashed a furor that continues unabated to this day. The anti-aging community has heralded growth hormone as the ultimate anti-aging therapy, while the conventional establishment continues to insist that growth hormone therapy is unproven and risky.

Anti-aging physicians are not the only ones prescribing growth hormone therapy, however. Growth hormone is a readily available, FDA-approved drug. It is given to children with growth disorders, and lately even to *healthy children who are simply of short stature.* (In my opinion, the purely cosmetic use of growth hormone in children who have not even finished growing renders the establishment's strident warnings about the use of growth hormone in aging adults almost ridiculous.)

Growth hormone injections are also standard treatment for adults with a clinical diagnosis of growth hormone deficiency due to pituitary failure or disease. It is widely accepted that growth hormone deficiency in adults causes premature aging, the symptoms of which are reversed when growth hormone injections are given. So what is the controversy all about? The controversy centers around the clinical definition of "deficiency."

With the exception of estrogen, the conventional medical community considers age-related hormonal decline to be normal, and therefore takes no action to correct it. Low levels of other hormones such as DHEA, thyroid, testosterone, and growth hormone are not treated unless (or until) a full-blown disease such as adrenal failure, hypothyroidism, or pituitary disease is diagnosed.

By the standards of anti-aging medicine, however, when a low hormone level has a negative impact on health, it is considered and treated as a *deficiency*. It doesn't matter to me whether that deficiency is the "normal" condition of the aging human. When we can improve health and function by restoring hormone levels to optimal levels, it makes sense to do so. This is the essence of *functional medicine*—the goal of which is to restore function and not necessarily to treat disease.

The subjects in the Rudman study were not growth-hormone-deficient by conventional standards. Their hormone levels were normal for their age. During the course of the study, however, the hormone status of the subjects rose from the low levels that are normal in older adults to higher levels typical of young, healthy adults. As their hormones were restored to more youthful levels, they experienced the reversal of ten to twenty years of biological aging. Rudman's results—along with those of subsequent researchers—raise a clear and potent question: why should the benefits of hormone replacement be reserved only for those suffering from full-fledged pituitary disease?

Since that landmark study, further clinical trials have continued to document the impressive benefits of growth hormone as an anti-aging therapy. A three-year Danish study showed that the anti-aging effects seen in the Rudman study can be sustained with long-term therapy, without adverse effects.

Other studies have shown that growth hormone can restore internal organs to a more youthful state, including the lungs, kidneys, liver, and spleen. Throughout life, the functional (or parenchymal) tissue found in all the major organs and glands is slowly replaced with nonfunctional fibrous and fatty tissue. Growth hormone reverses this process by increasing the parenchymal mass, or functional tissue. In short, growth hormone helps restore the entire body to more youthful function.

ADDING GROWTH HORMONE TO AN ANTI-AGING PROTOCOL

Throughout the past three chapters, we've been following the progress of my patient Brian. Over the course of several months, Brian had been renovating his health and his lifestyle. With every change, he felt more energized, fitter, and more motivated to take the next step. Brian began by cleaning up his diet and instituting an aggressive program of nutritional supplementation that was based on his particular needs and risk factors. These are the steps outlined for you in Part III.

As you have read, we also implemented a complete regimen of hormone replacement (including DHEA, testosterone, and thyroid hormone). As his hormone profiles improved, Brian felt increasingly energized and buoyant. He became more active, his weight began to drop, and his confidence soared.

Thrilled with the changes he felt as a result of his program, Brian was ready to take his anti-aging efforts to a higher level. At the beginning of our time together, I had given Brian some information about growth hormone to read, and told him that it was an option we could consider. Brian was excited about the benefits that growth hormone can offer but also had some questions about the risks. Together, we evaluated whether this powerful therapy was right for someone in his situation.

USING GROWTH HORMONE SAFELY AND SANELY

Although growth hormone has an almost magical ability to rejuvenate the human body, it is a mistake to view it as a magic bullet against aging. Unfortunately, we have seen the emergence of drive-through growth hormone clinics that inject growth hormone as if it were Botox. Growth hormone is not simply internal plastic surgery, and it is not a quick fix for obesity or other health problems.

> **!** Growth hormone should always be administered as part of a comprehensive anti-aging program. A healthy diet, exercise plan, and lifestyle help to balance and modulate the effects of growth hormone in the body. Growth hormone also works in synergy with the other hormones to produce its effects. The best results by far are seen in those who use growth hormone as an integral part of a total hormone replacement program.

Who Is a Candidate for Growth Hormone?

Measuring the level of growth hormone in the body is tricky. Growth hormone is released in pulses, or surges, by the pituitary gland. Typically, the pituitary will release five or six pulses of HGH per day, with the largest release right before sleep. In older people, the pituitary may release only two or three pulses per day. The constant rise and fall in growth hormone makes it difficult (but not impossible) to get a reliable measurement.

Typically, we use a different, more easily measured hormone called IGF-1 (insulin-like growth factor 1) as a surrogate marker for growth hormone. IGF-1 is the agent by which growth hormone actually achieves its effects in the body. The release of growth hormone from the pituitary gland stimulates the liver to produce IGF-1, which then goes on to affect the function of cells in the muscles, bones, and organs.

While growth hormone levels are volatile, the levels of IGF-1 in the body remain more nearly constant, making them more convenient and less expensive to test. Under normal circumstances (more about that in a moment), IGF-1 levels give us a fairly good idea of growth hormone activity. If IGF-1 levels are low, it suggests that growth hormone secretion is also low. When administering growth hormone therapy, we monitor IGF-1 levels to gauge the response and modulate the dosage.

Target IGF-1 Levels

Normal range	Optimal range
114–492 ng/mL	200–300 ng/mL

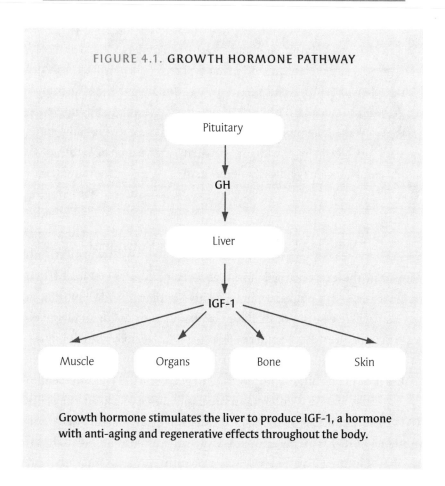

FIGURE 4.1. GROWTH HORMONE PATHWAY

Growth hormone stimulates the liver to produce IGF-1, a hormone with anti-aging and regenerative effects throughout the body.

! As with all of the other hormones we have discussed, more is not necessarily better, and this is especially true for growth hormone. The goal is to use the smallest dosage of growth hormone necessary to achieve the optimal balance of hormones.

It is very common to see low IGF-1 levels as people get older. This reflects the normal, age-related decline in growth hormone production. And in fact, when first we tested him, Brian's IGF-1 levels were 98 ng/mL (nanograms per milliliter). But, as I explained to Brian, it's not quite that simple.

The use of IGF-1 as a surrogate measure of growth hormone activity has some problems. It assumes, of course, that the two hormones always track one another (that is, that high IGF-1 levels always indicate high growth hormone levels, and low IGF-1 levels always mean low growth hormone levels). But this is not always the case. Just a bit more endocrinology will allow you to appreciate some of the higher level complexities of growth hormone therapy.

The secretion of growth hormone by the pituitary gland is regulated by the hypothalamus. When the hypothalamus senses that the level of growth hormone in the blood is too low, it releases a hormone called growth-hormone-releasing hormone (GHRH). This hormone, in turn, stimulates the release of growth hormone in the pituitary gland. When the levels of IGF-1 are high enough, the hypothalamus begins to secrete a different hormone, called growth-hormone-inhibiting hormone (GHIH), which tells the pituitary to decrease the production of growth hormone.

The growth hormone feedback loop works much the way you use the gas and brake pedals to control the speed of your car. By monitoring your speed on the speedometer and applying the gas and brakes accordingly, you maintain your desired speed. In this analogy, the hypothalamus is watching the speedometer (the level of growth hormone). If growth hormone is low, the hypothalamus steps on the gas by releasing GHRH. If growth hormone is high, the hypothalamus steps on the brakes by releasing GHIH.

This regulating feedback loop is the same sort of mechanism that we have seen in other hormone systems, including the thyroid (discussed above) and the adrenal glands (discussed in Chapter 2). Although the mechanisms look fairly straightforward on paper, things get a bit more complicated in the body, where dozens of different systems have to interact and interface.

For example, we know that high cortisol levels (due to stress and aging, as discussed in Chapter 2) can cause an increase in IGF-1 levels. When IGF-1 levels are high, it sends a message to the hypothalamus to inhibit the release of growth hormone. So if you are under a lot of stress, your growth hormone production may be inappropriately sup-pressed because your IGF-1 levels are elevated. Diabetics and over-weight people also tend to have high IGF-1 levels, which suppress growth hormone release.

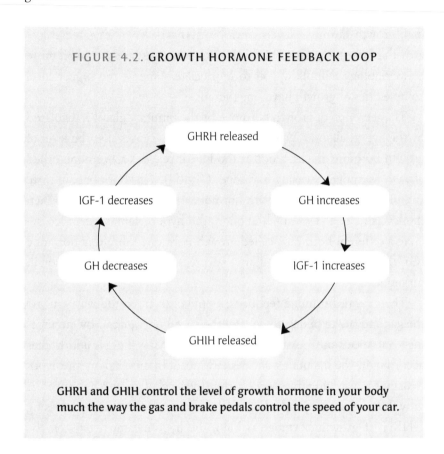

FIGURE 4.2. **GROWTH HORMONE FEEDBACK LOOP**

GHRH released

GH increases

IGF-1 decreases

IGF-1 increases

GH decreases

GHIH released

GHRH and GHIH control the level of growth hormone in your body much the way the gas and brake pedals control the speed of your car.

Exercise, on the other hand, increases growth hormone but at the same time lowers the level of IGF-1 in the blood. In young, healthy ath-letes, for example, the serum (blood) levels of IGF-1 are typically quite low even though growth hormone levels may be optimal. People who are fasting or restricting their caloric intake also experience a surge of growth hormone but a drop in IGF-1. As you can see, there are many circumstances in which the level of IGF-1 does not accurately indicate the level of growth hormone.

Growth Hormone and Life Expectancy

All of this is significant because there is some research showing that high IGF-1 levels may reduce life expectancy. It's important to understand that reduced life expectancy has not been observed in those taking growth hormone therapy, but it has been seen in those who have high IGF-1 levels for other reasons. Because growth hormone therapy tends to raise IGF-1 levels in the body, however, this is obviously a concern that must be addressed. Are we trading quantity of life for a higher quality of life? It's a fair question, but I do not think this is the case.

We know that low growth hormone levels are associated with increased mortality, and growth hormone therapy clearly has anti-aging effects. And we've also seen that IGF-1 levels can be elevated by unhealthy conditions such as stress, inactivity, obesity, and disease. The association between high IGF-1 and decreased life expectancy may in fact simply reflect the decreased life expectancy associated with stress, obesity, and diabetes.

Nonetheless, it underscores the importance of integrating growth hormone therapy into a balanced, healthy anti-aging lifestyle, not as a stand-alone quick fix. When you also take steps to reduce stress, eat a healthy diet low in sugar, and get proper sleep and exercise, you create the conditions that enable your body to utilize growth hormone to its greatest effect, and avoid the conditions that unnaturally elevate IGF-1 levels. The anti-aging lifestyle outlined in Chapter 12 is the ideal complement to growth hormone therapy.

Because I knew that Brian was following a healthy, anti-aging lifestyle and still had suboptimal levels of IGF-1, he was a good candidate for growth hormone therapy. Having weighed the pros and cons, he ultimately opted to add growth hormone to his regimen.

Using Growth Hormone

Growth hormone is an extremely complex protein molecule that is too large to be absorbed through the digestive tract. Therefore, growth hormone must be administered by injection (although with very small needles). In the earliest days of growth hormone therapy, patients would receive injections once or twice a week. As you recall, however, the pituitary gland secretes growth hormone in bursts, resulting in several small surges of growth hormone throughout the day. We now administer growth hormone in much smaller dosages, once or twice a day. This allows us to mimic more closely the behavior of the pituitary gland.

Brian began a program of growth hormone injections, which he learned to administer himself, using a low dose twice a day, six days a week. After six weeks, his IGF-1 level had increased from 98 to 242 ng/mL. Although he had already been pleased with the results of his anti-aging program up until that point, Brian couldn't believe how profound a difference the growth hormone made. "I feel invincible again," he said.

Brian is now in his third year of growth hormone therapy, and his IGF-1 levels have remained constant in the mid-200s. He continues to inject growth hormone twice a day, five days a week. Every five months, he takes three or four weeks off. This regular break ensures that the natural function of his pituitary gland is not suppressed by the supplemental hormone. And of course, Brian has continued all the other elements of his anti-aging program and lifestyle.

At 50 years of age, Brian is trim, fit, and youthful-looking. People guess him to be in his late 30s, but it is not just his appearance that creates this impression. He is simply *charged up,* overflowing with energy and enthusiasm for work, play, and for his family. Brian's wife, Beth, has been amazed and inspired by the physical, mental, and emotional transformation in her husband. Not wanting to be left behind, she recently began an anti-aging program of her own, much to Brian's delight. The two have been a very inspiring example of how anti-aging medicine can make it possible to reclaim youth and vitality in midlife.

Are There Side Effects?

The side effects that have been associated in the past with higher-dose growth hormone therapy include carpal tunnel syndrome, arthritis, high blood pressure, and heart problems. Most of these are due to fluid retention and are temporary, disappearing as the body adjusts to the therapy. When side effects persist, a reduction in the amount of growth hormone (or discontinuation of therapy) leads to complete reversal of symptoms.

As growth hormone therapy has evolved, we have developed more sophisticated protocols that allow us to use even lower dosages than those used in studies such as the Rudman study—without reducing the effectiveness of the therapy. In my practice, I have consistently seen excellent results with dosages equivalent to 1 IU (international unit) per day, either all at once or divided into twice-daily injections. Among my patients who choose growth hormone, even minor side effects have been almost nonexistent.

Is Growth Hormone Safe?

In the early days, growth hormone was extracted from the pituitary glands of cadavers, which raised the fear of problems such as Creutzfeldt-Jakob disease (a relative of mad cow disease). Today, we can synthesize this hormone using modern biotechnology techniques, in a completely pure form that is identical to the molecule produced in the human pituitary gland.

There have also been questions about whether the use of growth hormone may increase the risk of cancer. The only evidence for this comes from children and young adults who were given growth hormone to treat growth disorders and who then had a higher rate of certain cancers as adults.

It's important to note that the dosages used in these cases are up to ten times the dosages used today in anti-aging therapies. The connection between cancer and growth hormone has also been observed only in patients who received therapy before 1985. (In the mid-1980s, synthetic forms of the hormone became available, and the use of growth hormone from cadavers was halted.)

To date, there is no conclusive data that connects the use of low-dose synthetic growth hormone with an increased risk of cancer. In my opinion, the positive effect of growth hormone on the overall health of the body, including the function of the immune system and other organs, is far more likely to decrease your chances of cancer and other diseases as you age. It remains, however, an unanswered question that must be carefully considered by each potential user.

Is Growth Hormone Therapy Right for You?

The conventional medical establishment frequently applies a double standard to anti-aging and alternative therapies. With pharmaceutical drugs, the benefits are stressed while the risks are downplayed. But with alternative therapies, the benefits are dismissed while the risks are blown out of proportion. Nowhere is this more true than with hormone replacement.

In my opinion, many of those throwing rocks at the anti-aging medical community are living in glass houses. While they rail against the dangers of growth hormone and the "quacks" who prescribe it, they continue to prescribe dangerous FDA-approved drugs to their patients without any meaningful discussion of the known side effects and risks of these medications.

Whether it is an FDA-approved drug or a controversial anti-aging therapy (growth hormone is both), I believe that you have the right to make your decision based on all available information, not a selective or biased picture.

Virtually everyone over the age of 40 has suboptimal growth hormone levels, and the earlier growth hormone replacement is initiated, the greater the benefits. But are the obvious benefits of growth hormone injections worth the potential risks? Ultimately, each person must reach his or her own conclusion based on a complete understanding of the evidence as well as the unanswered questions that remain. In this chapter, I have tried to give you an in-depth understanding of the pros and cons of growth hormone therapy.

Personally, I believe the anti-aging effects of growth hormone are so profound and so beneficial to your long-term health that the benefits far outweigh the possible risks. In addition, I firmly believe that when growth hormone is properly used, according to the guidelines I've outlined in this discussion, the risks are minimized. I not only offer growth hormone therapy to my patients as an option but also personally use growth hormone injections as part of my own anti-aging regimen.

If you have an aversion to needles, you might find growth hormone therapy difficult. But the biggest obstacle for most people considering growth hormone therapy is the cost. While anyone can be taught to self-inject the hormone so that the therapy can be administered at home without the need for a doctor's office visit, the cost of the drug itself remains quite high and is not generally covered by insurance when used for anti-aging purposes. Although still quite expensive, the costs of growth hormone therapy have decreased substantially over the last ten years and may continue to go down with more widespread use.

If you think that growth hormone injections may be for you, I encourage you to consult with a qualified anti-aging physician for an evaluation. (The appendix lists some resources for locating qualified physicians.) Beware of clinics that dispense growth hormone with little or no testing or medical follow-up, and of those who give growth hormone injections as a stand-alone therapy, without any consideration of diet, nutrition, lifestyle, and the balance of other hormones. As we have seen, the effectiveness of growth hormone therapy is maximized and the risks minimized when it is used in a complete and balanced anti-aging program.

Alternatives to Growth Hormone Injections

Growth hormone injections supply an exogenous (from outside the body) source of hormone. While injectable growth hormone remains the gold standard in terms of proven efficacy, there are a plethora of products on the market that contain no actual growth hormone but claim to stimulate the endogenous (internal) secretion of growth hormone by your own pituitary gland. Such products are commonly referred to as *secretagogues.*

When taken in sufficient quantities, the amino acids arginine, lysine, and ornithine have been shown to raise growth hormone levels. (Amino acids are the building blocks that make up proteins.) For years, athletes and bodybuilders have been taking amino acids before working out, in an effort to enhance the exercise-induced surge of growth hormone. This practice, known as stacking, is not the same as taking steroids or other illicit performance-enhancing drugs.

With the growing interest in growth hormone as an anti-aging therapy, the use of amino acids to stimulate growth hormone is gaining popularity outside the world of professional sports and bodybuilding. Most secretagogues contain one or more of these amino acids, along with herbs and glandular extracts intended to stimulate the growth hormone pathway.

While there is evidence that various nutrients (see box below) are effective in enhancing growth hormone release, there are no published, placebo-controlled clinical trials to prove that any of these proprietary secretagogue "cocktails" are effective. Some manufacturers have conducted their own clinical trials, yielding rather spectacular results. But the evidence has yet to be independently verified or corroborated.

To the extent that they are effective, an advantage of a secretagogue (in addition to the reduced cost) is that any increase in growth hormone is naturally regulated by the body's own feedback mechanisms, with no possibility of overstimulation. This effectively removes any concern of side effects or risk associated with growth hormone injections.

On the other hand, the dosages of amino acids required to stimulate the release of growth hormone are fairly high—enough to cause stomach discomfort, nausea, and diarrhea in a significant number of people. If you try the GH-releasing protocol, start with one-quarter the recommended dosage and gradually increase the amounts to the recommended level. Studies have also shown that the effectiveness of amino acids as growth hormone secretagogues is highly variable and tends to be less effective in older people.

I have had patients who have used secretagogues and felt that they made a definite difference in their energy, stamina, and overall well-being. You may find that a nutritional approach yields noticeable benefits for you as well.

SUBSTANCES KNOWN TO INCREASE GROWTH HORMONE RELEASE

> L-arginine (2,000–3,000 mg)
> L-glutamine (500–1,000 mg)
> L-ornithine (2,000–6,000 mg)
> Lysine (250–600 mg)
> Glycine (2,000–6,000 mg)
> Niacin (250–500 mg)

Take nutrients once a day on an empty stomach, ideally before bed or exercise. The effectiveness of these nutrients may be enhanced by taking choline (2,000–3,000 mg) and pantothenic acid (1,000–2,000 mg) at the same time.

! Because growth hormone depletes potassium and opposes the actions of insulin, diabetics should use GH-releasers with care. L-arginine and L-ornithine sometimes reactivate latent herpes virus infections. Therefore, persons who have ever had ocular or brain herpes should not use these nutrients.

Finally, there is a bewildering array of sprays, drops, and tablets that claim to provide actual human growth hormone. As a consumer, you need to know that it is illegal to dispense human growth hormone without a prescription. Products sold on the Internet or by mail order cannot by law contain any physiologically active amount of GH.

! Any true growth hormone product being sold without a prescription may be black-market, unregulated, and therefore unsafe.

Increase Growth Hormone Naturally

Certain aspects of your lifestyle can also be modified to maximize the natural release of growth hormone. You'll find all of these discussed in more detail in the anti-aging diet and lifestyle recommendations in Part III. It is no coincidence that the habits that promote health and longevity are those that increase growth hormone secretion. The two are inextricably linked.

➤ Exercise promotes the secretion of growth hormone, providing yet another good reason to exercise regularly. To maximize the effects of exercise on growth hormone release, do not eat for two hours beforehand. If desired, take growth-hormone-releasing nutrients before exercise (see box above).

➢ Fasting also stimulates the release of growth hormone. Extended fasts should be done only with a physician's supervision, but most people can safely fast for twenty-four hours at a time, up to once a week, without difficulty. (Be sure to drink plenty of water.) Even a twelve-hour fast can help to increase growth hormone production. Try not eating between 8 p.m. and 8 a.m. most days.

➢ Avoid highly processed foods containing refined white flour and sugar. These foods cause a quick rise in blood sugar, followed by a surge of insulin. Both can suppress the release of growth hormone.

➢ Take steps to reduce stress. In addition to the other aging effects of stress (see Chapter 2), it causes an increase in IGF-1, which suppresses growth hormone release.

POWERFUL AGENTS FOR CHANGE

Many of my patients are themselves physicians, most of them specialists in other types of medicine. All of them could order their own blood tests, prescribe their own medications, and monitor their own results. But they understand that they will get better results by working with someone who specializes in anti-aging medicine. As I have said, hormone replacement of any kind, including growth hormone, is like brain surgery: it's not something you want to perform on yourself. While this remark usually gets a laugh, it is also very serious advice. I include it here not as a pro forma disclaimer but as a heartfelt recommendation to you.

The hormone therapies we have discussed in these chapters are powerful agents for change. They should be used with intelligence, sensitivity, and care. Not only do I want you to be safe, but I also want you to get the best possible results! With the help of a qualified anti-aging professional, hormone modulation can help you to achieve a stronger, healthier, and more youthful body, no matter what your age. In the next and final chapter of Part I, we'll focus on an equally important challenge: defending your brain and intellect from the destructive forces of aging.

CHAPTER 5

Maximum Brainpower for Life

*There is a fountain of youth: it is your mind, your talents,
the creativity you bring to your life. When you learn to
tap this source, you will have truly defeated age.*
—SOPHIA LOREN

WHEN I WORK WITH patients on anti-aging programs, I spend considerable time talking with them about their concerns, expectations, and goals related to getting older. I ask them what aspects of their health they are satisfied with and what they are dissatisfied with. I have noticed a subtle thread that runs through all of the answers.

Tina, 66, mentioned that increasing forgetfulness made her feel anxious about traveling alone, something she had done with pleasure for years. Nora, 50, was bothered by a persistent "fuzziness" or "brain fog." Famous among her colleagues for having an almost photographic memory of project details, Nora feared that she was losing her sharpness, and with it her reputation in the advertising world. At 47, Brian felt he had lost his ability to focus and concentrate at work. He worried about losing ground to the "young Turks" who were taking over the software industry.

These remarks could easily get lost in the midst of more concrete concerns such as high cholesterol or joint pain or cancer prevention, but I take them quite seriously. Even a minor loss of cognitive function is a serious matter, and one that can cause a great deal of emotional distress. Our minds are the thing that make us most uniquely us, the means by which we interact with the world around us and make our mark in that world. The thought that this might somehow slip away from us as we get older is very disturbing.

One of the greatest fears that people have about getting older is losing their independence and self-determination. This fear was poignantly played out in the public consciousness by the plight of former president and Alzheimer's victim Ronald Reagan. He was once one of the most powerful men in the entire world, yet before his death his disease rendered him unable to think, act, or speak for himself. In the later stages of the disease, he reportedly had little memory of his own personal family history, much less the part he played on the world stage.

It's not just the fear of Alzheimer's disease that haunts us (although this tragic disease is becoming epidemic as our population ages). Even a slight erosion of our current mental powers feels very threatening. And so we may joke about "senior moments" when we can't think of our neighbor's name or remember whether we dropped off the dry cleaning. But our laughter rings a bit hollow. We joke to cover our embarrassment but also to quiet the gnawing fear that these minor slips are actually the beginning of a gradual slide into increasing fogginess and confusion. It's not an irrational fear, either. Short-term memory loss is usually the first sign of age-related mental decline.

THE AGING BRAIN

The brain is subject to the same aging process that affects the rest of the body. The brain's biochemistry and metabolism change as we get older. The structural integrity of the brain cells is compromised, and the cells function less effectively. Neurons shrink and stiffen, chemical messengers become less plentiful, and vital connections are lost.

The aging brain starts to lose its ability to access stored information and process new information. It becomes more difficult to recall names and phone numbers. Words become elusive as language-processing centers atrophy. Reaction time slows, and the ability to make quick, effective decisions is impaired. The capacity to focus on and solve complex challenges is diminished.

Just like all of the other aspects of aging we have discussed, however, the aging of the brain is not an inevitable feature of growing older. We can take steps to maintain the brain's youthful biochemistry and metabolism. We can provide nutrients that preserve youthful brain cell structure and behavior. We can enhance the ability of the brain to process and transmit information.

While the approach is multifaceted, the principle is simple: by protecting the brain from the changes associated with aging, you can grow older without losing your intellectual agility and mental sharpness. In fact, research is now showing that a healthy brain can continue to grow and learn throughout your entire life span.

PRESERVING PEAK BRAIN FUNCTION FOR LIFE

When they first take steps to enhance brain function, a substantial number of people realize that they have never actually experienced peak brain function before. Many are surprised by a completely new level of mental acuity and keenness. Even younger patients report newfound reserves of concentration, motivation, and problem solving. Learning and retention require less effort. Memory and recall are sharpened. Many even report new levels of insight about their work and personal lives. It is an exciting transformation to witness, and even more exciting to experience. With the dawning of the information age and the dominance of service-oriented companies, brainpower is essential to keeping us vital, productive, and competitive. It's what keeps you in the game.

Our ability to enhance brain function throughout life grows out of an increasing understanding of how the brain works. As we learn more about the biochemical and energy-producing processes that underlie our thinking and memory, we have greater opportunity to support and enhance those processes. Using a combination of lifestyle and behavioral changes, diet, supplements, and in some cases pharmaceutical drugs, we aim to:

1. Increase circulation and oxygenation to the brain

2. Enhance energy production in the brain

3. Promote neurotransmitter production

4. Maintain the structural integrity of the neuronal membranes

5. Increase the size and complexity of the neuronal network

6. Protect the brain from oxidative damage

I'll briefly discuss each of these aspects of brain function individually, along with the most effective tools to maximize them. Later in the chapter, I'll outline a six-step program that combines all of these strategies into an integrated program for maximum brain health and function. You will see that your brainpower program is really the culmination of everything we have talked about to this point, incorporating all of the anti-aging therapies discussed in earlier chapters. The same steps that promote a healthy, youthful body help to promote a strong and vital brain. And the effects can be absolutely dazzling.

Enhancing Blood and Oxygen Flow to the Brain

The brain is a hungry organ. Although it accounts for only 2 percent of your total body weight, it uses one-quarter of your body's oxygen supply and one-half of your body's glucose in order to supply its extraordinary energy needs. Although its nutrient and energy needs are huge, the brain—unlike the heart and other muscles—cannot store nutrients, oxygen, or energy for future use. As every paramedic and emergency room doctor knows, brain cells begin to starve and die if the flow of oxygen and nutrients is interrupted even for a few minutes. Oxygen, glucose, and other nutrients reach the brain via the blood, so one of the most important ways to maintain cognitive vitality is to ensure excellent blood flow to the brain.

Aerobic exercise can help to increase the number and size of the blood vessels to the brain, which greatly increases the supply of oxygen and nutrients. Recent studies conducted at the University of Maryland show that physical exercise can prevent the loss of cognitive powers as you age. The studies compared the cognitive performance of older and younger subjects who were either sedentary or physically fit. With the younger subjects, physical activity did not have very much impact on their cognitive scores. But among the older subjects, the level of physical activity had a dramatic effect on the level of mental acuity.

The sedentary older subjects performed much more poorly on tests that measured reaction time, problem-solving abilities, and other cognitive skills than the three other groups. The active older subjects, however, were comparable to the younger subjects in their cognitive performance. Regular exercise therefore helps you maintain not only physical fitness, but mental fitness as well.

The flowing characteristics (rheology) of your blood also affect how efficiently it circulates throughout the brain and the body. Youthful red blood cells have two important characteristics, both of which increase their oxygen-carrying capacity: they are very elastic, and they are slippery. They move easily through the body, passing through the smallest capillaries with ease. This is especially important in the brain, where much of the dense gray matter is nourished by a vast network of tiny blood vessels.

As we age, the characteristics of the blood can change. The red blood cells tend to lose their elasticity and become increasingly sticky. When the blood is thick and sludge-like, it has more difficulty passing through tiny capillaries, and the aging brain suffers from oxygen deficit as a result. I call this "thick-blood syndrome." It is like trying to lubricate an engine with thick, sludgy 50-weight oil, when what you want is thin, slippery 10-weight motor oil.

Nutrients that enhance the flowing characteristics of the blood can increase the flow of blood (and oxygen) to the deepest and most vital areas of the brain—the centers of emotion, mood, libido, and short-term memory. **Vitamin E** and **fish oil** both help to keep your red blood cells slippery and elastic and your blood flowing freely. Both are a foundational part of your supplement program, outlined in Chapter 11.

Ginkgo biloba is an herbal triple whammy, enhancing brain function in a number of complementary ways. First, it has been shown to en-hance circulation in general, and specifically to improve the flow of blood to the brain by dilating the blood vessels.

Second, ginkgo keeps platelets from sticking together, which keeps the blood thin and slippery. Ginkgo works by the same anticoagulating mechanism as aspirin, inhibiting the formation of platelet aggregation factors (PAF). It thus provides you with the same benefits as low-dose aspirin, only with a host of ancillary benefits. Third, it is a powerful antioxidant. We will see why this is so important in a moment.

Over forty clinical studies report that ginkgo can improve symptoms of age-related cognitive decline, such as memory problems, confusion, and fatigue. It has even been shown to help slow the progression of Alzheimer's disease. Ginkgo is widely used in Germany as a pharma-ceutical treatment for dementia.

The effects of increased blood flow to the brain can make a dramatic difference in your cognitive function in a surprisingly short period of time. One study showed that a single large dose of ginkgo extract was enough to significantly improve the subjects' scores on tests that mea-sured short-term memory. The effects of ginkgo are more pronounced in older subjects than in younger ones, which underscores the fact that ginkgo works specifically on age-related changes in blood flow and brain function.

Increasing Energy Production in the Brain

Once the oxygen and glucose have been delivered to the brain cells by the blood, they must be converted into a form of energy that can be used in the cells. As you probably remember from high school biology, plants manufacture energy through photosynthesis, which transforms energy from the sun into a form of energy that can be used in the plant's cells.

Through a similar process, our bodies create cellular energy by transforming glucose into a chemical form of energy called ATP. Every cell in the body requires ATP as its energy source. But of all the cells in the body, the brain cells have the highest requirements for ATP. Unlike other cells, however, brain cells have no capacity to store ATP and no ability to "borrow" ATP from neighboring organs. This makes the brain exquisitely vulnerable to cellular energy deficit.

Energy deficit in the brain has been implicated in neurological diseases such as Alzheimer's, Parkinson's, and Huntington's. But long before these diseases appear, cellular energy deficit in the brain undermines your ability to think quickly and clearly. At the most fundamental level, even depression and fatigue have their roots in this loss of energy production.

The transformation of glucose into ATP takes place in the mitochondria, tiny energy factories found in each cell. As we get older, the size and number of the mitochondria decrease. The remaining mitochondria become less efficient at producing ATP. This loss of mitochondrial function is thought to be a major contributing factor to the aging of the body in general and particularly of the brain.

The reduction in energy production in the brain leads to symptoms such as memory loss and reduced cognitive function. The fatigue and failure of the mitochondria also lead to a buildup of cellular debris, which eventually kills brain cells. Brain cells are not as readily replaced as other cells in the body are, so the loss of brain cells is a serious problem. Eventually, when enough brain cells have died, it leads to symptoms of dementia or senility.

Certain nutrients have the ability to increase the function of mitochondria and to prevent and reverse age-related mitochondrial fatigue. **Carnitine,** for example, is a vital amino acid that helps to promote the production of ATP in the mitochondria. Carnitine's effects on energy metabolism throughout the body can help mobilize stored fat, increase lean muscle mass, and increase the energy efficiency of the brain and heart. However, carnitine does not cross the blood-brain barrier (BBB) very efficiently.

In order to maximize the effects of carnitine in the mitochondria of the brain cells, it is often given as **acetyl-L-carnitine (ALC),** a fat-soluble form of the nutrient that is readily absorbed across the BBB. This keeps the brain's energy stores of ATP high and protects against cell death.

CROSSING THE BLOOD-BRAIN BARRIER

Brain cells are extremely sensitive to chemicals that may be circulating through the bloodstream. These include natural chemicals, such as hormones and nutrients, as well as unnatural chemicals, such as pharmaceutical drugs or environmental toxins. The blood-brain barrier is a special protective organization of cells that prevents large molecules and potentially damaging substances from entering the brain tissue from the blood.

Many of the nutrients circulating in the blood do not cross the BBB, making brain nutrition tricky. Nutrients that readily cross the BBB—such as ALC—are particularly valuable in preserving brain function.

Research studies with aging lab animals have shown that supplementation with ALC reverses the age-related decline in mental functioning, improving the memory, learning ability, and problem-solving abilities of the animals. In a study on several hundred healthy seniors, Italian researchers confirmed the effects of ALC on aging humans. The doctors reported that "every measure of cognitive function" was improved through the use of ALC, noting that ALC also led to an improvement in mood and emotional well-being. I was particularly intrigued by a recent study that found that acetyl-L-carnitine reduced age-related hearing loss by preserving the mitochondrial function in the inner ear and the auditory nerves.

The second nutrient that is vital to the production of cellular energy is **coenzyme Q_{10} (CoQ_{10})**. The cell's ability to "breathe" (transport electrons in and out of the mitochondria) is limited by the amount of CoQ_{10} available. Your body synthesizes its own CoQ_{10}, which is one of the most abundant nutrients in the body. As we grow older, however, the amount of CoQ_{10} in the body can drop by as much as 50 percent.

This antioxidant has a particular affinity for organs with high energy demands, such as the brain and heart. When taken as a supplement, it seems to concentrate specifically in the cells of the heart and the brain, protecting the mitochondria from damage-causing free radicals and toxins. CoQ_{10} can restore energy production in weakened brain cells to nearly normal levels, preventing cell death.

Increasing Neurotransmitter Function

Your ability to process, store, and access information is dependent on the ability of your brain cells to communicate with one another. Cell-to-cell communication is dependent on an adequate supply of chemicals called neurotransmitters.

The neurotransmitters occupy the spaces between the brain cells, the synapses, and carry the electrical impulses emitted by the brain cells across these synaptic gaps to adjacent brain cells. When the levels of neurotransmitters decline, as they do with age and in certain neurological diseases, brain function is diminished.

Scientists have identified sixty or so different neurotransmitters, including adrenaline, dopamine, serotonin, and GABA. Each of these has specific roles in controlling mood, alertness, movement, coordination, sensory interaction, and other cerebral functions. Adrenaline and dopamine are stimulating or energizing neurotransmitters, for example, whereas serotonin and GABA are calming or tranquilizing. The most abundant of all the neurotransmitters, and the most essential to memory function, is acetylcholine.

To increase the efficiency of cell-to-cell communication, we want to increase the level of acetylcholine in the brain. But, like carnitine, acetylcholine has a hard time making it through the blood-brain barrier. So instead, we use **phosphatidylcholine (PC),** a precursor nutrient that contains the building blocks that the brain needs to manufacture acetylcholine. When taken as a dietary supplement, PC helps to increase brain levels of this critical neurotransmitter and enhance cellular communication. PC is one of the most commonly used memory-enhancing nutrients.

Dimethylaminoethanol (DMAE) is another precursor to acetylcholine, one that readily crosses the blood-brain barrier. Inside the brain, DMAE works with PC to increase acetylcholine levels. DMAE is widely used in Europe as a memory-enhancing drug.

Maintaining the Integrity of Brain Cell Membranes

Neurotransmitters are the biochemical carrier pigeons that carry messages from one neuron to the next. They deliver their messages by plugging into the receptor sites in the membrane that encases each cell. When the membranes are healthy and flexible, the receptor sites are reinvigorated and cell-to-cell communication is enhanced.

Cell membranes are primarily made of lipids, or fats. The most important of these is **phosphatidylserine (PS),** which constitutes about 70 percent of the cell membrane. As we get older, the level of PS in the brain cells drops, and the cell membranes become brittle and less permeable. This impairs the ability of the cell to absorb nutrients and receive messages from neurotransmitters.

When PS is taken as a nutritional supplement, it can restore the amount of PS in the brain cell to youthful levels, enhancing cell-to-cell communication. In a study of 150 seniors suffering from age-associated memory loss, half the subjects were given PS and half were given a placebo for twelve weeks. At the end of that time, those taking PS had improved performance on tests of memory and learning compared with those who had taken the placebo. Interestingly, the subjects who had the most difficulty with memory at the beginning of the study were the ones who had the best response.

Increasing the Size and Complexity of the Neural Network

Cognitive function is somewhat like a public transportation system. A good mass transit system has multiple bus and/or subway lines that crisscross the entire city. If one route is blocked, there are plenty of backup routes. If a bus or subway car breaks down, there are replacement vehicles available. All the vehicles have plenty of gas.

Your brain contains billions of neurons. Each neuron has arms, called dendrites, which reach out to other neurons to create information pathways. In a healthy brain, the neurons have many dendrites, connecting each neuron to tens of thousands of other neurons. This vast network of dendritic connections is like a well-developed transportation system.

There are multiple routes for the information to travel. This allows the brain to process information quickly, to learn, synthesize, and remember information efficiently, and to attend to multiple different tasks at the same time.

As we get older, the infrastructure of our neural network thins out. The neurons themselves shrink in size, and the number of connections between the brain cells is fewer. The reduced complexity and richness of the neural network causes delays and interruptions in information processing. Our learning ability, recall, reaction time, and logic and language centers all suffer as a result.

In other words, our mental mass transit system becomes less efficient. We have fewer buses, the buses don't have as much gas, and they are traveling only a few routes. Breakdowns and closed roads are common. It takes a lot longer for passengers to get where they want to go. Some never arrive.

The best way to maintain a healthy, complex neural network is to challenge and exercise your brain as you get older. Learning, problem solving, and memory exercises can stimulate the formation of new neural pathways. Games such as bridge or chess, word games, and puzzles are all terrific "mental aerobics," literally exercising the brain and keeping the connections strong and vital. By maintaining a complex network of connections, virtually no processor speed is lost as you get older.

Preventing Oxidative Damage

The brain cells are especially vulnerable to oxidative damage from free radicals, unstable molecules that corrode the membranes and mitochondria of cells. (We'll be discussing free radicals and the damage they do in more detail in the next chapter.)

The production of ATP in the mitochondria creates an enormous number of free radicals inside the cell. In order to prevent damage to the DNA of the neurons, the free radicals must be neutralized by antioxidants. The fatty membrane surrounding each neuron is also a preferred target for oxidation by free radicals. Several of the agents discussed above, including ginkgo, CoQ_{10}, and vitamin E, help to fight free radical damage in the brain. **Alpha-lipoic acid,** another powerful anti-oxidant with specific brain-protective properties, is discussed in more detail in the next chapter.

YOUR BRAINPOWER PROGRAM

Now, let me show you how I build a brainpower program that addresses and supports all of these different aspects of brain function. The program takes a multilevel approach, incorporating all of the anti-aging therapies and strategies that we have discussed so far—from stress reduction to hormone balance to proper diet and nutrition. Each step helps to set the stage for and reinforce the next level.

SIX STEPS TO MAXIMUM BRAINPOWER

1. Basic nutritional support
2. Physical exercise
3. Hormone balancing
4. Mental exercise
5. Stress reduction
6. Targeted brain nutrition

Step One: Basic Nutritional Support

The first step of any anti-aging program is to make sure that the body's basic nutritional needs are being met. Few Americans get the nutrients they need in sufficient quantities from the foods they eat, which undermines the body's function at every level.

Your cognitive function, in particular, is directly affected by your nutritional status. People who have a higher intake of B-complex vitamins and antioxidants such as vitamins A, C, and E consistently perform better on tests of cognitive function. The B vitamins are critical to the function of the central nervous system and the synthesis of neurotransmitters. Studies have shown that when the body has low levels of B vitamins, cognitive function suffers. Furthermore, supplementation with B vitamins quickly leads to improvement in memory and other neurological functions, and can protect against brain aging.

Antioxidant nutrients are needed to prevent premature aging of the brain from free radical damage. Researchers have found that the ability of older people to recall names, recognize faces, and summon up vocabulary is directly related to the intake of antioxidant nutrients.

Essential fatty acids (EFAs) are absolutely vital for brain power. They help maintain the flexibility and vigor of the brain cell membranes, enhancing nerve and brain function. The most important EFAs are eicosapentaenoic acid (EPA) and docosahexaenoic acid (DHA). Both are found in fish oil, which, as mentioned above, also helps to promote blood flow to the brain.

In Chapter 11, I will detail the basic nutrient regimen that forms the foundation for your complete anti-aging program. By implementing this basic regimen, you will be getting the B-complex vitamins, antioxidants, and essential fatty acids needed for optimal brain function.

BLOOD SUGAR AND THE BRAIN

Maintaining steady blood sugar levels is also important to healthy brain function. Refined sugars and highly processed foods, which unfortunately make up a large part of the standard American diet, cause a sharp rise in blood sugar. This sudden increase in blood sugar triggers a surge of insulin from the pancreas, which clears the sugars from the blood. This "sugar rebound" effect not only leaves you feeling fatigued and depleted but also deprives the brain of the fuel it needs to function optimally. The dietary recommendations in Chapter 12 explain how to maintain even blood sugar levels by choosing foods that release their energy into the bloodstream slowly and evenly. These dietary guidelines support your program for cognitive vitality.

Step Two: Physical Exercise

Aerobic exercise helps to keep your brain sharp, primarily by increasing the flow of blood and oxygen to the brain. Even moderate exercise increases brain wave activity. Studies have shown that older people who are more physically active have a greater ability to tune out distractions and focus their attention.

Exercise also counteracts the aging effects of stress, discussed in Chapter 2, and promotes the release of growth hormone. In Chapter 12, we'll discuss how to structure an exercise program to yield maximal anti-aging benefits for body and mind. At a minimum, make sure that each day includes some type of physical effort, whether it is a brisk walk, an hour in the garden, or a more organized sport or fitness activity. The effects of exercise on mood and mental clarity are immediate, and the age-proofing effects on the brain are long-lasting.

Step Three: Hormone Balance

Brain function is intimately tied to hormone balance. Brain tissue is rich with receptors for estrogen, testosterone, and growth hormone, all of which promote the production of neurotransmitters. The brain is also sensitive to stress hormones, which can damage and age brain cells. With age, the levels of estrogen, testosterone, and growth hormone tend to decline, while the levels of cortisol increase, resulting in brain aging and loss of cognitive function.

As part of your anti-aging program, I recommend that you have your hormone levels evaluated by a qualified anti-aging specialist (see also Chapter 10 on medical testing). A program of bioidentical hormone replacement, as detailed in Chapters 3 and 4, will help to preserve a youthful, healthy body and mind. As we have seen in the previous two chapters, the effects of a hormone modulation program almost always include a marked improvement in mental clarity and energy. This sets the stage for a more targeted and intensive program for brain aging.

Step Four: Mental Exercise

Although the brain is not a muscle, it responds to mental exercise the way muscles respond to physical exercise. To activate the language centers of the brain, learn a new language, read music, write poems or essays, or solve crossword puzzles and other word games.

Exercise the logical, problem-solving parts of your brain with games of strategy such as chess or bridge. Give your memory a workout by memorizing phone numbers instead of programming the speed dial on your phone. Memorize song lyrics, poems, or short shopping lists. Make an effort to meet new people and try new things. The more you stretch and challenge your brain, the more vital it becomes.

Learning increases blood flow to the brain and stimulates the brain to increase the number and complexity of neural connections. It also promotes the production of new neurons. Scientists used to believe that brain cells were incapable of reproducing. You may have learned in school that once brain cells are lost, they are lost forever. But recent discoveries have shattered this long-held notion. We now know that lost brain cells can in fact be regenerated at any age! Although brain cells do not reproduce as readily as other types of cells, experiments with lab rats show that older rats that are required to learn complicated mazes produce chemicals in the brain that encourage the formation of new brain cells. This amazing ability is further enhanced by combining learning with physical activity.

This breakthrough in our understanding of the brain's regenerative capacity means that it is never too late to learn, to increase the size and complexity of your neural network, and to slow and even reverse the effects of aging on the brain.

Step Five: Reduce Stress

As we discussed in Chapter 2, stress raises cortisol levels, which leads to premature brain aging and even neurological disease. In addition to regular exercise, which helps to lower cortisol levels, be sure that each day includes a few moments of genuine relaxation. Meditation, gentle stretching, listening to music or relaxation tapes, breathing exercises, yoga, and prayer are all powerful stress-reducing practices that will enhance your cognitive vitality. Specific stress reduction techniques are discussed in more detail in Chapter 12.

Step Six: Targeted Brain Nutrition

The ultimate step toward maximum brainpower is a program of nutritional supplements specifically focused on enhancing the function of the brain from a variety of angles. These nutrients can be purchased separately or in combination formulas from health food stores or through mail order sources. This "cognitive cocktail" has produced excellent results in my patients.

NUTRIENTS FOR COGNITIVE ENHANCEMENT

> **Phosphatidylcholine** (1,200–6,000 mg per day). Provides essential precursors for the synthesis of acetylcholine, an important neurotransmitter.

> **DMAE** (100–300 mg per day). Works with phosphatidylcholine to increase acetylcholine levels.

> **Ginkgo biloba extract** (120 mg per day). Enhances blood flow to the brain, prevents platelet aggregation (clotting), and protects neurons from free radical damage.

> **Acetyl-L-carnitine** (1,000–2,000 mg per day). Enhances energy production in the mitochondria and promotes neurotransmitter production.

> **Coenzyme Q$_{10}$** (100–200 mg per day). Enhances energy production in the mitochondria and fights free radical damage.

> **Phosphatidylserine** (100–300 mg per day). Maintains the integrity of brain cell membranes, enhancing cell-to-cell communication.

I think of these nutrients as a "first-pass" approach to cognitive vitality. The program is easy to implement and produces substantial results. For those who want a more intensive approach to cognitive vitality, I have a "second-pass" protocol that is more complex but can offer even richer results. The second pass involves a class of drugs known as nootropics, or "smart drugs," discussed in the following section.

SMART DRUGS

The development of bona fide smart drugs opens the door to a very exciting future. Not only do these agents help to prevent the cognitive decline that is associated with aging, but they can actually improve your cognitive function and vitality at any age. Imagine being able to summon more mental energy, creativity, speed, and even intelligence to bring to your daily life. It's an incredible opportunity for medicine to improve lives and even the world, by allowing us to interact, create, and contribute at a higher level.

Some of these drugs have not yet been approved for use in the United States, although they are widely used in Europe and elsewhere throughout the world. As we will discuss below, European drugs such as adrafinil, modafinil, and piracetam can be imported by anti-aging physicians for use in the United States. However, the relative difficulty of obtaining these valuable drugs means that they are not widely used.

Other drugs, such as L-deprenyl and hydergine, have been approved in the United States, but not necessarily to improve mental performance or to prevent age-related cognitive decline. Although physicians have the freedom to use approved drugs for applications other than their approved uses (a practice known as *off-label use*), the failure of the FDA to affirm the value of these drugs to improve neurological function in healthy individuals means that their use as anti-aging agents is also regrettably limited.

THE OFF-LABEL USE OF PRESCRIPTIONS

Off-label usage of approved prescription drugs is actually fairly common. This perfectly legal practice provides a valuable opportunity for knowledgeable physicians to push beyond the sometimes needlessly conservative views of U.S. drug regulators.

Off-label use of drugs is common in cancer treatment; a government survey found that up to one-quarter of cancer drugs were prescribed off-label. Doctors who work with difficult-to-treat pediatric diseases such as autism have also had success using approved drugs for unapproved applications.

Often, off-label use leads to the official recognition of new uses for drugs. For example, sildenafil citrate, better known as Viagra, was originally developed to treat heart pain until users noticed unexpected benefits. Minoxidil, also known as Rogaine, was originally developed to treat high blood pressure.

L-Deprenyl

L-deprenyl (also known by its generic name, selegiline) is approved in the United States for the treatment of Parkinson's and Alzheimer's diseases. These diseases of the brain are both characterized by low levels of the neurotransmitter dopamine.

Normally, dopamine in the brain is broken down by an enzyme called monoamine oxidase (MAO). Deprenyl is an MAO inhibitor. It helps to keep dopamine levels high by blocking the dopamine-clearing action of the MAO enzyme. (More specifically, deprenyl is an MAO-B inhibitor and does not have the problems associated with older MAO-A inhibitors that were used primarily as antidepressants.)

Even in those without these serious diseases, however, dopamine levels typically decline as we get older. Raising the level of dopamine in the brain to youthful levels with deprenyl has a natural mood-enhancing effect and a pronounced effect on libido. It also acts to prevent oxidative damage to brain cells. Animal studies have shown that deprenyl improved age-related memory loss and significantly extends maximum life span.

A review of deprenyl's proven benefits, published in the *Journal of the American Geriatric Society,* concluded with the following proposal (italics added for emphasis):

> We propose that the healthy population be maintained on 10–15 mg deprenyl weekly starting at age 45 in order to combat the age-related decline of the [neurotransmitter-producing] neurons. Prophylactic deprenyl medication seems to offer a reasonable prospect of *improving the quality of life in the later decades, delaying the time of natural death and decreasing the susceptibility of age-related neurological diseases, like Parkinson's disease and Alzheimer's disease.*

Although the conventional medical community in the United States has unfortunately ignored the evidence supporting deprenyl as a potent anti-aging therapy, it is widely used in Europe to prevent age-related senility. I use this amazing drug extensively as part of a cognitive enhancement protocol. Side effects with deprenyl are both rare and minor.

In my own practice, I use slightly more aggressive dosages of deprenyl than those recommended in the article quoted above. For anti-aging purposes, I have found that 2 to 3 mg per day works well for those in their 40s, 4 to 5 mg per day for those in their 50s, and 5 to 6 mg for those in their 60s and older. (By comparison, the usual dosage for Parkinson's and Alzheimer's patients is 10 mg per day.)

 Deprenyl should not be taken with antidepressants such as Prozac unless under the specific advice of a physician.

Hydergine

Hydergine is a bit of a strange case. It has been used in Europe and other countries for over forty years and has been shown in multiple clinical trials to improve memory, cognitive function, alertness, and mood. To its credit, the FDA has approved hydergine for the *treatment* of age-related cognitive decline in the elderly (although its use as a brain-*protective* agent in people under 60 is still considered an off-label use). But there's an ironic twist to the hydergine story. Although it is the closest thing we have to an FDA-approved "smart drug," hydergine has been virtually ignored by the conventional medical community.

In Europe, hydergine is prescribed in dosages of 9 to 18 mg per day and has been shown to be highly effective at these levels. In America, however, the recommended dosage is only 3 to 6 mg per day. There is virtually no dosage at which hydergine becomes toxic, and side effects are rare and mild, so there is no obvious rationale for limiting dosages to these low, ineffective levels.

Studies using hydergine at low dosages found only mild or minimal effects on cognitive function, causing researchers to dismiss it as "ineffective." This is ridiculous science. If you used only one-sixth of the amount of yeast called for in a recipe, you can hardly conclude that yeast is not an effective leavening agent when the bread rises very slowly.

Conventional doctors in the United States were also turned off to hydergine by widely cited research showing that it is of little value as a treatment for Alzheimer's disease. Although the symptoms of early Alzheimer's disease may resemble those of age-related cognitive decline, the two conditions are very different. To conclude that hydergine is ineffective in preventing brain aging on the basis of its inability to treat Alzheimer's disease is, once again, absurd. You might as well conclude that because sunscreen cannot remove freckles, it is of no value in preventing skin cancer.

Despite the illogical response of the conventional medical community to hydergine, it is highly valued and widely used by anti-aging practitioners to protect the brain against aging and cognitive decline.

How Hydergine Works

An extensive body of research on hydergine demonstrates multiple mechanisms by which it protects the brain from aging. It addresses virtually all of the goals that we set out at the beginning of this chapter.

> ➢ Hydergine increases the flow of blood and oxygen to the brain and increases the utilization of glucose for energy.

> Hydergine protects brain cells from damage due to decreased or insufficient oxygen supply. It is used in many countries as an emergency treatment for strokes or accidents that could interrupt the oxygen to the brain. In these cases, hydergine can buy valuable time, preserving brain cells until the oxygen supply can be restored.

> Hydergine enhances the energy metabolism of brain cells, preventing age-related shrinkage of the mitochondria.

> Hydergine promotes healthy levels of various neurotransmitters. By decreasing the levels of monoamine oxidase (MAO), an enzyme that breaks down dopamine, it helps to maintain higher dopamine levels. It also enhances serotonin levels.

> Hydergine stimulates the growth of dendrites at the end of each neuron, which increases the size and speed of the neural network.

> Hydergine prevents free radical damage to brain cells and helps to prevent the buildup of lipofuscin, a toxic by-product of cellular metabolism that typically accumulates in brain cells with age, impairing their function.

Using Hydergine to Maintain Youthful Brain Function

Laboratory studies have demonstrated that animals who receive hydergine beginning in middle age maintain healthy brain activity as they age, compared with untreated animals, which display cognitive decline as they age. Scientists have concluded that hydergine could help prevent the sequence of brain changes that leads to Alzheimer's disease (but would be of little value as a treatment once Alzheimer's disease was established).

A landmark study on otherwise healthy elderly subjects suffering from age-related cognitive decline showed that supplementation with hydergine led to increased cognitive scores, memory, learning, and recall. These results, published in the *Journal of the American Geriatric Society* in 1971, have been confirmed by countless other clinical trials.

After decades of use around the world, hydergine has an excellent track record of safety.

Hydergine is frequently combined with low-dose deprenyl to boost cognitive function and protect against brain aging. It is highly synergistic, meaning that it is more potent when combined with other smart drugs, and also enhances the actions of other agents. When used along with other cognition-enhancing agents, the dosage should be kept to 5 to 10 mg per day. In a small number of patients, hydergine causes mild stomach upset, but this is easily avoided by using coated tablets or liquid preparations that are absorbed under the tongue (sublingually).

PREVENTING AND TREATING NEUROLOGICAL DISEASE

The protocols outlined in this chapter are designed to prevent brain aging and to help you to maintain your cognitive vitality as you get older. Many of these protocols, which keep the brain healthy and youthful, are also potent protection against the changes that lead to serious neurological diseases such as Alzheimer's disease and Parkinson's disease. In Part II, we will be focusing on additional protocols that reduce your risk of these and other diseases of aging.

Please also consult the LEF Disease Prevention and Treatment database under the headings of "Alzheimer's Disease" and "Parkinson's Disease" for protocols that may slow the progression or improve the symptoms in those suffering from these diseases.

European Smart Drugs

Other nootropics, such as piracetam, adrafinil, and modafinil, enjoy widespread use in Europe as cognition-enhancing and anti-aging drugs. Although there is little question of their safety, efficacy, and medical value, the FDA has not seen fit to approve them for use in the United States.

Piracetam

Piracetam was the very first of the nootropic drugs and is still among the most popular of the cognition enhancers. Three decades of research and widespread use in Europe have firmly established its benefits and actions. Although it is not a stimulant, many people describe a feeling of being "more awake" after taking piracetam. I find that it increases mental clarity and focus.

One of the most interesting things about piracetam as a cognition enhancer is its documented effects on higher cortical functioning. It seems to concentrate in the frontal lobes of the brain, which is where our most advanced cognitive functions take place. It has been shown to improve concentration, learning, creativity, memory, and even measures of intelligence.

It is also unique among smart drugs for its documented ability to increase the transfer of information between the left and right hemispheres of the brain, across the bundle of nerves called the corpus callosum. It is the coordination and integration of the two hemispheres that produces the highest level of brain activity and creativity. It is widely used in Europe to treat dyslexia, a learning disability linked to a malfunction in the brain's language processing centers.

On a structural level, piracetam protects the brain from damage due to an insufficiency of oxygen. In fact, it has been used on expeditions to Mount Everest to prevent cognitive changes due to low oxygen levels at very high altitudes. It is also administered to stroke victims to prevent neurological and functional damage to the brain following a stroke.

At a functional level, piracetam can increase the number of neurotransmitter receptors on brain cells by 30 to 40 percent. At the same time, it blocks the effects of some sedatives in the brain, including alcohol. In Europe, it is used to treat alcoholism and certain kinds of drug-resistant depression.

As part of its actions in preventing brain aging and deterioration, piracetam protects brain cells against free radical damage and the buildup of the toxic metabolic by-product lipofuscin. If you have ever seen liver spots on someone's hands, you have seen the effects of lipofuscin on skin cells. In the brain it is far more serious.

Despite all the evidence and its long track record of safe and beneficial use in Europe, the FDA has not approved piracetam as a drug in the United States. But it has (illogically) placed piracetam on a short list of drugs that can be obtained in bulk by pharmacists and used to make customized formulations according to a physician's specifications. It can be obtained with an enlightened doctor's prescription—or from offshore sources (see page 152).

Piracetam is typically used in doses of 2,400 mg per day. It is remarkably fast-acting, producing a noticeable effect in thirty to sixty minutes. There is research that suggests that the effects of piracetam are made much more potent when it is given in combination with hydergine, and vice versa (hydergine's potency is enhanced when used with piracetam). When these agents are used together, the dosages of each are reduced to compensate for the potentiating effect.

Adrafinil and Modafinil

The two drugs adrafinil and modafinil are "cousins," both developed by the same French laboratory, and both belonging to a new class of drugs called eugeroics. The word is coined from the Greek and means "good arousal." Originally developed as a treatment for narcolepsy and other sleeping disorders, these safe and nonaddictive drugs have taken their place as the newest smart drugs.

Eugeroics have a unique ability to enhance vigilance and can allow you to maintain an intense state of concentration and alertness for long periods of time without fatigue. Unlike caffeine, ephedrine, or other stimulant drugs, eugeroics do not interfere with sleep patterns or cause cardiovascular side effects such as an acccelerated heartbeat. With eugeroics there is not a high followed by a low, but merely a sustained wakefulness. People taking eugeroics report that they can easily remain alert for long periods of time but have no trouble falling asleep when they wish to.

Eugeroics work by stimulating the receptor sites for norepinephrine (also called noradrenaline). This is the neurotransmitter that is primarily responsible for alertness and the sleep/wake cycle, but it also plays a role in attention, memory, and learning functions.

A clinical trial tested the effects of modafinil on people who were kept awake for sixty straight hours. Throughout the test, the subjects completed various questionnaires and tests designed to measure cognitive function. The subjects using modafinil had virtually no degradation of brain function throughout the test, whereas the scores among the placebo group gradually declined and the subjects had difficulty remaining awake.

Modafinil is now used by the military corps of many countries (including, by some reports, our own) to keep soldiers awake and vigilant for long periods of time. Although prolonged sleep deprivation is never desirable, there are circumstances when it is unavoidable, and alertness may be a matter of life and death. (Military operations and medical residencies come to mind.)

In these extreme circumstances, eugeroics are a much safer option than the amphetamines that have been used for this purpose. Side effects from the drugs are virtually nonexistent (although prolonged or frequent sleep deprivation has its own hazards).

For most people, however, eugeroics simply offer the opportunity to enjoy a higher level of intellectual and mental function in their normal activities. For this purpose, a single 100 mg dosage of modafinil in the morning will provide a feeling of alertness and focus throughout the day, without caffeine jitters or afternoon crash. For those who need to maintain a high degree of alertness throughout the evening, a second dose can be taken in the afternoon.

Adrafinil is simply an earlier version of modafinil. It offers the same benefits but is less potent, requiring dosages of 300 mg at a time to be effective. It also has a slightly higher profile of side effects, including a temporary elevation in liver enzyme levels with sustained use. Modafinil is a more refined version of the drug and appears to be without these side effects.

There is still a high demand for adrafinil, however, largely because it is far less expensive than modafinil (about one-fifth the cost). Obviously, where cost is the deciding factor, adrafinil may be preferable.

! Those using adrafinil on a continuous long-term basis should have their liver enzymes evaluated periodically. Because the effect on the liver is reversed when the drug is discontinued, adrafinil can be used intermittently without risk.

Obtaining Offshore Drugs

The FDA allows American citizens to legally import for personal use drugs that are legal in other countries, under certain restrictions. Unfortunately, these restrictions are rather arbitrarily interpreted and enforced. Access to foreign drugs can be unreliable, subject to the FDA's favor or disfavor.

There are numerous offshore pharmacies that sell smart drugs such as piracetam, adrafinil, and modafinil to Americans. Certain FDA-approved prescription drugs (such as deprenyl and hydergine) are also available at substantial savings through offshore pharmacies. You can find them on the Internet and in the classified sections of health publications, but there can be difficulties. If the source you are ordering from runs afoul of the FDA, for example, by violating regulations about advertising and promotion, you may find your order impounded by the government. There is also a possibility of unknowingly purchasing bootleg or counterfeit drugs.

I recommend that you obtain these medications through an anti-aging physician, who can ensure the reliability and authenticity of the source as well as advise you and monitor your dosages as part of a comprehensive program. Alternatively, work with an established and trusted distributor and be prepared for possible delays or interruptions in availability.

For additional information and resources, refer to the LEF Disease Prevention and Treatment database under the heading "Age-Associated Mental Impairment," or consult the Life Extension Foundation Web site at www.lef.org.

ACCESS UNDER ATTACK

At the time of this writing, the availability of nutritional supplements in Europe, the United States, and other countries is threatened by proposed changes in dietary-supplement standards by the Codex

Alimentarius Commission, the United Nations organization that develops international food regulations. As with the FDA here in America, the governing body that oversees the Codex is a highly politicized group under undue influence from commercial interests. The changes being proposed in the Codex clearly place the interests of the international pharmaceutical companies above the rights and interests of ordinary people. The Life Extension Foundation has always been an outspoken advocate for your right to obtain information and products that can improve your health, winning several important lawsuits against the U.S. federal government. For information about these victories, as well as current issues such as the controversy over the Codex Alimentarius, log on to LEF's Web site at www.lef.org, and click on "consumer alerts."

AN ADVANCED COGNITIVE AND ANTI-AGING PROTOCOL

As you may recall, one of Brian's primary goals in beginning an anti-aging program was to function at a higher level at work and in his personal life. When I first met with him (he was 47 at the time), he described a feeling of slowing down, of running out of steam.

"I've got this business that I've spent the last ten years building. But I'm running out of gas at the end of the day," he told me. "My partner and I have a dozen people working for us now. They're depending on me, and I'm afraid I'm going to let them down. I'm losing my motivation. I'm not enjoying my work. I'm not enjoying my life. I've got to do something."

You've seen Brian's progress unfold throughout the previous chapters. The first step was a foundational program of nutritional supplements (antioxidants, essential fatty acids, minerals, and a range of other nutrients) to start to rebuild his nutritional status. I also recommended some dietary and lifestyle changes, such as those described in Chapter 12.

The next time I saw him he was already feeling better. He felt he was thinking a bit more clearly, feeling a modest improvement in energy. I began to work on balancing his hormone levels with hormone replacement therapy. As you've already read in the previous chapters, we addressed the deficiencies in his testosterone and thyroid levels and began growth hormone therapy.

At this point, Brian was already a different person compared to the tired, burned-out man who had first sought my help. He couldn't believe the difference that the program had made in such a short period of time. "I'm feeling so much better," he reported. "I'm not dragging at the end of the day. A month ago, I found myself wondering how I was going to be able to keep on doing this for another fifteen years. Now I actually look forward to work!" He said his staff had also noticed a big difference in his mood. I'm sure his clients felt the change as well.

At this point in his program, we started working on an aggressive program of nutrients to help boost his cognitive powers and enhance his focus, concentration, memory, and even libido. We started with some of the nutrients in the "first pass" cognitive cocktail detailed earlier in the chapter:

> Phosphatidylcholine (3,000 mg)
> Phosphatidylserine (100 mg)
> Ginkgo biloba (60 mg)
> CoQ_{10} (100 mg)

We then added some "second pass" agents to build up an even richer program:

> Piracetam (2,400 mg)
> Deprenyl (2 mg)

On particularly long days or on days when he needs exceptional focus, Brian adds to his morning regimen:

> Adrafinil (300 mg)

The addition of the brainpower nutrients brought Brian's anti-aging program to a new peak. In addition to a more youthful appearance and increased health, vitality, and virility, he also feels sharper and more in control and notices greater mental clarity. The difference—both in the way he feels and in the way he comes across—is incredible. It has made it possible for him to be more successful in his business and to take on new projects. At 47, he had been ready to throw in the towel and accept the "inevitable" decline of middle age. Now he's a vibrant, energetic guy who is completely enjoying his life.

This is the type of transformation that awaits you as you begin your own personal anti-aging revolution. In this first section of the book, we've looked in detail at therapies that rejuvenate your body and mind. These are the tools that will help you extend the prime of life into what used to be considered "old age."

You've also seen how these therapies have worked for patients such as Brian, Tina, Nora, and others. Your program, of course, will be unique, customized to your individual needs and goals. The creation and implementation of your individualized anti-aging program is the subject of Part III of this book. But first, there is another topic that requires our attention. As we take steps to maintain our youthful vitality as we get older, we also want to take care that that bright future is not dimmed or diminished by disease. Avoiding the diseases of aging is the focus of Part II.

STOPPING DISEASE AT THE CELLULAR LEVEL

Now that we are able to grow younger as we age, we need to do everything we can to ensure that we're around to enjoy our extended prime. That means preventing life-shortening and life-limiting diseases such as cancer, heart disease, diabetes, Alzheimer's, arthritis, and age-related eye disease.

The Life Extension Foundation has made several vital discoveries in the area of disease prevention—identifying key cellular processes that are at the root of diseases most likely to affect us as we get older. Now, instead of playing catch-up once symptoms arise, we can take action that will stop disease before it starts.

In Part II, you will learn how to identify key risk factors that may increase your susceptibility to disease—and then take steps to reduce the threat. Basic preventive protocols are outlined here, along with targeted programs for specific concerns.

CHAPTER 6

Curtailing Oxidation: Rust-Proofing Your Cells

If you rest, you rust.
—HELEN HAYES

HALF A CENTURY AGO, Dr. Denham Harman secured his place in medical history by proposing the free radical theory of aging. As familiar as we are today with free radicals and their damaging effects, it's hard to imagine how revolutionary Harman's theory was in its day. At that time, aging was widely thought to be a mechanical issue—brought on by a lifetime of wear and tear on the body's parts. The idea that aging might be caused or accelerated by molecular or biochemical reactions was completely new. It represented a critical shift in our thinking about how bodies age—a shift that ultimately led to the anti-aging revolution that LEF has spearheaded.

Generations of scientists have followed in Harman's path, exploring the role of free radicals in aging and disease and the effectiveness of antioxidants as a way to forestall both. We have learned that free radical damage is a chief contributor to the most common diseases of aging, including cancer, heart disease, diabetes, Alzheimer's disease, and even arthritis. And we have seen that antioxidant nutrients have protective and preventive benefits against all these diseases.

In the years since Harman's groundbreaking work, we have learned that free radical damage is only one of many factors that drive the aging process, not the single cause of aging. Nonetheless, preventing free radical damage remains a cornerstone of my program for preventing disease and forestalling the aging process.

THE CASE AGAINST FREE RADICALS

Harman had noticed that the degenerative changes of aging (loss of function, increased susceptibility to disease, etc.) were similar to the changes seen when organisms are exposed to radiation. Radiation sickness is largely the result of unstable molecules called free radicals that are generated in the body when it is exposed to radiation. A radiation-triggered onslaught of free radicals can quickly disrupt the functioning of cells and tissues, causing severe symptoms and even death. Harman's idea was that the gradual degeneration that happens as we age might be caused by free radical damage that accumulates slowly over the course of a lifetime.

Scientists knew that certain substances could protect against radiation damage by neutralizing the free radicals and limiting their damaging effects. These substances were called *antioxidants.* Harman reasoned that if aging was also the result of free radical damage, antioxidants might be able to slow down the aging process.

To test his theory, he administered a variety of antioxidant chemicals to lab mice. He observed that as the mice got older, those that were protected with antioxidants remained more youthful in their behavior and appearance than did the untreated mice. Moreover, the mice treated with antioxidants lived significantly longer than the untreated control group.

In other experiments, Harman showed that antioxidants helped to keep mice healthy even when they were fed a nutrient-deficient synthetic diet. And mice that were genetically prone to cancer were protected from the disease when they were fed antioxidants. In other words, Harman's work suggested that antioxidants offer specific protection against two of the primary causes of aging and disease in humans: a poor diet and genetic influences.

These early experiments showed that by slowing aging and preventing disease, antioxidants could increase the life expectancy, or average life span, of an animal. Some of Harman's work even suggested that antioxidant nutrients might be able to extend the maximum possible life span of an organism. The antioxidant revolution was under way.

What Exactly Is a Free Radical and Where Do They Come From?

Free radical is a term for a molecule that has one or more unpaired electrons orbiting around it. Free radicals may be as small as a single atom or may be larger, more complex molecules. While there are different types, all free radicals have one thing in common: an unpaired electron creates an unbalanced electrical charge, which the free radical seeks to correct by finding another electron to restore its equilibrium.

In their search for electrons, free radicals may steal electrons from stable molecules that happen to be close by. This can set off a chain reaction, as the newly destabilized molecule tries to replace the electron it lost by stealing one from a neighbor, and so on. A cascade of molecular destruction is set in motion. The damage spreads from cell to cell, much the way rust spreads on metal, only faster.

Alternatively, a free radical may simply latch on to an electron from a neighboring molecule and attempt to share an electron with its host. In the case of a biological molecule such as a protein or enzyme, the addition of the free radical can deform the host molecule in such a way that it can no longer function correctly.

Given the damage they can do, it is easy to think of a free radical as some sort of dangerous germ or enemy intruder. But the truth is that free radicals are the natural and inevitable by-product of our oxygen-based metabolism.

When the mitochondria in each of our cells produces ATP, the cellular energy that fuels life itself, copious numbers of free radicals are produced. When our white blood cells engulf and destroy viruses or bacteria, free radicals are created as a critical part of this defense process. When we exercise, the heart and other muscles are bathed in the free radicals that are produced by our increased respiration and energy use. When the liver detoxifies chemicals, free radicals are produced. And every time we step outdoors and feel the warm sun on our skin, the UV radiation generates free radicals in our bodies.

In short, free radicals are the normal consequence of life as an oxygen-powered organism. As stress researcher Hans Selye once observed, the complete absence of stress is death. Likewise, the complete absence of free radical activity would mean the end of life. But at the same time, free radicals can disrupt the structure and function of our cells. Fortunately, the body has an elegant system that allows it to maintain a balance between the oxidative processes that power life and the mechanisms that defend cells from free radical damage.

Antioxidants are your body's natural defense against free radicals, protecting your tissues and organs from oxidative damage by mopping up free radicals before they can attack vulnerable cells. These specialized compounds sacrifice themselves by donating an electron to stabilize the free radical. Having parted with an electron, the discharged antioxidant is either broken down into a harmless compound (like water) or recharged with a new electron and returned to the workforce. This system prevents the domino effect of progressive electron stealing and spares the surrounding cells and tissues from damage.

OXIDATIVE STRESS HASTENS THE AGING PROCESS

To the extent that the body has a sufficient supply of antioxidant nutrients, free radical damage is kept to a minimum. If, however, the antioxidant reserves are insufficient to handle the amount of free radical activity being generated in the body, those free radicals will begin to attack healthy cells and tissues. The body slips into a state of oxidative stress.

Oxidative stress begins at the molecular and cellular level, with free radical activity impairing cell membranes, DNA, enzymes, protein synthesis, and mitochondrial function. The damage quickly progresses to the structural and functional level, compromising blood vessels, nerve cells, skin, muscles, and organs. Eventually, the cumulative injuries lead to premature aging and chronic and degenerative disease.

Cell membranes, which are high in fatty acids, are a favorite target for free radicals. As the cell membrane is damaged, it begins to have difficulty maintaining the integrity of the cell's contents. Toxins leak into the cell, and nutrients and water leak out of it. The cell becomes dehydrated and weakened and may die. Oxidative stress can lead to the buildup of the cellular debris called lipofuscin, discussed earlier. Lipofuscin deposits have also been linked to both macular degeneration and Alzheimer's disease.

Inside the cell, free radicals prey on the delicate structure of the DNA molecule. Stealing electrons from DNA can quickly create mutations and errors in that cell's copy of the DNA sequence that instructs the cell on how to behave. The cell may cease to function properly, die, or mutate into a cell that grows too quickly (a cancer cell).

As they travel through the blood, free radicals also oxidize fats (cholesterol) in the blood, making the cholesterol stickier and more likely to build up in blood vessels. Free radical damage to the blood vessel walls further increases the risk of heart disease, stroke, and Alzheimer's disease.

Free radicals will attack the body's proteins as well, denaturing (deforming) the enzymes that your body needs to carry out cellular repair and maintenance. Free radicals can oxidize the structural proteins in the skin, leading to wrinkles, discolorations, and skin cancers. When free radicals are unleashed in the cartilage tissue that lines the joints, it can lead to joint pain and osteoarthritis. Oxidative damage also is to blame for the development of age-related cataracts.

In this, Harman's theory was largely correct: free radical damage is a major contributor to most age-related degenerative conditions and diseases.

Who Is at Risk of Oxidative Stress?

We are all exposed to free radicals, but certain factors increase the risk of oxidative stress. Risk factors include:

➢ **Poor diet.** Those with a low intake of antioxidant nutrients are at increased risk of oxidative stress. In general, the modern diet of processed foods contains only a tiny fraction of the antioxidants that would have been consumed on a daily basis by our ancestors.

➢ **Age.** Free radical damage increases with age, as the body's antioxidant reserves tend to decline as we get older. The digestive system becomes less efficient at extracting and absorbing antioxidant nutrients. Additionally, genetically programmed changes in cellular function lead to a slowing in the body's own manufacture of antioxidant nutrients.

➢ **Intense exercise.** Athletes are at an increased risk of oxidative stress because of the high numbers of free radicals created in the muscles, lungs, and heart during strenuous exercise. Anyone who spends a great deal of time outdoors will also have an increased oxidative burden from exposure to UV radiation from the sun.

➢ **Exposure to toxins.** Those who are exposed to environmental pollutants such as smog, cigarette smoke, pesticides, or other industrial or agricultural toxins will have an increased oxidative burden. In our industrialized society, heavy exposure to these environmental pollutants in our air, food, and water supplies is unfortunately the norm.

➢ **Illness.** Those with chronic illnesses, infections, inflammation, or disease also have elevated levels of free radical activity. Extra protection is needed to minimize the effects of oxidative stress during illness.

Measuring Oxidative Stress

There are a number of medical tests that can evaluate your level of oxidative stress and/or your antioxidant status. We can measure the level and activity of various antioxidants in the blood. We can test the urine for metabolites that indicate the amount of unchecked free radical activity. There are genetic profiles that evaluate an individual's inherent capacity to combat oxidative stress. We can even look at blood cells under a microscope for evidence of membrane disruption or other indicators of oxidative stress.

If you have one or more risk factors that place you at particular risk of oxidative stress, such as heavy exposure to pollutants or toxins, chronic inflammatory conditions, autoimmune disease, serious illness such as cancer, or being an elite athlete, you may want to consider oxidative stress testing as a way to ensure that your antioxidant program is aggressive enough to handle the oxidative stress you are under. For most people, however, the regimen of antioxidant nutrients outlined below will provide adequate protection against oxidative stress.

REDUCING EXPOSURE TO FREE RADICALS

As we have seen, many of the free radicals in our body are the unavoidable by-product of our metabolism. But some of our exposure to free radicals is under our control. Limiting your exposure to avoidable sources of free radicals can help to reduce your risk of oxidative stress. For example:

> Avoid unprotected exposure to the sun, which causes free radical damage to the skin (leading to skin cancer and premature aging).

> Limit your exposure to agricultural chemicals by eating organic foods and drinking purified water. This reduces the toxic load on your liver and reduces free radical generation.

> Chronic inflammation can also generate free radicals. Reducing inflammation (the subject of Chapter 7) helps to reduce free radical damage in the body.

> Avoid breathing in vapors from oil paint, gasoline, cleaning chemicals, and other volatile chemicals, which generate free radical activity in the lungs and brain.

➢ Use a dechlorinating showerhead to reduce the amount of chlorine being absorbed through the skin.

➢ Keep your distance from microwave ovens when they are operating, at least three feet.

➢ The newer-generation flat-screen LCD computer monitors protect you (and your eyes) against harmful emissions.

By reducing your exposure to these free radical promoters, you can reduce oxidative stress somewhat. The other tool we have in reducing oxidative stress is to increase the amount of antioxidants available in the body to quench free radical activity before it harms other tissues. Supplements help to close the gap between the body's antioxidant needs and its available supply.

PROTECTING AGAINST OXIDATIVE STRESS

In order to win games, a football team needs a roster of strong players with a variety of different talents. You wouldn't want an entire team of linebackers any more than you'd want an entire lineup of quarterbacks or placekickers. Each position plays an important role in winning the game. Likewise, your body relies on many different antioxidant compounds to protect its various cells and tissues from the many sources of free radical activity. Each antioxidant has unique sources, actions, pathways, and targets. Working together as a team, they provide a thorough defense.

One of the ways antioxidants work together is by recharging or recycling one another. For example, a molecule of vitamin E might give up one of its electrons in order to stabilize a free radical. A molecule of vitamin C can then recharge that molecule of vitamin E by providing a new electron. Vitamin C then is recharged by the antioxidant glutathione, and so on.

Chemically, this electron swap meet is called the redox cycle, because it involves a combination of reduction and oxidation reactions. The redox system of mutual protection and regeneration is one of the reasons that we need a variety of different antioxidants in order to have a strong antioxidant defense team.

THERE IS NO DOUBT: ANTIOXIDANTS PROTECT YOU AGAINST DISEASE

Studies have shown over and over again that those who take in more antioxidant nutrients, either from dietary sources or with supplements, have reduced risk of heart disease, various kinds of cancer (including breast, prostate, bladder, ovarian, and others), cataracts, and skin aging.

However, there have also been some recent studies claiming that antioxidants failed to protect against disease—or even slightly increased the risk of death. Proclamations from these researchers that antioxidants are "useless" or even "harmful" have caused a lot of confusion among the general public. In each case that I have looked into, I found that the studies were poorly designed, poorly analyzed, or simply inconclusive.

In 2004, for example, the *Annals of Internal Medicine* published an analysis of nineteen unrelated studies, which found that vitamin E supplements slightly increased the risk of death. When the report made headlines, several patients called my center to see if they should discontinue taking their supplements. Absolutely not! What the major media outlets failed to include in their coverage was the fact that many of the patients in those particular studies were already gravely ill with diseases including cancer, heart disease, Alzheimer's disease, and other deadly conditions. Some of the studies weren't even evaluating the effects of vitamin E, but of a multivitamin supplement that contained vitamin E. As several commentators noted, the conclusion by these researchers that vitamin E supplementation was responsible for any deaths in these patients was inappropriate, even absurd.

When viewed as a whole, the medical research over the last half century leaves little doubt that antioxidants, whether consumed in foods or as supplements, offer powerful protection from premature disease and aging. The best and most effective strategy is a diet with plenty of antioxidant-rich foods, combined with a supplementation program containing a broad spectrum of antioxidant nutrients.

THE ESSENTIAL ANTIOXIDANTS

Many of the antioxidants we need are manufactured in our cells. But some antioxidants cannot be manufactured in the body and must be obtained from external sources. These are known as *essential nutrients* and include vitamin C, vitamin E, beta-carotene, and selenium.

Vitamin C

Although British sailors knew in the eighteenth century that some substance in oranges and limes could prevent the ravages of scurvy (hence they were called "limeys"), it wasn't until 1932 that scientists were able to isolate and identify this compound as vitamin C. The chemical name for vitamin C, ascorbic acid, is derived from the word *antiscorbutic,* which means "antiscurvy."

Vitamin C (also known as citric acid) gives foods a characteristically tart taste and is widely used as a natural preservative to prevent oxidation of prepared and packaged foods. It is found naturally in fruits and vegetables, especially citrus fruits, tropical fruits (guava, kiwi, papaya, mango), tomatoes, peppers, and melons.

Vitamin C is used throughout the body for cellular and metabolic functions such as building bones, cartilage, and skin. As an antioxidant, it plays a special role in preventing free radical damage to DNA. Because it is not stored in the body, vitamin C is rapidly depleted and needs to be replenished through regular intake of the vitamin. For antioxidant protection, the recommended amount is 2 to 4 grams (2,000 to 4,000 mg) per day.

The Vitamin C Paradox

Dr. Linus Pauling, nutritional pioneer and two-time Nobel laureate, is perhaps most closely associated with his work with vitamin C. Building on the work of Frederick Klenner (who showed that high-dose vitamin C could alleviate polio) and Irwin Stone, Pauling promoted the theory that very high doses of vitamin C could prevent and cure a multitude of diseases.

Today, many nutritionally oriented physicians use vitamin C at extremely high dosages for specific therapeutic purposes such as viral infections or cancer. Under a doctor's close supervision, vitamin C can be administered orally in amounts of 10 to 20 grams, or even larger amounts, up to 30 to 60 grams, when given intravenously.

But in this case, the vitamin C is not being used as an antioxidant to mop up free radicals. Instead, it is thought to act as a pro-oxidant, destroying bacteria, viruses, and even cancer cells by oxidizing them. Large doses of vitamin C can actually increase the free radical burden in the body, increasing the body's requirement for other antioxidants. Although it can be a very effective therapy, high-dose vitamin C (either oral or intravenous) should be administered only by a qualified physician.

Vitamin E

Vitamin E is a fat-soluble vitamin that plays a special role in preventing the oxidation of cholesterol in the blood and protecting the cell membranes from free radical damage. This makes vitamin E of particular importance in the prevention of heart disease and stroke. It also enhances immune function.

In large-scale studies, supplementation with vitamin E has been found to reduce the risk of heart disease and heart attack, to lower the risk of prostate, breast, and colon cancer, and to protect against the development of Alzheimer's disease.

Vitamin E is stored in the fatty tissues of the body, including the skin, and helps to protect the skin from UV-induced free radical damage. It also helps to protect the eyes against free radical damage that can lead to cataracts.

There are two families of vitamin E, the tocopherols and the tocotrienols. Each family is divided into at least four different forms (alpha, beta, delta, and gamma). Although most vitamin supplements (and most clinical research to date) use only the alpha-tocopherol fraction, more recent studies show that a mix of tocopherols and tocotrienols offer much greater protection against free radical damage. Natural forms are also preferred over synthetic forms (tocopheryls). For antioxidant protection, the recommended amount is 400 to 1,200 IU (international units) per day.

Beta-carotene

Beta-carotene is one of the carotenoids, a huge family of antioxidant nutrients that were first found in carrots, hence their name. Other fruits and vegetables, particularly yellow-orange ones such as sweet potatoes, squash, mangoes, and papayas, are also good sources, as are the leafy green vegetables.

Your body uses beta-carotene to manufacture vitamin A, a fat-soluble vitamin. In addition to being a powerful antioxidant, vitamin A helps to maintain the health and function of the retina, repair tissues, and fight infection. People who consume more carotene-rich foods have higher levels of beta-carotene and vitamin A in their blood and also have a lower risk of lung and colon cancer. This protective effect is seen in both smokers and nonsmokers.

However, a large study in Finland was halted several years ago when it was discovered that smokers who took beta-carotene supplements actually had a higher incidence of lung cancer than smokers who did not take the supplements. This result was confounding to many researchers. Smokers tend to be lower in antioxidant reserves than nonsmokers because of the increased free radical burden created by smoking. This is presumed to be one of the reasons that smokers suffer higher rates of cancer. It follows logically that antioxidant supplements such as beta-carotene would be of particular benefit to smokers.

Some have suggested that a chemical in cigarette smoke may actually degrade beta-carotene into a harmful compound, which might explain the results of the Finnish study. Researchers are still searching for other answers to this seeming paradox, but it appears that, once again, balance is the key.

Foods that contain beta-carotene also contain a wide variety of other carotenoids, including alpha-, gamma-, and delta-carotenes, as well as zeaxanthin, cryptoxanthin, lycopene, and lutein. Of all of the carotenoids, beta-carotene is by far the most potent precursor of vitamin A, and it is the one that was singled out for research as a possible cancer preventive. But those who eat foods high in beta-carotene are also consuming a lot of these other carotenoids as well. It appears that these other dietary antioxidants play an important role in cancer prevention.

! When taken as a dietary supplement, beta-carotene should be taken with other carotenoids and antioxidants. This is particularly important for smokers. For antioxidant protection, a mixed carotenoid supplement providing 5,000 to 10,000 IU of beta-carotene is recommended.

Vitamin A can also be taken as a supplement, but it is one of a few vitamins with a somewhat low threshold for toxicity. Excessive amounts over time can lead to symptoms including headaches, dizziness, hair loss, blurred vision, or dry, scaly skin. High-dose vitamin A can also lead to liver damage. Vitamin A can safely be taken in amounts up to 5,000 IU per day.

Selenium

Selenium is an antioxidant mineral that breaks down harmful peroxide radicals into harmless water and oxygen molecules. A large body of evidence shows that selenium is a powerful anticancer nutrient. In those with low selenium levels, the risk of many kinds of cancer (including colon, breast, ovarian, prostate, and lung) is increased. Supplementation with selenium has been shown to reduce the incidence of prostate, lung, colon, and skin cancers.

The amount of selenium in the foods you eat will vary greatly according to the soil in which it was grown. The selenium in meat and seafood likewise relates to the amount of selenium in the food supply of the animal. The recommended supplement dosage is 200 mcg per day. The preferred form of selenium is selenomethionine, derived from cruciferous vegetables such as broccoli.

THE ANTIOXIDANTS YOUR BODY MAKES

In addition to the essential antioxidants derived from external sources, our cells also manufacture important antioxidants. These include coenzyme Q_{10}, glutathione, and alpha-lipoic acid. The body's production of these nutrients can slow down as we age—one of the many genetically programmed changes in cell function that contribute to aging. We can compensate for the age-related decline in cellular antioxidants with nutrient supplements.

Coenzyme Q_{10}

Coenzyme Q_{10}, also known as ubiquinone, is the most abundant of the cellular antioxidants. (The name *ubiquinone* stems from the word *ubiquitous,* which means "present everywhere.") In addition to being a powerful antioxidant itself, CoQ_{10} helps to preserve higher levels of vitamins C and E in the body.

CoQ_{10} is particularly important in protecting the tissues of the brain and heart, organs that have very high energy needs and are exposed to large numbers of free radicals. As cellular production of CoQ_{10} declines with age, the heart and brain are increasingly vulnerable to free radical damage.

Taking CoQ_{10} as a supplement can restore the levels of this nutrient in tissues where cellular production has waned. Studies show that

CoQ_{10} supplementation reduces oxidative stress and also increases cellular levels of vitamins C and E. A good baseline protection against oxidative damage is provided at a dose of 50 to 200 mg per day. For those with specific issues such as heart disease, up to 400 to 600 mg per day may be recommended.

Glutathione

Glutathione (GSH) has a specific role in protecting immune cells from free radical damage. White blood cells patrol the bloodstream on the lookout for intruders such as bacteria, viruses, or cancer cells. When it encounters a pathogen, the white blood cell disables it by oxidizing it. In the process, free radicals are created, which then pose a threat not only to the surrounding tissues but also to the white blood cells themselves.

Glutathione acts as a sort of bodyguard for the white blood cells, neutralizing the free radicals that are created by the immune cells in the line of duty. Glutathione also helps to recycle vitamins C and E through the redox cascade. Glutathione is also the most important detoxification pathway in the liver.

Like other cellular antioxidants, the level of glutathione in the cells tends to decline as we get older, and low glutathione levels are found in those with degenerative diseases such as heart disease, Alzheimer's, and Parkinson's disease.

Taking glutathione as a supplement is problematic because much of the glutathione molecule is broken down in the digestive system before it can be absorbed by the cells. However, taking antioxidant nutrients such as vitamin C and alpha-lipoic acid helps to increase the manufacture of glutathione in the cells.

You can also help your body produce more glutathione by supplying amino acids that act as building blocks for it. Glutathione is made up of three different amino acids: glutamine, methionine, and cysteine. Of these, cysteine is the one most likely to be in low supply. Cysteine can be taken as N-acetylcysteine (NAC), a form that is well absorbed. NAC is itself a potent antioxidant and can help to promote glutathione production in the cells. Whey protein powder is another source of cysteine that has been shown to promote glutathione production.

To encourage glutathione production, take 500 mg of NAC or 1 to 2 scoops of whey protein blended with juice or milk daily.

Alpha-lipoic Acid

Alpha-lipoic acid (ALA) is a multitalented player on the antioxidant team, notable for being soluble in both water and fat. ALA promotes energy production in the mitochondria, protects the mitochondrial membranes from oxidative damage, and protects the body against poisonous heavy metals such as cadmium, arsenic, and lead. ALA is particularly protective of brain cells, shielding them from oxidative damage and also protecting the brain against the effects of insufficient oxygen (such as in a stroke).

In the antioxidant defense system, ALA is a consummate team player. It increases the level of glutathione available to the cells and helps to recycle vitamins C and E. Alpha-lipoic acid also appears to take up the slack if other antioxidant levels are low. Studies show that ALA completely protects against the symptoms of vitamin E deficiency.

ALA also has an unusual ability to improve the body's response and utilization of glucose, and it is widely used in Europe to treat diabetes and prevent diabetic complications. Its antioxidant effects are particularly helpful in protecting diabetics from oxidative damage to the nerves and heart. For this application, the dosages used are between 300 and 1,200 mg per day.

For antioxidant protection, the recommended supplement dosage is 250 to 500 mg per day, taken in two or three divided doses throughout the day.

CELLULAR ANTIOXIDANTS AND FATIGUE

Although oxidative damage has long been linked to cancer, heart disease, and skin aging, some researchers have advanced an intriguing new theory about free radicals and fatigue. Dr. Jay Lombard of Cornell Medical School and his colleague Dr. Christian Renna believe that oxidative stress and/or impaired production of cellular antioxidants may underlie chronic fatigue and other conditions characterized by low energy states.

As we've already seen, cellular energy production creates a large number of free radicals, and brain cells produce and use more energy than any other type of cell. If there were a deficiency of antioxidants in the brain tissue, brain cells could be heavily damaged by free radicals.

But the brain appears to have a protective mechanism that senses the antioxidant reserves available to quench free radicals. Lombard and Renna's theory proposes that when there are not sufficient antioxidants in the body, the brain lowers its energy production in order to create fewer free radicals and protect itself from free radical damage.

By enhancing the levels of cellular antioxidants (CoQ_{10}, alphalipoic acid, and glutathione), the signal can be sent to the brain that it is safe to increase energy production. I have seen aggressive antioxidant nutrition produce phenomenal results in patients suffering from fatigue syndromes.

THE ANTIOXIDANTS YOU DON'T NEED TO TAKE

In addition to the antioxidant nutrients, the body's defense against free radicals relies on several antioxidant enzymes that are manufactured by the body. The three most important antioxidant enzymes are superoxide dismutase (SOD), peroxidase, and catalase.

Unlike antioxidant nutrients, which neutralize free radicals by donating electrons, the antioxidant enzymes simply break free radicals into pieces and recombine them into harmless compounds. SOD, for example, converts dangerous superoxide radicals to hydrogen peroxide molecules. The hydrogen peroxide molecules are then further converted into water by the catalase enzyme.

The enzymes themselves remain unchanged and, unlike antioxidant nutrients, do not have to be recharged or replaced. While antioxidant nutrients can be depleted by large numbers of free radicals, the antioxidant enzymes can continue to disarm as many free radicals as needed.

You can buy SOD as a nutritional supplement, but you will notice that I don't include it or other enzymatic antioxidants in my supplement recommendations. Your body should produce all the enzymatic antioxidants it needs, as long as you supply it with the necessary cofactors. Your body needs certain minerals, including zinc, copper, manganese, and iron, to regulate the production of antioxidant enzymes. If you are deficient in copper, for example, it can lead to decreased SOD activity in your cells and result in oxidative damage. But at the same time, copper is itself an oxidizing compound that creates harmful free radicals. And iron, which is needed to activate the antioxidant enzymes catalase and peroxidase, is also a strong oxidant.

The body is designed to maintain a delicate balance between its pro-oxidative functions and its anti-oxidative defenses. That's why it is so important to have a complete and balanced supplement program. Copper, manganese, and zinc enhance SOD activity, while vitamin E, beta-carotene, and ALA protect the body from copper-induced free radicals. Alpha-lipoic acid also breaks down excess iron, helping to protect against its oxidizing tendencies.

ARE YOU GETTING SUFFICIENT PROTECTION?

The table below gives recommended amounts for the most important antioxidants and several cofactors. While many of these nutrients are found in multivitamin formulations, most multivitamins do not contain sufficient amounts to protect against oxidative stress. Supplement your multivitamin with individual nutrients as needed to bring the total daily intake up to the levels recommended below.

ANTIOXIDANT PROTECTION PROGRAM

Essential antioxidants	Suggested dosage	Notes
Vitamin C	2,000–4,000 mg	Vitamin C can be taken as tablets or as a crystalline powder dissolved in water or juice. A buffered form can prevent stomach upset for those very sensitive to acidic foods.
Vitamin E	400–1,200 IU	Choose a blend of natural (not synthetic) tocopherols and tocotrienols.
Beta-carotene	5,000–10,000 IU	Take a mixed-carotenoid supplement.
Selenium	200 mcg	
Cellular antioxidants		
Coenzyme Q_{10}	50–200 mg	Coenzyme Q_{10} is best absorbed when taken with foods or supplements that contain fats (such as a vitamin E or fish oil capsule).
Alpha-lipoic acid (ALA)	250–500 mg (up to 1,200 mg for those with or at risk of diabetes)	Maximize the effectiveness of ALA by dividing the dose into two or three doses throughout the day, or by taking an extended-release formula.
N-acetylcysteine, to promote glutathione production	500 mg	As an alternative, take 1–2 scoops of whey protein powder.

ANTIOXIDANT PROTECTION PROGRAM, cont.		
Antioxidant cofactors		
Zinc	35 mg	
Copper	2 mg	
Manganese	5 mg	
Iron	Only as needed	

! Iron tends to build up in the bodies of men and nonmenstruating women, creating an oxidative threat and contributing to heart disease. Most adult men and postmenopausal women do not need supplemental iron and should choose nutrient formulations without iron.

MAXIMIZING ANTIOXIDANTS IN YOUR DIET

Although I believe that supplementation is essential in order to get sufficient antioxidant protection, that is not to say that antioxidant-rich foods are not important. Fruits and vegetables, which are high in antioxidant vitamins and minerals, also contain a rich variety of antioxidant phytochemicals, including the flavonoids, catechins, and carotenoids. People who consume more fruits and vegetables have much lower rates of disease.

Scientists are still in the process of identifying the countless different phytochemicals and discovering how they contribute to health, but it appears that these natural chemicals are an important part of the body's antioxidant defense network. Some multivitamins now include phytonutrient complexes and food extracts in their formulations, but because no standards have been established, dosages vary greatly and can be quite minimal.

We also don't completely understand all of the ways in which these nutrients work together synergistically. In addition to taking vitamin supplements, be sure to enhance your diet with a wide variety of fresh fruits and vegetables to maximize your intake of these natural protective chemicals in their naturally occuring combinations.

Antioxidant phytochemicals	Known functions	Food sources
Proanthocyanidin, Resveratrol, Pycnogenol (OPC)	Protect tissues from free radical damage, particularly the heart and skin	Grapes, berries
Indoles (I3C and DIM)	Cancer preventive	Kale, cabbage, broccoli
Lycopene	Prevents cancer, especially of the prostate	Tomatoes and tomato products, red grapefruit, watermelon
Lutein, zeaxanthin	Protect against macular degeneration and breast cancer	Spinach, dark leafy greens (lutein); corn, peaches, mangoes, persimmons (zeaxanthin)
Catechins	Protect cell membranes, shield tissues from UV radiation and carcinogenic chemicals	Black and green tea

PROTECTING YOUR SKIN
FROM PREMATURE AGING

Antioxidants have become the latest thing in cosmetics and skin care products, and for good reason. As you probably are aware, the changes in the skin that accompany aging (lines, wrinkles, age spots, and skin cancer) are accelerated by exposure to UV radiation. When UV rays hit the skin, enormous numbers of free radicals are produced in the skin, setting off a chain reaction of tissue damage. Free radicals alter the DNA of skin cells, laying the ground for future skin cancers. They also wreak havoc on the collagen matrix that supports the skin. Damage to the collagen matrix causes the skin to become loose, lined, and more subject to the pull of gravity.

Consuming antioxidant nutrients through the diet and supplements can help protect your skin cells from sun damage. Putting certain antioxidant nutrients directly onto the surface of the skin can also have extraordinary effects in preventing and even reversing signs of aging in the skin.

Vitamin E is a valuable skin protective nutrient. However, when applied directly to the surface of the skin, the tocotrienol form of the vitamin is much better absorbed and utilized in the cells than the tocopherol form. Topical use of CoQ_{10}, vitamin C, and alpha-lipoic acid can also help to repair skin aging. Many skin care products advertise antioxidant nutrients, but few contain anything more than trace amounts. Look for products that use antioxidant nutrients in concentrations of 1 to 5 percent. Vitamin C products should use a fat-soluble form of the vitamin (ascorbyl palmitate). Products containing a blend of several antioxidants can yield better protection by exploiting the synergistic properties of different antioxidant nutrients. Vitamin C, although very effective when used topically, can be very unstable.

Protecting the body, inside and out, from the damaging effects of oxidation is one important hedge against aging and disease. But preventing age-related disease requires a multifactorial approach. The next chapter explores the surprising role that chronic inflammation plays in the development of age-related disease, along with strategies to protect yourself against this potent risk factor.

CHAPTER 7

Cooling Inflammation: Disease-Proofing Your Body

Old age is like everything else. To make a success of it, you've got to start young.
—THEODORE ROOSEVELT

A T 60 YEARS OLD, Ben was starting to worry about what the future might hold for him. Ten years earlier, Ben had had a serious heart attack. He hadn't had any further cardiac events, but he knew his blood pressure and cholesterol levels were still in the danger zone. He was haunted by the possibility of another, perhaps fatal, heart attack.

He also knew that, statistically, his chances of developing serious diseases such as cancer or Alzheimer's disease were getting higher every year. But now the statistics were starting to take on a more personal face. Ben and his wife had just made the agonizing decision to move his mother-in-law, who was suffering from Alzheimer's disease, into a long-term care facility. While this was going on, a close friend of the family was diagnosed with cancerous polyps in his colon and began chemotherapy.

Shaken by these upsetting events, Ben came to see me, wanting to know what he could do to take control of his destiny. "I don't need to look like I'm 25 again," Ben told me. "I just want to stay healthy. I want to be there for my wife and kids. I don't want them visiting me in the hospital or nursing home in ten years—or even in twenty years."

After a complete evaluation, I told Ben that there was much that we could do to help him live longer and healthier. As he already knew, his cholesterol and triglycerides were high, something we could certainly work on. But there was something else in his blood work that concerned me even more. Although he had no obvious inflammatory conditions such as arthritis, Ben had very high levels of C-reactive protein and fibrinogen in his blood. Elevated levels of these proteins suggest an unhealthy state of systemic inflammation.

INFLAMMATION AS A HIDDEN CAUSE OF DISEASE

The research on the dangers of systemic inflammation is still not widely recognized. It is a much bigger factor in the diseases of aging than most people—or even their doctors—realize. In fact, it now appears to be a primary risk factor for cancer, Alzheimer's disease, and heart disease. This is a very important discovery because, as you will see in this chapter, inflammation is a highly treatable, correctable condition.

Understanding and controlling systemic inflammation is critical to disease prevention and life extension. By reducing systemic inflammation, you will slash your risk of heart disease and many types of cancer in half. (It will also greatly lessen the aches and pains of arthritis and other inflammatory conditions.) Perhaps most significant of all, controlling systemic inflammation may ultimately prove to be the key to preventing Alzheimer's disease.

INFLAMMATION CAN ALSO HELP YOU

At its most basic level, inflammation is a defensive reaction to a specific infectious agent, toxin, or injury. The inflammation response is turned on (and then off) at the cellular level by a variety of pro- and anti-inflammatory chemicals called cytokines. The heat of a fever, the swelling of a sprain or toothache, the redness of a sore throat or a sunburn—all are indications of pro-inflammatory cytokines at work, disabling pathogens and repairing damaged tissue.

Right after a serious injury or surgery, for example, the levels of inflammatory chemicals in your blood are elevated. Once the healing process is under way, the inflammation subsides, and the levels of inflammatory chemicals in the blood return to normal.

But far too many of the patients I see have a lot of inflammatory chemicals in their blood, for no obvious medical reason. This is an indication of systemic inflammation, a chronic state of low-grade inflammation throughout the body. Inflammation can be driven by constant exposure to toxins in the environment, poor dietary choices (such as the standard American diet), poor nutrient status, or the persistent presence of bacteria in the blood. As we age, our cells also tend to produce more inflammatory chemicals than they do when we are younger.

While systemic inflammation is a common phenomenon, we are just now beginning to understand the implications, thanks in large part to the Life Extension Foundation's leadership in this area.

FINDING THE SMOKING GUN

C-reactive protein and fibrinogen are two proteins that act as indicators, or markers, of the degree of inflammation present in the body. While these are not included in every routine blood test, they are often included in more comprehensive blood work panels.

Fortunately, these inflammation markers—along with scores of other health statistics—were measured in several very large and high-profile studies, including the Physicians' Health Study of twenty-two thousand men and the Women's Health Initiative involving forty thousand women. Analysis of these data now reveals that those with elevated levels of C-reactive protein or fibrinogen have several times the incidence of heart disease, heart attack, and stroke as those with lower levels. Even slight elevations of these inflammation markers can double the risk of heart disease, even in those who have no other risk factors for heart disease, such as high cholesterol.

Cardiovascular disease is the number one killer of both men and women, accounting for more than four in every ten deaths. The

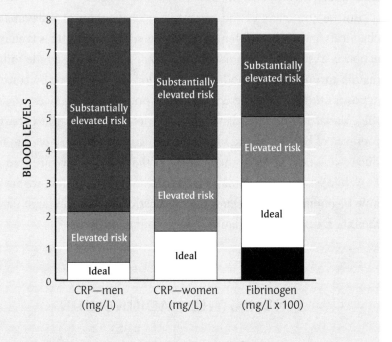

FIGURE 7.1. EFFECT OF INFLAMMATION MARKERS ON RISK
OF HEART ATTACK

As levels of C-reactive protein and fibrinogen in the blood
rise, the risk of heart attack increases.

connection between inflammation and heart disease alone is compelling enough to make controlling systemic inflammation a high priority. But C-reactive protein and fibrinogen are not just cardiac risk factors. Researchers are now seeing inflammation as a central agent in the development and progression of both cancer and Alzheimer's disease.

Unfortunately, the conventional medical community has been slow to tune in to the importance of testing for and treating systemic inflammation. Until they do, millions will continue to suffer and die unnecessarily.

MEDICAL CONDITIONS
ASSOCIATED WITH INFLAMMATION

> Cancer
> Heart disease, heart attack, stroke, congestive heart failure
> Alzheimer's disease
> Allergic conditions including sinusitis, eczema, and asthma
> Autoimmune conditions including lupus, psoriasis, fibromyalgia, and rheumatoid arthritis
> Pancreatitis
> Kidney failure
> Osteoarthritis, bursitis, tendinitis
> Surgical complications, including poor wound healing

NSAIDS: BUILDING THE CASE
AGAINST INFLAMMATION

Scientists at the Life Extension Foundation were among the first to suspect systemic inflammation as a major cause of aging and disease. The fact that several large-scale studies documented a clear link between inflammation markers and heart disease was the foundation of the theory. The fact that people who use nonsteroidal anti-inflammatory drugs (NSAIDs) have much lower risks of many diseases was the next big piece of evidence.

Aspirin, ibuprofen, and other NSAIDs are a standard remedy for headaches, fever, muscle aches, and other relatively minor complaints. Because they are inexpensive and seen as relatively harmless (more about that in a moment), NSAIDs are taken daily by millions of arthritis sufferers. Whether or not this is a good idea, the fact that NSAIDs are so widely used has created a very large body of data that can be used to test the validity of the inflammation theory of disease.

Sure enough, when you sift through the data on NSAID users, they strongly suggest that the use of these anti-inflammatory drugs is highly protective against diseases that have been linked to inflammation. This would seem to confirm the theory that inflammation not only is present in these diseases but may actually be a key factor in their development.

People who take aspirin regularly have a substantially lower risk of many kinds of cancer, including breast cancer, esophageal cancer, colorectal cancer, and prostate cancer (especially the metastatic form of the disease). Given that inflammation is now known to be a factor in cancer growth, it seems possible that NSAIDs protect against cancer at least in part by reducing inflammation. This protective effect is more significant than you might imagine. Aspirin users have:

> 50 percent lower risk of dying of colon cancer
> 60 percent lower risk of prostate cancer
> 40 to 50 percent lower risk of breast cancer (and in those who do develop breast cancer, the tumors are smaller and less invasive)
> 90 percent lower risk of esophageal cancer (in one study involving fourteen thousand subjects, occasional aspirin use reduced the risk by 90 percent, and among those who used aspirin regularly, there were no cases of esophageal cancer whatsoever)

When you consider that about 150,000 Americans die every year from these four types of cancer alone, the potential to reduce those numbers by 40, 60, or even 90 percent is staggering.

You might be wondering whether low-dose aspirin therapy, such as that prescribed to protect against heart disease, is enough to protect against cancer. Taking one baby aspirin every day (or one regular aspirin tablet every other day) has been shown to substantially reduce the risk of heart attack and stroke. Unfortunately, this low dosage does not seem to be enough to provide significant protection against cancer. Across the various studies, the general trend is that people who take regular doses of aspirin more frequently (on a daily or near daily basis) and for longer periods of time (several years) have the most reduction of risk.

In the case of Alzheimer's disease, the protective effects of NSAIDs are equally stunning. If you have any personal experience with Alzheimer's disease, you know the anguish that this disease brings to both the sufferers and to their families. As Ben and his wife are painfully aware, there is at present no cure for Alzheimer's disease and only minimally effective treatments.

If you don't know anyone with Alzheimer's disease, you soon will. Half of all people 85 years of age and older suffer from it. Experts calculate that as the American population ages, ballooning numbers of Alzheimer's cases will single-handedly bankrupt our Medicare system.

Regular use of NSAIDs, however, appears to protect the brain from the changes associated with this disease. At least two dozen studies show that regular (daily or near daily) NSAID use can cut the risk of Alzheimer's by as much as 75 percent. The longer you have been taking NSAIDs and the earlier in life you started using them, the lower your risk of developing Alzheimer's disease. The best protective effect is seen with dosages of at least 800 mg of ibuprofen or 2.4 grams of aspirin per day. Again, the best theory is that NSAIDs protect against the development of Alzheimer's disease by reducing inflammation.

For more on alternative and experimental therapies for Alzheimer's disease, consult the LEF Disease Prevention and Treatment database, under "Alzheimer's Disease."

NONSTEROIDAL ANTI-INFLAMMATORY DRUGS

Standard NSAIDs (by prescription or over the counter)	COX-2 Inhibitors (by prescription only)
Aspirin (Bayer, Excedrin)	Celecoxib (Celebrex)
Ibuprofen (Advil, Motrin)	Valdecoxib (Bextra)
Indomethacin (Indocin)	
Naproxen (Aleve, Naprosyn)	

Acetaminophen (Tylenol) is not an NSAID. Although it is a pain reliever, it does not reduce inflammation and has not shown any protective effect against cancer, heart disease, or Alzheimer's disease. In fact, one study showed that Tylenol users had a 35 percent higher risk of Alzheimer's disease.

What About the COX-2 Inhibitors?

In the body, inflammation is mediated by a class of enzymes called cyclooxygenase (or COX) enzymes. COX-2 inhibitors are a newer type of NSAID, approved by the FDA in 2000. Their chief benefit is more selective action, which suppresses the inflammatory COX-2 enzyme without affecting the stomach-protective COX-1 enzyme. For this reason, the new COX-2 inhibitors are less likely to irritate and damage the stomach lining. (Standard NSAIDs block both COX-1 and COX-2 enzymes.)

Unlike the standard NSAIDs, which have been in widespread use for decades, we don't have nearly as much data on whether or not the newer COX-2 inhibitors can lower disease risk over the long term. Preliminary research suggests that COX-2 inhibitors, like the standard NSAIDs, may have benefits in the prevention and perhaps treatment of cancer and Alzheimer's disease. (See also "Novel Therapies for Cancer," page 191.)

We also don't yet fully know the risks of long-term use. Researchers have been concerned that COX-2 inhibitors may increase the risk of cardiovascular events. And in late 2004, one of the most popular COX-2 inhibitors (Vioxx) was taken off the market due to an increase in cardiovascular events in those using the drug for eighteen months or longer.

HOW INFLAMMATION DRIVES DISEASE

Now that the links between inflammation and disease have been more firmly established, the next challenge is to understand more exactly the ways in which inflammation contributes to disease. Many leading researchers are searching for the answers. Although this research is still in its infant stages, here are some of the most likely mechanisms:

> **Inflammatory chemicals kill brain cells.** Alzheimer's disease is characterized by the presence of plaques in the brain, and for a long time research has been focused (so far without success) on finding therapies to prevent the formation of these plaques. Alzheimer's disease is also characterized by significant inflammation in the brain, a condition that neurologist David Perlmutter has aptly described as "the brain on fire." This inflammation is now believed to be an immunological reaction to the plaques. In fact, it may be inflammatory chemicals, not the plaques themselves, that do the most damage to the surrounding brain tissue.

> **Inflammatory products thicken the blood.** The buildup of fibrinogen in the blood affects the flowing characteristics of the blood, making it sticky and thick. This "thick blood syndrome" makes it harder for the blood to circulate through the small blood vessels, resulting in heart pain (angina), muscle pain, weakness, foggy thinking, and fatigue.

> **Inflammation causes arterial plaques to break off.** In the case of heart disease, Harvard researcher Paul Ridker believes that inflammation plays a deadly role in destabilizing arterial plaques. In other words, it is inflammation that causes plaques to break free of the arterial walls and travel through the bloodstream, causing heart attacks or strokes.

> **Inflammation causes free radical damage.** The inflammatory response creates tremendous numbers of free radicals. For this reason, chronic systemic inflammation can dangerously deplete the body's reserves of antioxidant nutrients. As we saw in Chapter 6, without sufficient antioxidants, our cells are more vulnerable to mutations that can lead to cancer.

> **Inflammatory enzymes fuel cancer growth.** Cancer cells are programmed to produce large amounts of the inflammatory COX-2 enzyme. The levels of COX-2 enzymes in cancerous tissue can be up to 60 times greater than in healthy tissue. The cells then use this

enzyme as fuel for the rapid cell division that is cancer's deadly hallmark. A big part of NSAIDs' ability to prevent cancer and improve survival in cancer patients may have to do with the suppression of the COX-2 enzyme.

Frankly, we still have a lot to figure out about the exact mechanisms by which anti-inflammatory drugs and nutrients protect us from disease (although they clearly do). But the research is moving quickly, with new pieces falling into place every day. The recently discovered link between cholesterol-lowering drugs and a reduction in Alzheimer's disease is one such piece.

Statins: A Medical Riddle Is Solved

People who take certain cholesterol-lowering drugs (the statin drugs, which include Lipitor, Mevacor, Zocor, and Pravachol) have only about one-third the risk of Alzheimer's disease compared with the general population. High cholesterol was at one time considered to be a possible risk factor for Alzheimer's disease, and so it might make sense that people taking cholesterol-lowering medications would reduce that increased risk. But newer research shows that the effect seems to have nothing to do with reducing cholesterol.

People with normal cholesterol (who don't take statin drugs) have three times the risk of Alzheimer's disease as those who use statin drugs to keep their cholesterol down. What's more, people who are treated with other kinds of cholesterol-lowering drugs (but not statin drugs) have three times the risk of Alzheimer's disease as those who are treated with statin drugs.

It seems to be a paradox. But guess what else statin drugs do besides lower your cholesterol? *They also reduce inflammation.* Suddenly the apparent paradox makes perfect sense.

The LEF and other researchers theorize that statin drugs protect against Alzheimer's because they also reduce inflammation. And this in turn forces us to reconsider the role of statin drugs in protecting against heart disease. As we'll discuss in more detail in the next chapter, high cholesterol does not appear to be as big a risk factor for heart disease as we once thought. At the same time, inflammation is a much bigger factor than we knew. The true benefit of statin drugs for patients with heart disease may have more to do with their ability to reduce inflammation than their cholesterol-reducing actions.

NOVEL THERAPIES FOR CANCER

Recognizing the central role of inflammation in the cancer process, several forward-thinking scientists are advancing novel therapies using anti-inflammatory agents as cancer therapies. Dr. Nick Gonzales, for example, is doing very promising, FDA-approved clinical trials at Memorial Sloan-Kettering Cancer Center, using high-dose anti-inflammatory enzymes such as bromelain to treat cancer.

The LEF has also advanced a novel cancer protocol that uses COX-2 inhibitors and statin drugs as an adjunct to other, primary cancer-fighting therapies. Both drugs have been shown to interfere with the ability of cancer cells to proliferate. Perhaps more importantly, cancer patients taking these drugs have better survival rates.

Both COX-2 inhibitors and cholesterol-lowering (statin) drugs can have undesirable side effects and risks of toxicity, however. Later in this chapter, I recommend supplements and dietary strategies that can reduce inflammation without any unwanted side effects. For the purposes of disease prevention, these alternatives offer the best balance of risk and benefit. For people with cancer, however, the risks of taking anti-inflammatory drugs are probably outweighed by the potential benefits.

You can learn more about anti-inflammatory agents and cancer and the research supporting their use, by consulting the LEF Disease Prevention and Treatment database under "Cancer (Adjuvant) Therapy and Cancer Treatment."

HOW YOU CAN USE THIS EMERGING RESEARCH TO IMPROVE YOUR HEALTH TODAY

If you are someone who has taken NSAIDs or statin drugs, the drugs may have reduced your risk of cancer, heart disease, and Alzheimer's disease. If you are not currently taking these drugs, you might be wondering if you should start taking them as disease prevention, whether or not you need them otherwise.

Clearly, drugs that reduce inflammation can help to prevent many diseases of aging—an unexpected bonus for people taking NSAIDs and statin drugs. Then again, these drugs also have side effects. NSAIDs can tear up the lining of your stomach and cause pain and internal bleeding. In fact, bleeding due to NSAID use is a major cause of anemia in older people. Both NSAIDs and statin drugs also put a strain on your liver and in rare cases can even cause drug-induced hepatitis.

Quite honestly, all of these side effects and risks would be worth taking if there were no other way to get the profound disease-reduction benefits of these drugs. But there *are* alternatives. There are safer, nontoxic nutrient therapies that can reduce inflammation and, along with it, your risk of disease. If you have high cholesterol, you also have alternatives that can help you reduce your cholesterol without drugs, which are outlined in the next chapter.

Anti-Inflammatory Supplements

There are a number of nutrients that can powerfully reduce inflammation in your body without side effects. You will recognize many of these from Part I, where they were discussed in relation to other anti-aging benefits.

> **Nettle leaf extract** inhibits COX enzymes (as do NSAIDs) and also suppresses inflammatory cytokines.

> **Essential fatty acids,** including EPA, gamma-linoleic acid (GLA), and especially DHA, inhibit inflammatory cytokines and can reduce both C-reactive protein and fibrinogen.

> **Bromelain** is a protein-digesting enzyme found in pineapple. It reduces inflammation and breaks down fibrinogen.

> **Ginger** is a natural COX-2 inhibitor, suppressing the same inflammatory pathway that Celebrex affects. It also suppresses the formation of cytokines.

> **Curcumin** is the active ingredient in the spice turmeric. (It is not present in cumin.) It inhibits inflammatory cytokines and fibrinogen.

> **DHEA,** the anti-aging hormone discussed in Chapter 2, is also anti-inflammatory. As DHEA levels tend to decline with age, inflammation and disease increase. DHEA supplementation can suppress the activity of inflammatory cytokines and can lower C-reactive protein and fibrinogen.

> **Vitamin K,** discussed in Chapter 11 for its unique role in forestalling diseases of aging, also inhibits the production of inflammatory cytokines.

> **Ginkgo biloba extract** is discussed in Chapter 5 for its benefits in enhancing and preserving brain function and cognitive abilities. It also has anti-inflammatory actions and reduces excess fibrinogen.

These nutrients can be used in various combinations to reduce inflammation, as well as for their other benefits. Following is a basic anti-inflammatory regimen that is appropriate for most people. Because of their multiple actions in the body, ginkgo, vitamin K, and DHEA need to be used with care in some situations. (Please refer to the individual chapters cited above for dosage guidelines and safety precautions for these nutrients.)

BASIC ANTI-INFLAMMATION PROTOCOL

Nutrient	Dosage per day
Nettle leaf extract	900 mg
Fish oil capsules *or* DHA capsules	3,000 mg 1,000 mg
Bromelain	2,000 mg
Ginger *or* curcumin	900 mg 900 to 1,800 mg

The comprehensive anti-aging program that we will develop in Part III includes many of these anti-inflammatory nutrients as well. For most people, the nutrient regimen recommended in Chapter 11 will be sufficient to protect against systemic inflammation, without the need for a separate protocol like the one above.

In Ben's case, for example, I prescribed a supplement regimen similar to the one described in Chapter 11. It included 2,000 to 3,000 mg a day of fish oil capsules, DHEA, and ginkgo. I also recommended some changes in his diet, similar to those outlined below and in Chapter 12. For him, these things were enough to produce profound anti-inflammatory benefits. When we retested his blood, we saw some spectacular reductions in his inflammation markers, along with improvements in many other areas.

If, however, his inflammation markers had still been elevated, I would have added one or more additional nutrients from the protocol above. When customizing your own program, blood tests will offer the most accurate gauge of whether or not your regimen has succeeded in reducing any systemic inflammation that may exist.

TRACKING INFLAMMATION
WITH BLOOD TESTS

There are some very specific (and expensive) blood tests that can measure the levels of individual inflammatory cytokines, such as interleukin-6 (IL-6), interleukin-1 beta (IL-1β), and tumor necrosis factor alpha (TNF-α). If any of these are abnormally high, it indicates some sort of inflammatory process.

More commonly, we use less expensive tests that measure the levels of the inflammation markers C-reactive protein and/or fibrinogen. For most people, these simpler tests are more than sufficient to reveal whether inflammation is a risk factor. For maximum protection against diseases associated with inflammation, levels of these markers should be as follows:

> C-reactive protein: less than 0.5 mg/L
> Fibrinogen: less than 300 mg/dL

When I first tested his blood, Ben had a C-reactive protein level of 1.6 mg/L and a fibrinogen level of 647 mg/dL. Both markers were three times higher than they should have been, at levels that increased Ben's risk of heart attack by about 300 percent.

After just twelve weeks on his anti-aging program, we tested his markers again and found that his CRP had dropped to 0.6 mg/L, just over the target; even more impressive, his fibrinogen had dropped to a healthy 206 mg/dL. (There were improvements in many other areas as well.) Ben was delighted to see that the program he'd adopted had produced such quantifiable effects. In a very short period of time, Ben had lowered his risk of having a second heart attack by two-thirds. He'd also greatly reduced his risks of cancer and Alzheimer's disease.

FIGURE 7.2. EFFECTS OF ANTI-INFLAMMATORY REGIMEN (BEN)

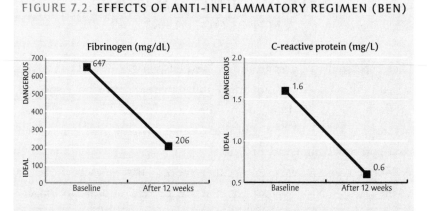

Anti-inflammatory nutrients reduced Ben's fibrinogen and C-reactive protein levels to ideal ranges in about twelve weeks.

Evaluating and Reducing Your Risk

Because systemic inflammation is dangerous, often silent, and easily treated, I highly recommend that you have your inflammation markers tested as part of an initial risk evaluation. As discussed in more detail in Chapter 10, an initial risk evaluation not only highlights areas of particular concern but also gives you a baseline for comparison.

The next step is to begin taking anti-inflammatory nutrients. Even if you don't have elevated inflammation markers, you will benefit from ongoing nutrient support to prevent systemic inflammation from taking hold. You can use the basic anti-inflammation protocol on page 194. Ideally, however, you will use anti-inflammatory nutrients as part of a more comprehensive anti-aging regimen such as the one outlined in Chapter 11.

If your initial blood work reveals elevated inflammation markers, you may wish to repeat your blood tests after eight to twelve weeks, to be sure that the program you have implemented has been sufficient to reduce your risk of inflammation-driven disease. Because each body responds differently, there is no recipe that will work for everyone. If inflammation continues to be an issue for you, you and your medical advisor will want to fine-tune your program by adding additional anti-inflammatory nutrients or increasing the amounts of the nutrients you are taking.

THE ANTI-INFLAMMATORY DIET

What you eat on a daily basis has a big impact on every aspect of your health, including the level of inflammation in your body. The following dietary modifications can—among other things—help protect you from excessive inflammation. You'll no doubt notice that the anti-inflammatory diet has a lot in common with the anti-aging diet that is discussed in more detail in Chapter 12.

General principles:

> **Emphasize monounsaturated fats.** Certain fats, specifically those found in fish, olive oil, nuts, seeds, and avocados, are converted into compounds that promote the production of anti-inflammatory chemicals. Other fats, chiefly those found in meats and dairy products, promote the production of pro-inflammatory chemicals.

> **Eat low on the glycemic index.** Carbohydrate foods that cause a quick rise in insulin also promote inflammation. The glycemic index is a rating system that calculates the impact of various foods on your production of insulin. Foods high on the glycemic index, such as white bread, pasta, rice, sweets, and fruit juices, tend to promote inflammation. Choosing carbohydrates that are low on the glycemic index, such as whole grains and fresh vegetables, will help to reduce inflammation.

> **Avoid foods rich in arachidonic acid.** Arachidonic acid is a fatty acid that is a precursor to pro-inflammatory cytokines. Foods such as eggs and organ meats are particularly high in arachidonic acid and are considered inflammation-promoting. These foods have other healthful benefits, however, and can be eaten in moderation, except by those for whom inflammation is a particular problem.

ANTI-INFLAMMATION DIET GUIDELINES

Foods to enjoy	Foods to avoid
Salmon and other fatty fish	Fatty cuts of red meat
Avocado	Egg yolks
Olive oil	White bread and pasta
Nuts and seeds	Potatoes
Fresh vegetables and fruits	Fruit juices
Whole grains, including oatmeal	White rice and rice cakes

THE CONNECTION BETWEEN YOUR HEART AND YOUR GUMS

In addition to avoiding inflammation-producing foods and taking anti-inflammatory supplements, be sure to take good care of your teeth. Gum disease is a highly inflammatory condition that has consequences far beyond the mouth. The inflammatory cytokines that accompany gum disease can contribute greatly to the problems associated with systemic inflammation. People with gum disease are much more likely to suffer from heart disease, for example. Regular flossing and professional dental care vastly reduce your risk of periodontal disease. As unlikely as it may sound, flossing your teeth is a crucial part of your disease prevention and life extension regimen.

 A treatment protocol for gum disease is found in the LEF Disease Prevention and Treatment database, under "Gingivitis."

REDUCING INFLAMMATION
CAN SAVE YOUR LIFE

The insidious thing about systemic inflammation is that it so often has no symptoms or signs. Ben, for example, was completely unaware of the degree to which his health was jeopardized by systemic inflammation. Once identified, the inflammation in Ben's body was quickly resolved by the anti-aging and inflammation-reducing program he adopted. In the process, Ben's risks, along with his anxiety about the future, were dramatically reduced.

Likewise, your anti-aging program (see Part III) will include screening for indications of systemic inflammation, as well as anti-inflammatory nutrients and lifestyle measures to reduce and prevent inflammation and its consequences.

At LEF, we know that the key to beating disease is to respond to early signs of cellular dysfunction, long before the first sign or symptom appears. While full-blown disease is often unstoppable, the cellular mechanisms that begin the disease process are relatively easy to influence. By quenching these tiny sparks, we can prevent the fires from igniting.

CHAPTER 8

Protecting Your Heart and Brain by Enhancing Methylation

It is what we think we know already that often prevents us from learning.
—CLAUDE BERNARD

THIRTY YEARS AGO, MEDICAL students learned about amino acids—including one called homocysteine—when they took organic chemistry. But as doctors, they wouldn't have paid the least attention to homocysteine levels in their patients. Today, we know that too much homocysteine in the blood is one of the most potent risk factors for heart attack and stroke. In fact, high homocysteine levels are even more significant than high cholesterol levels, as we will discuss later in this chapter. Homocysteine is not just a cardiovascular risk factor, either. High homocysteine levels have also been linked to Alzheimer's disease, osteoporosis, Parkinson's disease, depression, and many other conditions.

Reducing homocysteine to safe levels is therefore another key aspect of my disease prevention protocol. You may have noticed, however, that this chapter isn't titled "Reducing Homocysteine" but "Enhancing Methylation." This is because high homocysteine is really just a warning flag: it tells us that your body is not methylating properly. Although the term may be unfamiliar, proper methylation is absolutely essential to your health.

Your body depends on methylation to detoxify carcinogens and other poisons, to repair damaged DNA, to form new cells, and to manufacture important anti-aging hormones. When your ability to methylate is impaired, all of these important functions are impeded, leading to accelerated aging and degenerative diseases such as heart disease, Alzheimer's, cancer, diabetes, and others.

Here's the good news: enhancing methylation is fairly easy to do. With a few basic nutrients, you can support this critical biochemical process, protecting against premature aging and substantially reducing your risk of disease. Unfortunately, most people do not have an adequate intake of methylation-promoting nutrients. As a result, inadequate methylation is one of the primary preventable causes of premature aging and disease.

WHAT IS METHYLATION?

Chemically speaking, methylation is the transfer of a *methyl group* (one atom of carbon attached to three atoms of hydrogen) from one molecule to another. Your body depends on this biochemical exchange for some of its most critical functions. Methylation takes place millions of times a day, in every cell of your body.

Methyl donors are compounds that supply the methyl groups needed for methylation. *Methylating factors* are nutrients that help with the methylation process by providing enzymes that detach the methyl groups from the methyl donors and reattach them to other molecules. Figure 8.1 on page 202 shows a common methylation reaction, illustrating how these players all work together to complete the methylation cycle.

In this example, the cycle begins with methionine, an amino acid that we get from meat, fish, dairy products, eggs, and whole grains. Methionine donates its methyl group in order to promote necessary chemical reactions in the body. Once it has lost its methyl group, methionine is then further reduced to another compound called homocysteine. With the help of methylating factors (vitamin B_{12} and folic acid), homocysteine is recycled back into methionine by acquiring a new methyl group from another donor.

The methylation process, therefore, requires an abundant supply of methyl donors as well as an ample supply of methylating factors. In

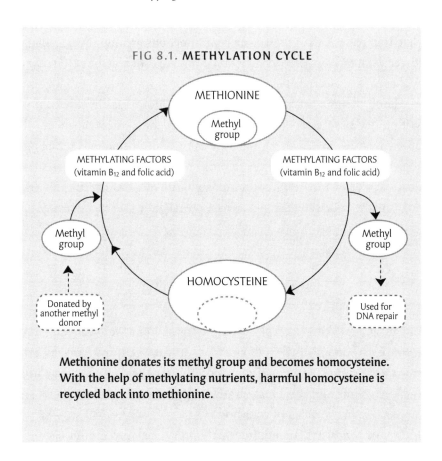

FIG 8.1. **METHYLATION CYCLE**

Methionine donates its methyl group and becomes homocysteine. With the help of methylating nutrients, harmful homocysteine is recycled back into methionine.

addition to methionine, other important methyl donors include choline, trimethylglycine (TMG), and S-adenosyl-methionine (SAM-e). Methylating factors include vitamin B_{12}, folic acid, and zinc.

Methyl Donors	Methylating Factors
Methionine	Vitamin B_{12}
Choline	Folic acid (folate)
Trimethylglycine (TMG)	Zinc
S-adenosyl-methionine (SAM-e)	

If your body runs low on methyl donors or methylating factors, the body's essential detoxification and repair functions are impaired. Among other things, the body begins to have difficulty keeping up with the job of recycling homocysteine back into methionine. The accumulation of homocysteine in the blood is a clear danger signal that methylation is impaired. It is also a direct threat to your health in and of itself.

THE DANGERS OF HOMOCYSTEINE

The connection between homocysteine and disease was first proposed in 1968 by Harvard pathologist Kilmer McCully. McCully argued persuasively that elevated levels of homocysteine are a far more accurate and meaningful predictor of cardiovascular disease (the number one killer of Americans) than cholesterol. High cholesterol, he argued, was not a primary cause of heart disease but a secondary factor.

McCully pointed out that cholesterol begins to build up inside blood vessels only if the blood vessel walls have been damaged. Lowering cholesterol may slow the accumulation of cholesterol deposits on the walls of the damaged arteries, but it does nothing to stop the initial damage from occurring. As such, focusing heart disease prevention efforts on lowering cholesterol is like trying to prevent rain with an umbrella.

Homocysteine, on the other hand, provokes a destructive cascade of chemical reactions in the endothelial cells that line arterial walls. The damage done to the arterial walls then encourages the formation of cholesterol deposits.

The presence of homocysteine in the blood also interferes with the body's ability to break down fibrinogen. As we saw in Chapter 7, high fibrinogen levels make the blood sticky and thick, and therefore more likely to form dangerous blood clots. By lowering homocysteine levels, we can prevent damage to arteries and reduce the incidence of clots, blockages, heart attacks, and strokes. Lowering cholesterol, McCully pointed out, would then be a secondary concern.

Because McCully's theory challenged the prevailing dogma about cholesterol and heart disease, it was met with enormous resistance. His work was originally discredited, and he lost his position at Harvard University's medical school. For almost two decades, the Life Extension Foundation stood virtually alone in its recognition of the importance of his research, recommending as early as 1981 that members take steps to lower homocysteine.

On the other hand, it took the medical establishment almost twenty years to acknowledge the validity of McCully's work. Hundreds of studies and papers have now confirmed McCully's original thesis that homocysteine is an independent risk factor for heart disease. High homocysteine levels greatly increase your risk of having a heart attack or stroke. And if you have heart disease, elevated homocysteine increases your risk of death from any cause.

In 1997, scientists writing in the *New England Journal of Medicine* went so far as to state that elevated homocysteine (not cholesterol or high blood pressure) is "the strongest modifiable predictor of overall mortality [death from any cause] and mortality due to cardiovascular disease among patients with . . . coronary artery disease."

But the implications of McCully's work extend far beyond the health of your heart. Remember that elevated homocysteine is a red flag for impaired methylation, a process that is critical to virtually every system and function of the body. Researchers have found that elevated homocysteine levels are correlated with an astonishing variety of age-related illnesses and conditions.

CONDITIONS ASSOCIATED WITH ELEVATED HOMOCYSTEINE LEVELS

> Alzheimer's disease
> Cognitive decline
> Chronic fatigue/fibromyalgia
> Osteoporosis
> Diabetic retinopathy (blindness)

> Parkinson's disease
> Depression
> Low thyroid function
> Inflammatory bowel syndrome

Homocysteine may even play a role in cancer formation. Abnormal methylation is one of the distinguishing features of cancer cells. In fact, research has shown that methylating factors can heal cancerous lesions in laboratory animals.

Homocysteine may contribute to cancer formation by increasing free radical activity. In a dangerous downward spiral of cause and effect, oxidative stress can also impair the methylation process. The combined and additive effects of impaired methylation and oxidative stress may be the link between homocysteine and cancer.

The Ongoing Search for Answers

Because the mainstream was slow to recognize the importance of McCully's work, research on homocysteine is still in its infancy. Although we have a good idea how homocysteine works in the promotion of heart disease, we don't know as much about the mechanisms that connect it to other conditions. In many cases, we know only that the connection exists. That is, people with certain diseases have significantly higher concentrations of homocysteine than healthy people, and otherwise healthy people with high homocysteine have an increased risk of becoming ill in the future.

We may eventually discover that the toxic effects of homocysteine itself contribute directly to some of these disease states. For example, it may be that homocysteine contributes to age-related cognitive decline by damaging the tiny blood vessels in the brain, leading to impaired blood and nutrient flow to the neurons.

In other cases, it may be that homocysteine is not a direct cause but rather a signal that the body is dangerously undermethylated. We know, for example, that Alzheimer's disease is characterized by a severe disruption in the methylation pathways of the brain, and this may explain why Alzheimer's patients have such high homocysteine levels. It also suggests that enhancing methylation may help to prevent the development of Alzheimer's disease.

Despite all we do not yet understand about the effects of homocysteine toxicity and the multiple roles of methylation, it is clear that enhancing methylation (and reducing homocysteine) is a powerful way to guard against premature aging and disease.

WHERE DOES CHOLESTEROL FIT IN?

You may now be wondering why it is that you continue to hear so much about cholesterol and so little about methylation (and inflammation) as risk factors for heart disease. As we have seen, methylation and inflammation are both potent risk factors for heart disease as well as for many other diseases of aging. Both can be effectively managed with nonprescription nutrient therapies, vastly reducing the risk of disease. And therein lies part of the answer.

Because cholesterol was once thought to be the chief culprit in the development of heart disease, pharmaceutical companies spent millions to develop drugs to reduce cholesterol. In an effort to protect that investment, they now spend millions on marketing and advertising. They continue to market the cholesterol theory of heart disease to doctors and have now started advertising the drugs directly to patients, employing emotion-laden commercials about grandchildren and golden wedding anniversaries. The influence that this marketing has on the beliefs and behavior of the medical community is greater than you might imagine.

While homocysteine levels are a very strong predictor of future heart disease risk, the association between cholesterol and heart disease is not as clear. The fact is that many people with high cholesterol don't get heart disease and many people with perfectly normal cholesterol levels die of heart attacks or strokes. In fact, basic cholesterol screening fails to identify about 50 percent of those with acute coronary syndromes.

Still, you've probably seen advertisements or read articles stating that "studies show that lowering cholesterol can help prevent heart disease." Here's the truth. In an analysis of twenty-two major clinical studies conducted in 1992, the number of studies that showed a benefit from lowering cholesterol was about the same as the number of studies showing no benefit whatsoever. In fact, when the data from all twenty-two studies were considered together, the authors concluded that "lowering cholesterol does not reduce mortality and is unlikely to prevent coronary heart disease."

However, that wasn't the most astonishing thing that the authors found. They then examined the medical literature at large and found that the studies that showed a benefit from cholesterol-lowering drugs were *six times more likely to be cited by other researchers* than the studies that showed that the drugs were of no benefit. In other words, the medical literature reflects a profound and self-perpetuating bias toward cholesterol-lowering medications, with researchers quoting only pro-drug studies and ignoring the rest.

Old Habits Die Hard

The fact that cholesterol-lowering drugs continue to be among the most-prescribed medications has far more to do with pharmaceutical companies' propaganda than it does with medical reality. Most recently, pharmaceutical companies have funded an advertising blitz to promote the results of the so-called Heart Protection Study, a large trial conducted at Oxford University and funded in part by one of the leading drug makers.

The study found that cholesterol-lowering drugs reduced the risk of death among subjects who were at increased risk of cardiovascular disease. But as we have already discussed in the previous chapter, there is reason to believe that the beneficial effects of cholesterol-lowering drugs have more to do with the reduction of inflammation than with the reduction of cholesterol. In fact, studies repeatedly show that the majority of those taking cholesterol-reducing drugs fail to achieve cholesterol readings in the target range.

Not only are the benefits arguable, but cholesterol drugs also come with a substantial risk of side effects, including disruption of sleep, muscle aches, nausea, headaches, heartburn, and mood changes. The drugs dangerously deplete the body of its reserves of CoQ_{10}, an antioxidant with specific heart-protective benefits, and occasionally cause severe liver damage. With the availability of natural therapies that can balance cholesterol levels, the many risks that accompany these drugs are usually not justified.

Later in this chapter, we will discuss natural therapies for cholesterol reduction. But in terms of reducing your risk of disease, enhancing your methylation rate and thus lowering the level of homocysteine in your blood is far more important. Unfortunately, no one is funding a multimillion-dollar advertising campaign to bring this to your attention.

HOW WELL ARE YOU METHYLATING?

As we saw above, the level of homocysteine in the blood is a useful indicator of how well the body is methylating. When homocysteine levels are low, we can be reasonably sure that the methylation cycle is working well. When homocysteine is high, it signals that methylation is impaired, and the risk of disease is elevated.

With the increasing recognition of McCully's work, homocysteine testing is becoming more common. However, once again, there is a big discrepancy between the level of homocysteine considered to be "normal" and the amount that can be considered ideal. After all, heart disease is so common among Americans that it approaches the statistical norm for those over 50.

According to a recent survey, the average homocysteine level among Americans is 10 mcmol/L (micromoles per liter), squarely in the accepted "normal" range of 5 to 15 mcmol. But the American Heart Association's own research shows that your risk of heart disease begins to increase as soon as your homocysteine levels climb above 6.3 mcmol/L.

The average American, with a "normal" homocysteine level of 10

Risk of Coronary Artery Disease

Blood homocysteine (mcmol/L)	Risk Level
6.3 or lower	No increased risk
10	2 times more likely
15	4 times more likely
20	8 times more likely
25	12 times more likely

mcmol/L is in fact at twice the risk of heart disease as someone with a homocysteine level of 6.3 mcmol/L or lower. By the time a patient's homocysteine levels reach 15 mcmol/L, enough to be considered "elevated," he or she is already at four times the risk. And, of course, elevated homocysteine increases your risk not only of heart disease but of many other conditions as well.

Given that enhancing methylation is simple and inexpensive, there is no reason to accept any level of risk. If your homocysteine level is even slightly elevated, you can take steps to bring it down with the nutritional therapies described below. If you have had your homocysteine tested and been told that your level was "fine," you may want to ask for the actual reading, to ensure that you are not at risk because of some laboratory's idea of "normal."

Enhancing Methylation and Reducing Homocysteine

If your diet includes meat, you most likely have a plentiful supply of methionine as a methyl donor. However, many Americans are deficient in the nutrients that act as methylating factors. As you will recall, these include vitamin B_{12} and folic acid.

Processed foods, which are a dietary mainstay, are notoriously low in B vitamins, especially B_6 and folic acid. Excessive intake of fats and sugars also depletes our stores of these nutrients. And with increasing age, vitamin B_{12} deficiency often becomes a problem due to decreased absorption of nutrients during digestion.

Research shows that high homocysteine levels are almost always correlated with low blood levels of vitamin B_{12}, folic acid, and vitamin B_6. (Strictly speaking, vitamin B_6 is not a methylating factor. It helps remove homocysteine from the blood by a different mechanism, by converting it into the harmless amino acid cysteine and ultimately into the valuable antioxidant glutathione.)

Supplementation with these three nutrients is usually effective in keeping homocysteine levels out of the extreme risk category. But to ensure that homocysteine is kept at the safer, lower threshold, I also recommend the addition of another methyl donor, trimethylglycine, to further lower homocysteine levels.

Trimethylglycine (TMG) is a methyl donor that helps to remethylate homocysteine back into methionine. The *tri-* refers to the fact that TMG carries three methyl groups, making it a very potent methyl donor. A starting dosage for TMG (which is also called betaine) is 750mg.

The Importance of Testing Your Blood

As noted above, homocysteine levels among the general American population average 10 mcmol/L. By comparison, the Life Extension Foundation conducted a survey of LEF members who had had their blood tested for homocysteine. Foundation members, who are typically quite aggressive about nutritional supplementation, scored significantly better than the American average, with 90 percent of those tested having homocysteine levels below 10 mcmol/L.

However, the survey results contained a significant surprise. While LEF members had homocysteine levels that were significantly lower than the average population, almost two-thirds of the members (62 per-

Basic Pro-methylation Protocol

Folic acid	800–1,600 mcg
Vitamin B$_6$	100 mg
Vitamin B$_{12}$	500–1,000 mcg
TMG	750 mg

cent) still had levels above 6.3 mcmol/L. The fact that so many LEF members were still at an increased risk of disease due to elevated homocysteine, despite a much higher than normal intake of nutrients, underscores the critical importance of blood testing for homocysteine.

Individual needs for methylating nutrients can vary greatly. Certain lifestyle factors, such as a high intake of meat, excessive coffee drinking, or smoking, can elevate homocysteine levels and increase the need for methylating nutrients (especially folic acid and vitamin B$_6$). Some people require higher levels of methylating nutrients because of disease conditions or genetic factors that impair methylation.

Ensuring adequate methylation is far too important to leave to chance. For many people, the basic methylation protocol is effective in reducing homocysteine to desirable levels. But for a significant number, it is not enough. Testing allows you to adjust your intake of nutrients to reflect your body's needs.

Victor, a longtime LEF member, was well aware of the importance of taking nutritional supplements, including pro-methylation nutrients. His regimen included 500 mg of TMG and 4,000 mcg of folic acid, along with other nutrients. But a homocysteine blood check showed that Victor's homocysteine remained above 11 mcmol/L, placing him at significantly increased risk.

Working with an anti-aging medical specialist through the Life Extension Foundation, Victor increased his TMG to a total of 6,000 mg and added additional vitamin B$_6$ to his nutrient program. Another blood test two months later showed a homocysteine level of less than 6 mcmol/L.

Advanced Methylation Protocol

If after implementing the basic pro-methylation protocol your homocysteine levels remain high, an anti-aging physician can work with you to tailor your regimen. Nutrient amounts can be increased, under a doctor's supervision, until homocysteine is at a safe level.

Jeff, a 60-year-old LEF member with a history of heart disease, had been taking methylating factors, including vitamins B_6 and B_{12} and a high dose of folic acid. Despite this regimen, Jeff continued to suffer from symptoms of heart disease, including angina. When his blood was tested for homocysteine, his doctor was surprised to see that Jeff's homocysteine levels were an extremely high 18 mcmol/L. Obviously, Jeff is someone whose individual need for methylating nutrients is very high. Jeff's doctor added 6,000 mg of TMG to his regimen and retested his blood after four weeks. After just one month, Jeff's homocysteine levels had fallen to 4 mcmol/L.

Other people may need additional nutrients such as choline or SAM-e in order to get the desired response. It can also be a matter of finding the nutrients that are most effective for you. Some people, for example, lack the enzyme that converts vitamin B_6 into its biologically active form. If you lack this enzyme, you may find that your homocysteine levels remain stubbornly high, despite taking the recommended amount of vitamin B_6. In this case, a more biologically active form of B_6, called pyridoxal-5-phosphate (P5P), can help. (If you are getting good results with the standard form of B_6, there is no reason to use the more expensive P5P form.)

ADVANCED PRO-METHYLATION PROTOCOL

A supervised, advanced protocol might include any combination of the following:

> TMG, up to 6,000 mg
> Folic acid, up to 10 mg (10,000 mcg)
> Vitamin B$_{12}$, up to 5,000 mcg
> Vitamin B$_6$, up to 250 mg
> SAM-e, up to 800 mg
> Choline, up to 5,000 mcg
> Pyridoxal-5-phosphate (P5P), up to 50 mg

Unlike many of the challenges we face with aging and disease prevention, enhancing methylation and lowering homocysteine is fairly easy to do. But it cannot be taken for granted that a one-size-fits-all regimen will do the trick. As these examples demonstrate, testing is the only way to ensure that you have found the regimen that works for you. Once you and your doctor have arrived at an effective formula, I recommend that you have your homocysteine levels retested annually.

DOES CHOLESTEROL EVEN MATTER?

Once you have taken steps to reduce homocysteine and enhance methylation, do you even need to worry about cholesterol levels? While the correlation between high cholesterol and heart disease is not as strong as we once thought, I won't go so far as to say that cholesterol doesn't matter at all. Very high (or very low) cholesterol is an indication that the body is out of balance. A holistic approach to health seeks to bring every part of the body's chemistry, including cholesterol levels, into optimal balance.

Many people have come to believe that the less cholesterol in your blood, the better off you are. But, in fact, cholesterol is an important and necessary substance. It is the basic material used for the synthesis of all the steroid hormones, including DHEA and testosterone. (The term *steroid* is, in fact, derived from chole*sterol*.) Cholesterol provides lipids needed to build healthy cell membranes. It also helps the body produce bile, which is needed for proper digestion of fats.

Cholesterol is not the enemy. You need a healthy amount of cholesterol in your body in order to function well and be healthy. Very low cholesterol levels can actually *increase* your risk of cancer, stroke, respiratory and digestive diseases. So with cholesterol, as with everything else, optimal health is a question of balance.

An ideal range for total cholesterol is between 160 and 180 mg/dL. If you are taking measures to lower cholesterol (whether pharmaceutical or the nutrient protocols outlined below), and you find that your cholesterol has dipped below 140 mg/dL, it may be a sign that you are overdoing it. I recommend that you discuss with your doctor whether to reduce your dosage slightly, allowing cholesterol levels to recover into the ideal range.

But balancing cholesterol is not just about lowering total cholesterol. Your body produces several different types of cholesterol, each with different functions. High-density lipoprotein (HDL) is often referred to as "good" cholesterol. Low-density lipoprotein (LDL) is sometimes referred to as "bad" cholesterol, because this is the type of cholesterol that tends to accumulate in blood vessels of those with heart disease.

The low-density form of cholesterol is also more prone to oxidation by free radicals, making it much more damaging and dangerous to blood vessel walls. Research shows that oxidized cholesterol (especially LDL) is a more potent risk for heart disease than cholesterol in general.

Balancing cholesterol profiles involves bringing all of these factors into optimal ranges and ratios with each other. The following chart shows ideal values for different blood lipids as well as some of the ratios that I have developed to evaluate the balance of various elements. (Please see Chapter 10 for additional lipid tests.) To calculate a ratio, the first value is divided by the second. For example, if your LDL is 100 and your HDL is 50, then your LDL/HDL ratio is $100 \div 50 = 2$.

Blood Lipid Values		
	Normal reference ranges	*Optimal ranges*
Total cholesterol	100–199 mg/dL	160–180 mg/dL
HDL	35–150 mg/dL	50–120 mg/dL
LDL	0–129 mg/dL	80–100 mg/dL
Total/HDL ratio		3–4 (men) 2–3 (women)
LDL/HDL ratio		Less than 2

Balancing Your Cholesterol Without Drugs

In my experience, I have found that cholesterol can usually be balanced without the use of prescription medications. High-dose niacin (vitamin B_3) is usually a safe and effective therapy to reduce elevated cholesterol and triglycerides. The effective dosages can range from 500 mg to as high as 6,000 mg per day. In some people, these doses of niacin can produce a flushing of the skin, sometimes accompanied by an itching sensation. The so-called niacin flush is caused by the dilation of small blood vessels and is completely harmless and temporary, although some find it uncomfortable.

Niacin can be taken as niacinamide, which does not cause the typical niacin flush, but I have found that the niacinamide form is not as effective. I do not recommend long-acting forms of niacin because of an increased risk of liver damage. I prefer an intermediate-acting form of the nutrient, sold as Niaspan.

In order to minimize any discomfort from the flush, I recommend taking niacin at bedtime. Most people sleep right through any reaction that occurs. There are those, however, who find that the rush of blood and increased skin sensations from high-dose niacin provide a temporary enhancement of sexual response, and time their doses accordingly.

Niacin is metabolized through methylation and can increase the body's requirements for methylating nutrients. As a result, high-dose niacin therapy can increase homocysteine levels. When using high-dose niacin, it's important for your doctor to monitor your homocysteine levels as well as cholesterol levels and adjust your pro-methylation regimen accordingly.

Another important heart health nutrient is vitamin E, which has been found to reduce heart attacks by 77 percent in patients with heart disease. Vitamin E protects the heart in a number of ways. It helps to improve the flowing quality (rheology) of the blood, making it less sticky and less prone to clotting. Vitamin E also helps to prevent the oxidation of cholesterol in the blood vessels, which is critical to the prevention of heart disease.

Most vitamin E supplements contain a form of the vitamin known as alpha-tocopherol. However, there are a number of forms of this vitamin, including various other tocopherols, as well as the tocotrienol forms.

The tocotrienol forms of vitamin E, although much less commonly used, are actually far more active. They are more powerful antioxidants, being up to sixty times more potent in protecting against free radical damage. Tocotrienols also display a remarkable ability to lower both total and LDL cholesterol levels. This cholesterol-lowering benefit is not found with alpha-tocopherol (or any other tocopherol form). The effective dosage of tocotrienols to reduce cholesterol is 50 to 100 mg per day.

Cholesterol-Lowering Nutrients	
Niacin	500–2,000 mg (at bedtime, or divided into two doses at morning and nighttime)
Vitamin E (as tocotrienols)	50–100 mg

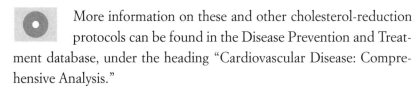

More information on these and other cholesterol-reduction protocols can be found in the Disease Prevention and Treatment database, under the heading "Cardiovascular Disease: Comprehensive Analysis."

KEEPING TRACK OF THE BIG PICTURE

In the last several chapters, we've been zeroing in on individual mechanisms (oxidative stress, inflammation, and undermethylation) that can lead to premature aging and disease. In each case, we've seen examples of individuals who have identified and reduced a particular risk factor.

But it's important to remember that in the highly complex human organism, nothing goes wrong—or is fixed—in a vacuum. In real life, of course, almost all of us will have some combination of overlapping factors that must be addressed. And the therapies we have discussed, when integrated into a comprehensive program, also work together synergistically in ways that cannot be reduced to simple equations.

My patient Ben, for example, had multiple risk factors when we began working together on his anti-aging program. As we saw in Chapter 7, Ben's biomarkers for inflammation (C-reactive protein and fibrinogen) were quite elevated but responded well to a program of anti-inflammatory nutrients. At the same time, however, his initial blood work also revealed high homocysteine levels as well as very high cholesterol levels.

Ben's previous heart attack was not surprising considering these many indications that his body was not functioning well on a cellular level. A previous doctor had prescribed cholesterol-lowering medications but had not addressed the homocysteine or inflammation issues. After a short time, Ben had discontinued the cholesterol drugs, preferring to find a nonpharmaceutical solution. Although I agreed with his decision not to use the drugs, we clearly needed to take aggressive steps to lower Ben's risk of future heart attack or stroke.

In addition to the inflammation-reducing protocol outlined in Chapter 7, Ben's nutritional regimen included extra vitamin B_{12} and folic acid to support methylation. His homocysteine levels began to drop in response, but Ben is an example of someone whose biochemistry is such that he requires more intensive nutritional support to keep his homocysteine at safe levels. With continued blood testing, we gradually increased the amounts of methylating nutrients until we found the regimen that worked for him

At the same time, I prescribed a regimen of high-dose niacin to bring down his cholesterol, along with a broad spectrum of antioxidants, including vitamin E and coenzyme Q_{10}, to prevent oxidation of cholesterol. All of this was in the context of a comprehensive and doctor-supervised program of hormonal support, vitamins, minerals, and other nutrients, similar to the program outlined for you in Chapter 11. Ben also made meaningful changes in his eating habits, his lifestyle, and even his psychological approach to life. All of these are discussed in Chapter 12.

As we tracked his progress with lab work over the next eight months, Ben's biomarkers for aging and disease improved dramatically. The following chart shows the improvement in his cholesterol levels.

Progression of Treatment: Ben			
Lipids	*Baseline*	*After 3 months*	*After 8 months*
Total cholesterol	312 (very high)	223 (high)	180 (ideal)
HDL	45 (fair)	40 (fair)	39 (fair)
LDL	231 (very high)	152 (high)	116 (fair)
VLDL	36 (high)	33 (borderline)	18 (ideal)
Triglycerides	182 (very high)	164 (high)	89 (ideal)

Ben didn't need to see the lab work to know that the program was working. As his body began to function more youthfully, he felt better and better. As he became healthier, his quality of life, both personally and professionally, soared.

Ben (and his doctors) had been focused for years on his cholesterol readings. But, as he learned, health, or the lack of it, is the cumulative result of many, many factors. Accordingly, your Anti-Aging Program will be an integrated and comprehensive program that supports the body from every possible angle.

CHAPTER 9

Preventing Glycation: Age-Proofing Your Organs

Old age is not for sissies.
—BETTE DAVIS

I N THE NEXT PART of this book, we are going to begin putting together your individualized anti-aging program, which will include medical testing to identify your risk factors, a customized nutritional supplement program, as well as some diet and lifestyle changes. In Chapter 12, when we discuss the ideal anti-aging diet, you will see that the first step is to reduce the amount of sugar and refined carbohydrates in your diet. A high-sugar diet (such as the typical American diet) can profoundly accelerate aging, in large part because it fuels a biochemical process called glycation.

Glycation is a chemical reaction in which molecules of sugar and protein get tangled up, resulting in deformed and nonfunctioning molecules. Glycated proteins then have a tendency to fuse together, a process known as cross-linking. As more and more cross-linking occurs, the tissues of the body become increasingly stiff and tough. Organs such as the heart, eyes, and skin, which must be flexible in order to function well, are particularly vulnerable to glycation damage as you get older.

The damage caused by glycation is irreversible. Just as an egg which has been hard-boiled can never be returned to its original state, once proteins in your body have been glycated, there is no way to repair them. Instead, glycated proteins begin to produce cellular toxins called advanced glycation end products, or AGEs. These toxic compounds bind to receptors in the surface of the cells, where they generate huge numbers of free radicals and promote inflammation.

Glycation is now known to be a primary factor in the development of many age-related diseases, including atherosclerosis, heart failure, Alzheimer's disease, complications of diabetes, cataract formation, and premature aging of the skin. Therefore, preventing glycation is a key aspect of my disease prevention program.

DIABETES-RELATED DAMAGE IS LARGELY DUE TO GLYCATION

The incidence of diabetes in this country is steadily increasing, driven in large part by our growing obesity problem. Millions of overweight Americans are already in the preliminary stages of developing diabetes, without even knowing it. Within ten years, today's obesity epidemic is likely to explode into a new and even more serious epidemic of newly diagnosed diabetes.

ARE YOU AT RISK FOR DIABETES?

Being overweight increases your risk for developing adult-onset (type 2) diabetes. But even if your weight is ideal, you could still be at risk or could even be in the early stages of diabetes without realizing it. With my patients, I routinely test fasting blood sugar levels to screen for diabetes risk. A fasting blood sugar level above 100 mg/dL suggests a predisposition toward diabetes that needs to be carefully monitored by your physician. Levels of more than 125 mg/dL indicate diabetes. (See also Chapter 10.)

I commonly see borderline readings (100–125 mg/dL) in new patients. These levels typically come down into acceptable ranges within a few months of implementing the anti-aging program. If you learn that you have slightly elevated fasting blood sugar (over 100 mg/dL) or are otherwise at risk of developing diabetes, the diet and exercise program outlined in Chapter 12 can help to reverse this trend.

At its most superficial level, diabetes is the body's inability to adequately control its blood sugar levels. Therefore, diabetics must carefully monitor and manage their blood sugar with strict dietary control and, sometimes, medication. It can be terribly inconvenient and unpleasant to live with diabetes. The real tragedy of diabetes, though, is in the serious, long-term complications of the disease, which commonly include heart and circulatory disease, kidney failure, and cataracts. Even for those who are careful to control their blood sugar levels, diabetes leads to a reduced life expectancy because of the greater incidence of heart disease and other complications.

In many ways, the progression of diabetes is actually a picture of accelerated aging. And in both diabetes and aging, glycation is responsible for much of the damage to the organs. Remember that glycation is fueled by the sugar in your blood. Because diabetics often have high blood sugar levels, their organs suffer more glycation-related damage at an earlier age.

Therapies that prevent or slow glycation should allow diabetics to live longer and healthier lives. In fact, diabetic mice that are given antiglycation therapies live longer. And in diabetic humans, antiglycation therapies have improved cholesterol profiles and reduced the formation of artery-hardening plaques. But glycation is a problem for everyone— not just diabetics. Finding ways to slow glycation will help us slow the aging process in nondiabetics as well.

LIMITING SUGAR CONSUMPTION
CAN SLOW GLYCATION

The typical Western diet is extremely high in sugar and other refined carbohydrates. This overconsumption of sugar promotes glycation like pouring gasoline on a fire, directly contributing to the modern epidemics of obesity, heart disease, and adult-onset (type 2) diabetes.

Glycation can never be completely prevented. But limiting your intake of sugary foods (including fruit juices and all sweetened beverages) and refined carbohydrates (including white flour, white rice, and pasta) can slow glycation and the formation of AGEs. We'll be discussing this at length in Chapter 12. In addition, there are a few natural and pharmaceutical compounds that can play an important role in slowing glycation and AGE formation.

NATURE'S ANTIGLYCATION THERAPY

Carnosine is a naturally occurring nutrient that appears to protect the body's proteins from glycation much the way antioxidants protect cells from free radicals. That is, carnosine offers itself as a target. Carnosine is very similar in structure to the proteins that are targeted by glucose for glycation. When glucose binds instead to carnosine, the other proteins are spared.

Carnosine also binds to previously glycated proteins that have accumulated in the tissues. These are then more easily broken down and disposed of by the body, sparing the body from further damage and cross-linking. This helps to keep the body's tissues and organs supple and youthful. Because of its ability to prevent glycation and the formation of AGEs, carnosine may be one of the most potent anti-aging compounds available today.

We get carnosine naturally from our diet, providing that we consume at least some meat protein. (Carnosine gets its name from the Latin word *carne,* meaning "meat.") Our bodies store carnosine in places where proteins are susceptible to glycation. It is found in particularly high levels in the muscle tissues and in the brain. But carnosine levels gradually drop with age. By age 70, the amount of carnosine in the muscle tissue may be less than 40 percent of youthful levels. This leaves our bodies more and more vulnerable to tissue and organ damage from glycation and AGEs.

Evidence for Anti-Aging Effects

Because we know that carnosine protects proteins from glycation, we would expect to see that carnosine would provide protection against glycation-related conditions. Indeed, in just the last few years, laboratory research has found that:

> Carnosine protects proteins in the eye against glycation and has been successful in treating and preventing cataracts in dogs and rabbits. Eye drops containing carnosine were highly effective in treating and preventing cataracts and vision loss in elderly humans.

> Carnosine has also been shown to protect the tiny blood vessels in the brain from damage that can lead to Alzheimer's disease and helps to protect the brain from the toxic effects of certain metals, particularly copper and zinc.

> Carnosine relaxes and dilates the blood vessels leading to the heart, increasing blood flow to the heart. It also enhances the heart's ability to contract and pump blood, offering protection against a common cause of fatal heart failure.

> Carnosine helps to prevent skin aging and wrinkles by inhibiting the cross-linking of collagen in the skin, preserving its elasticity. It has also been shown to speed the healing of wounds by promoting more youthful cell division.

➢ In addition to being a hedge against glycation, carnosine is also a potent antioxidant, particularly active against one of the most destructive types of free radicals, the hydroxyl (hydrogen-based) radical. Carnosine's antioxidant properties are particularly valuable in protecting delicate brain tissues from oxidative damage.

All of this evidence supports the theory that by preventing glycation we can delay the aging process and the progression of a multitude of age-related diseases. While there appear to be many natural substances that can protect against oxidation and prevent inflammation, carnosine is one of only a few substances known to protect against glycation.

Rejuvenating Aging Cells

Beyond its beneficial effects on specific systems of the body and various disease conditions, carnosine has displayed a tantalizing potential to rejuvenate aging cells and extend the life span of both aging cells and of aging animals.

Many of the cells in our body replace themselves by dividing periodically, creating new "daughter" cells. But each of these cells has a genetically programmed limit on how many times it can divide. Tissue culture studies show that normal cells stop reproducing after creating a certain number of generations.

As a cell gets close to the end of its reproductive life, it is said to be entering senescence, or old age. The function of a cell changes according to where it is in its life span. Older cells tend to be less active. They may be less vigilant in their defensive response to intruders or lazy in their production of hormones or enzymes. These cellular changes translate into some of the changes we associate with aging. As more and more of our dividing cells enter their senescence, we too may experience the symptoms of senescence, or old age.

Scientists have found that carnosine can rejuvenate aging cells in tissue cultures, restoring their appearance and function to that of more youthful cells. Elderly cells that were rejuvenated by carnosine lived an amazing three times longer than cells without carnosine. Some of the cells even experienced an enhanced ability to reproduce.

Interestingly, when the rejuvenated cells were removed from the carnosine-rich environment, they quickly assumed the appearance and behavior of aging cells. When they were given carnosine again, they were again rejuvenated. The implications for health and longevity are profound. When individual cells are rejuvenated in their function and behavior, it will have a rejuvenating effect on the entire organism.

Evidence for Life Extension

Carnosine appears to be linked to longevity in animals. In fact, the level of carnosine normally present in the muscle tissue of any given species is directly linked to the normal life span of that species. In other words, animals that have more carnosine in their muscles live longer than animals that have lower carnosine concentrations.

Researchers fed carnosine to mice that are specially bred to have a very short life span. These particular mice are considered old if they live to be 12 months old. In this experiment, the mice that were given carnosine were almost twice as likely to reach old age than the mice who did not receive carnosine. On average, the treated mice lived about 20 percent longer than the untreated mice (although none of the mice lived longer than the maximum life span for that breed, about 15 months). Moreover, the mice receiving carnosine remained more youthful-looking, with fuller, glossier coats and fewer skin problems. Carnosine also protected the mice against age-related changes in their brain biochemistry.

Realizing the Potential

Could carnosine offer the same anti-aging and life extension benefits to humans as it did to these mice? To date, there have been only limited human trials exploring the benefits of carnosine. There is no question that it is safe and nontoxic for humans, but we do not yet know its full potential to prevent disease and extend life span.

In order to prove the long-term efficacy of a substance such as carnosine on human beings, a study has to continue for decades and evaluate dozens of different aspects of health and aging. These types of studies are exceptionally expensive to conduct. As a natural substance, carnosine is not attractive to pharmaceutical research companies that seek to maximize their profits by developing patentable drugs. Carnosine has so far also failed to attract the attention of government-funded researchers.

There is no doubt, however, that preventing glycation is a critical step toward slowing down some of the physical changes that accompany normal aging and lead to disease. All the available evidence indicates that carnosine has the ability to powerfully inhibit glycation-related conditions and is exceptionally safe and nontoxic. As such, the Life Extension Foundation strongly recommends its use as part of a comprehensive anti-aging and disease prevention program.

The future may one day bring even better antiglycation agents (see below). For now, the accumulating evidence for carnosine makes it prudent to include it in our program.

Using Carnosine Effectively

Carnosine is a naturally occurring amino acid peptide found in meat. Unless you are a strict vegetarian, you consume some carnosine in your diet. Your body produces a special enzyme called carnosinase, which is specifically designed to break down carnosine. Much of the carnosine you take in through your diet is digested by carnosinase and broken down into amino acids, which can then be used as building blocks for other proteins as needed.

In order to protect your tissues and organs from glycation, you must raise the levels of free carnosine circulating in your bloodstream. To accomplish this, you need to consume enough carnosine that it cannot all be broken down by the available carnosinase enzyme. This allows some of the carnosine to enter the bloodstream intact.

An effective dosage of carnosine is 1,000 mg per day. By way of comparison, this is about the amount that you would obtain from eating 2 pounds of cooked ground beef. That's a lot of beef. Besides being impractical, a diet containing this much meat protein on a daily basis would be dangerously unbalanced. As we saw in Chapter 8, meat provides large amounts of the amino acid methionine, which can raise homocysteine levels. And as we will see in Chapter 11, a healthy anti-aging diet must contain a wide range of foods to maximize the benefits of food-based anti-aging nutrients.

Taking carnosine as a dietary supplement ensures a constant and sufficient amount of carnosine without the risks that accompany excessive consumption of meat. No toxicity has ever been observed with carnosine, even at dosages equivalent to thirty times the recommended dose. Carnosine has a relatively short half-life in the body, dissipating after several hours. Ideally, carnosine should be taken in divided doses, 500 mg in the morning and 500 mg in the evening, to provide more even protection.

ANTIGLYCATION DRUG THERAPIES

There are currently a handful of antiglycation drugs in development, and one drug that has been on the market in Europe for several years.

Aminoguanidine (brand name: Pimagidine) is an anti-aging drug that inhibits glycation by stabilizing glucose in the blood and preventing the binding of glucose to proteins. Animal studies show that aminoguanidine prevents enlargement of the heart in older animals and prevents stiffening of the arterial walls. Its effects on blood cholesterol and coagulation were also positive, reducing the binding of LDL cholesterol to the arterial walls and inhibiting the formation of blood clots.

One very interesting study at the University of Milan, done about twelve years ago, tested aminoguanidine on a small cadre of patients who were suffering from arterial blockages. These patients were so disabled by their condition that they were unable to walk even once around a quarter-mile track. After taking aminoguanidine, the patients had much better blood flow and were able to increase their walking distance by 50 percent. Some were able to more than double their exercise capacity.

Approved for use in Europe, aminoguanidine can be imported into the United States for personal use. (See "Offshore Drugs" in Chapter 5.) While it has not yet been approved by the FDA, it is currently being studied in clinical trials at the University of Washington. The trials focus on its ability to prevent complications from diabetes, particularly damage to the eye.

There is little evidence that aminoguanidine is more effective than carnosine. In fact, its side effect profile, while mild, is not as good as carnosine, which has virtually no side effects. Considering the expense and inconvenience of acquiring offshore drugs, there doesn't appear to be a compelling argument for the use of animoguanidine when carnosine is readily available, is better tolerated, and appears to be equally effective.

Alagebrium (formerly known as ALT 7111) is a newer drug under development by Alteon, the same company that developed aminoguanidine. Unlike aminoguanidine and carnosine, both of which *prevent* glycation and AGE formation, alagebrium attempts to *reverse* the damaging effects caused by AGEs by dissolving the bonds that hold AGEs together. If proven effective, this would obviously be a major anti-aging breakthrough.

Playing by the FDA'S Rules

In order to have a drug approved by the FDA, a company must first show that the drug is safe, with an acceptable risk and side effect profile. (Ironically, as we have discussed previously, there is a double standard applied to alternative and nutritional therapies. Nutritional supplements have been banned or restricted based on risks or side effects far milder than those of many approved pharmaceutical drugs.)

Once a drug is shown to be safe, it must then prove to be effective against some condition or illness. Alagebrium is clearly intended to be a multipurpose anti-aging therapy, but for reasons discussed above, it could take years of study and millions of dollars to prove this benefit.

Once a drug has been approved for any purpose, however, it can be prescribed by doctors for any condition as an off-label usage. Drug companies such as Alteon are sometimes forced to play a bit of a game in order to get their drugs approved. They design trials that they hope will quickly demonstrate some aspect of efficacy, even if it is not the main therapeutic intent of the drug. In this way, they can get the drug to market sooner, funding further research.

Alteon is currently involved in a number of clinical trials in an effort to win FDA approval. Studies are under way that researchers hope will demonstrate whether alagebrium can reduce blood pressure and/or reduce enlargement of the heart in older subjects, either with or without diabetes. This narrow look at one aspect of glycation may or may not give a good indication of the true value and benefit of the drug as it is intended to be used. But if the trial can demonstrate an effect that the FDA finds medically worthy, the drug can be made publicly available.

So far, alagebrium has proven to be extremely safe and well tolerated, with a minimum of side effects. However, the company has not yet been able to show compelling improvements in the conditions they have chosen to study. The short-term reductions in blood pressure have been minimal, and the studies have been too short to measure long-term effects.

All of this is a frustration to many in the anti-aging community who are anxious to have access to a substance that not only can prevent glycation-related damage but also may actually be able to reverse this damage, something that no other therapy has yet been able to do. I believe that research will ultimately produce more compounds to fight glycation and AGEs. For now, carnosine offers an excellent tool against this dangerous threat.

BEATING DISEASE AT THE CELLULAR LEVEL

In the last few chapters, we have discussed four key processes that lie at the heart of aging and most age-related diseases. Long before the first symptoms of disease are present, these silent cellular mechanisms can undermine the body's function and erode your health. By taking steps now to prevent oxidation, reduce inflammation, enhance methylation, and prevent glycation, you can improve your chances of living a long and healthy life.

In the next chapters, we will begin to integrate and implement all the anti-aging and disease prevention therapies we have explored up until this point, with a complete program of supplements, dietary recommendations, and lifestyle habits that will help you grow old without aging.

PART III

INDIVIDUALIZING YOUR ANTI-AGING PROGRAM

This is where the science gets personal. The following three chapters will show you how to develop and implement your own customized anti-aging and disease prevention program.

The program incorporates all of the therapies discussed in previous chapters, and more. Testing protocols and supplement regimens are outlined in detail, along with the essential components of the anti-aging lifestyle.

This personalized anti-aging program is your passport to a long and vibrantly healthy life.

CHAPTER 10

Medical Testing for Aging and Risk Factors

To be seventy years young is sometimes far more hopeful than to be forty years old.
—OLIVER WENDELL HOLMES

MEDICAL TESTING WILL BE an integral part of your successful anti-aging program. With nothing more invasive than a needle prick, we can gather an enormous amount of information that will make your program more effective.

Testing allows us to assess your aging status and identify risk factors for disease, customize your protocols, and monitor your ongoing progress and the effectiveness of your program. To implement an anti-aging program without benefit of this information is like driving with a blindfold on. If the road is perfectly straight and the car perfectly aligned, it might be possible to stay on the road and reach your destination. But you have a much better chance of getting there safely if you can see where you are going.

In this chapter, I will show you how all of the tests discussed in the previous chapters are best used to guide your anti-aging program. The testing protocols below are organized into three categories: hormone profiles, testing for reversible risk factors, and blood chemistry. For each category, I'll outline which tests should be included and what the target ranges are for each. Following the protocols are guidelines on when best to schedule your testing.

UNDERSTANDING YOUR TEST RESULTS

Your anti-aging physician will interpret your test results and determine what action needs to be taken based on this information. But in order to be an informed and active participant in your anti-aging program, you also need to understand the significance of your test results. A few words about medical testing in general will help to provide a context for the specific recommendations that follow.

The most important thing to understand about medical testing is the significance of the *reference range.* Your test results will be compared to a reference range indicating which values are considered to be "normal." The lab bases these reference ranges on the results of all the blood samples that particular lab has tested. The "normal" part of the range reflects the test results of healthy subjects. By healthy, they mean anyone who did not have a clinical diagnosis of a disease at the time of the test.

Health Is Not Simply the Absence of Disease

Our medical culture has become overly focused on diagnosing and treating *disease,* rather than promoting and preserving *health.* As a result, you are considered to be healthy right up until the point at which you are diagnosed with a disease. Of course, as we saw in Part II, full-blown disease is usually the last chapter of a very long story. Hormonal imbalances such as elevated cortisol may be observed years or decades before heart disease or osteoporosis is diagnosed. Protecting against inflammation while in your 30s and 40s may help prevent Alzheimer's disease in your 60s and 70s.

Everyone understands that it is much easier to stop an automobile that is going 30 miles an hour than it is to stop one that is speeding along at 75. So why would we wait until major health problems have developed before taking action?

As I discussed in Chapter 4, for example, thyroid function tests (discussed below in "Testing Hormone Levels") are ordered fairly routinely by conventional doctors. But most endocrinologists do not recognize or treat thyroid problems unless the level of TSH (thyroid stimulating hormone) is either so low that it indicates hyperthyroidism or so high that it indicates hypothyroidism. In other words, you may have all the symptoms of low thyroid function—fatigue, weight gain, increased susceptibility to infection, low body temperatures, cold hands and feet—and you might feel absolutely terrible. But unless your thyroid dysfunction is extreme enough to meet the clinical definition of thyroid *disease,* a conventional physician will consider you to be "healthy."

Not only will you continue to suffer from symptoms that could be alleviated with thyroid hormone therapy, but research shows that your doctor's failure to react may have even graver consequences. TSH levels of over 4.0 (still well within the "normal" range) increase your risk of future heart disease. And even moderately increased levels of 2.0 to 4.0 increase your risk of future thyroid disease.

Testing for Thyroid Function

TSH (mU/L)	Conventional medicine	Anti-aging medicine
Over 5.5	Clinical hypothyroidism	Underactive thyroid
4.0–5.5	"Normal"	Low thyroid function
2.0–4.0	"Normal"	Low thyroid function
1.0–2.0	"Normal"	Optimal
0.2–0.9	"Normal"	Borderline overactive thyroid function
Less than 0.2	Clinical hyperthyroidism	Overactive thyroid

The way cortisol tests are interpreted provides another example of the same sort of thinking. If a conventional doctor tests your cortisol levels, he or she is probably checking for either Cushing's syndrome (massive overproduction of cortisol by the adrenal glands) or Addison's disease (adrenal failure). Both diseases are relatively rare.

Once again, the standard reference ranges for cortisol levels reflect the disease-oriented bias of our medical system. As long as you are not suffering from Addison's disease or Cushing's syndrome, your tests results will indicate normal adrenal function—and most doctors will therefore take no action. But, as we have seen over and over again, there is a vital difference between *normal* and *optimal.*

As discussed in Chapter 2, even slightly elevated cortisol levels can promote heart disease, obesity, and diabetes and harm brain function. Normal adrenal function is not good enough for me. Unless your adrenal function is optimal, you are at increased risk of disease, not to mention the fact that you are aging more quickly than you need to.

Testing for Adrenal Function

Cortisol (mcg/dL)	Conventional medicine	Anti-aging medicine
Over 29	Cushing's syndrome	Cushing's syndrome
24–29	"Normal"	Accelerated aging
19–24	"Normal"	Accelerated aging
14–19	"Normal"	Accelerated aging
9–14	"Normal"	Optimal
5–9	"Normal"	Risk of adrenal exhaustion
0–5	Addison's disease	Addison's disease

Aging Is Normal, Anti-Aging Is Optimal

There's another problem with the reference ranges. The levels of anti-aging hormones such as DHEA, testosterone, and growth hormone decline markedly as we age. This is normal—in the sense that it happens to most people. However, it is also normal to lose muscle mass and gain fat as we go through middle age. It is common to feel increasing fatigue or become forgetful as we get older. It is common to see lowered immune response and weakened heart function in older people. In other words, *aging is normal.* But that doesn't mean it is desirable.

Anti-aging medicine offers another option. We do not have to live with the consequences of declining hormone levels. Instead, we can use hormone replacement to preserve optimal hormone levels. By restoring your DHEA levels to more youthful levels, for example, you can protect against bone loss and skin aging, reduce body fat, enhance sexual function, and boost immune function. Because we have the option to intervene with replacement hormones, the distinction between normal and optimal values is very important.

Normal vs. Optimal DHEA Levels (mcg/dL)

Sex	Age	Normal	Optimal
Male	18–30	125–619	250–450
	31–50	59–452	
	51–60	20–413	
	61–83	10–285	
Female	19–30	29–781	150–350
	31–50	12–379	
	Postmenopause	30–260	

Redefining Our Notions of Health

I have very high standards. To me, healthy does not mean "with no obvious signs of disease or illness" or "in pretty good shape for your age." To me, healthy means that your organs are operating at peak function and your immune system is strong and resilient—no matter what your age. From what I see, the "normal" person is really not very healthy at all.

The goal of this program is for you to enjoy *vibrant* good health throughout a long lifetime. That means that most of the standard reference ranges must be discarded in favor of optimal ranges. Please remember that the guidelines that follow cannot replace the input of a qualified anti-aging practitioner. Even the optimal values given here will not be right for every individual.

My repeated emphasis on the importance of working with a qualified physician is not meant to discourage or disempower you—quite the opposite. I want you to get the best results from your anti-aging program. In order to do that, you need to work with a doctor who understands the difference between *normal* and *optimal* and is willing to take preemptive action against aging.

If you have not yet found a medical advisor who will support you in your anti-aging quest, the resources listed in the appendix can help you locate an anti-aging physician. Now, on to the specific testing recommendations.

I.
TESTING HORMONE LEVELS

As we saw in Part I, hormones serve as biomarkers of the aging process, giving us an idea of your biological age. Chronologically, you may be 45 years old. But if you have the hormone profile of a 60-year-old, your body is going to feel, act, and look much older than its years. The same, of course, is true in reverse. By testing your hormone levels, we can customize a hormone replacement program that will restore your hormones to optimal, youthful levels.

Your hormone testing should include the adrenal hormones (cortisol and DHEA), sex hormones (testosterone, estrogens, and progesterone), thyroid hormones, and IGF-1 (as a marker for growth hormone). These tests are discussed in detail in Chapters 2, 3, and 4. The table on page 241 summarizes the standard and optimal reference ranges for women, and the table on page 242 shows the ranges for men.

Female Hormone Profile

Hormone	Normal reference range	Optimal range
DHEA-S (Chapter 2)	30–700 mcg/dL	150–350 mcg/dL
Cortisol (Chapter 2)	5–29 mcg/dL	9–14 mcg/dL
Estrogen (Chapter 3)	30–480 pg/mL	180–200 pg/mL (women under 50)
		60–120 pg/mL (women over 50)
Progesterone (Chapter 3)	300–26,000 pg/mL	2,000–14,000 pg/mL (women under 50)
		2,000–8,000 pg/mL (women over 50)
Total Testosterone (Chapter 3)	140–760 pg/mL	120–900 pg/mL
TSH (Chapter 4)	0.2–5.5 mU/L	1.0–2.0 mU/L
Free T3 (Chapter 4)	2.60–4.80 pg/mL	2.80–3.20 pg/mL
Free T4 (Chapter 4)	0.70–1.53 ng/dL	1.2–1.4 ng/dL
IGF-1 (Chapter 4)	114–492 ng/mL	200–300 ng/mL

Comparing Apples to Apples

If your hormone levels are not optimal, hormone replacement protocols such as the ones described in Part I will be a critical part of your anti-aging program. But before you begin comparing your test results to the numbers given here, you must be sure that you are comparing apples to apples. The meaning of your blood test results depends entirely on the reference range *of the lab that performed your test.*

Imagine, for example, that you and I each made a cake using the same recipe. We each used one cup of cherries, but the cherries you used were very sweet, and the ones I used were quite tart. We each used

Male Hormone Profile

Hormone	Normal reference range	Optimal range
DHEA-S (Chapter 2)	20–620 mcg/dL	250-450 mcg/dL
Cortisol (Chapter 2)	5–29 mcg/dL	9–14 mcg/dL
Total estrogens (Chapter 3)	40–115 pg/mL	Less than 100 pg/mL
Estradiol (Chapter 3)	21-50 pg/mL	Less than 40 pg/mL
Progesterone (Chapter 3)	300–1,200 pg/mL	1,500–2,500 pg/mL
Total testosterone (Chapter 3)	2,700–9,700 pg/mL	6,000–9,000 pg/mL
TSH (Chapter 4)	0.2–5.5 mU/L	1.0–2.0 mU/L
Free T3 (Chapter 4)	2.60–4.80 pg/mL	2.90–3.20 pg/mL
Free T4 (Chapter 4)	0.70–1.53 ng/dL	1.2–1.4 ng/dL
IGF-1 (Chapter 4)	114–492 ng/mL	200–300 ng/mL

three cups of the same flour, but the flour I used had less moisture in it because the humidity in my house is lower. I mixed mine by hand, but you used an electric mixer. Although we both used the same recipe and measured carefully, our cakes will look and taste very different. (Yours will be sweeter, moister, and lighter than mine!)

It's somewhat similar with testing labs. Although they may be testing for the same compounds, they use different equipment, different methods, different solvents or preservatives. The atmospheric conditions in the lab are different. As a result, two labs could test the same blood samples and come up with completely different numbers. This is why each lab must provide reference ranges—to supply the context that will enable your doctor to interpret your results. Accordingly, the optimal ranges given here are not absolute but relative to the accompanying reference ranges.

If the reference ranges provided with your test results are very close to the reference ranges in the charts on pages 241 and 242, the optimal ranges given will give you a good idea how close your result is to the optimal zone. (Remember also to check to see that the unit of measurement corresponds exactly.)

UNITS OF MEASUREMENT USED IN LAB TESTS

dL	deciliter	1 tenth of a liter
Eq	equivalent	the amount of a substance needed to react with 1 mole of hydrogen ions
g	gram	1,000 milligrams
L	liter	1,000 milliliters
mcmol (or μmol)	micromole	1 millionth of a mole
mEq	milliequivalent	1 thousandth of an equivalent
mg	milligram	1 thousandth of a gram
mcg	microgram	1 thousandth of a milligram
mL (cc)	milliliter (cubic centimeter)	1 thousandth of a liter
mm^3	cubic millimeter	1 thousandth of a cubic centimeter
mU (or mIU)	milliunit	1 thousandth of an International Unit
ng	nanogram	1 thousandth of a microgram
pg	picogram	1 thousandth of a nanogram

If the reference ranges for your lab tests are very different from the ones shown in the charts above, the numbers I've given as optimal will not necessarily apply to your test results. However, it is still possible to extrapolate to a certain extent. As a general rule, the optimal range is quite a bit narrower than the normal range. From the tables given here, you can see whether the optimal range occupies the center or the high or low end of the standard range. With cortisol, for example, the optimal range is at the lower end of the standard reference range. With DHEA, however, you want your levels to be at the high end of the reference range.

Evaluating Hormone Ratios

When looking at your blood tests, also keep in mind that achieving healthy ratios between various hormones is at least as important as hitting the target zone for any one particular hormone. Hormones work not in isolation but in an intricate balance with one another.

When I started working with my patient Nick, for example, his cortisol levels were dangerously high. As we discussed in Chapter 2, high levels of this stress hormone can accelerate the aging process and increase the risk of heart disease and other conditions. Accordingly, Nick began taking supplemental DHEA to balance his cortisol levels. He also enrolled in a stress management workshop to learn some relaxation techniques.

A year later, Nick's cortisol levels are still slightly above the target range. In his case, however, I am not concerned. Although his cortisol is a bit high, Nick's DHEA levels are quite robust, which protects him from the damaging effects of high cortisol. The fact that his DHEA/cortisol ratio is on target is more important than the level of each hormone.

Based on many years of clinical experience, I have developed a set of ratios that I use when interpreting hormone profiles. The key ratios, which are discussed in detail in the chapters on hormone replacement, are summarized on page 245. To calculate a ratio, divide the first value by the second. For example, DHEA ÷ cortisol = DHEA/cortisol ratio.

The Big Picture

When I review lab results, I am looking at more than the individual numbers. I look at the balances between various elements. I also examine each set of results in the context of previous testing, looking for the trends and patterns. And finally, I look at the big picture: Do all the test

Target Hormone Ratios for Women

DHEA/cortisol (Chapter 2)	15–25
Progesterone/estrogen (Chapter 3)	10–20
Total estrogen/estradiol (Chapter 3)	Less than 2.5
Total testosterone/estrogen (Chapter 3)	2–5

Target Hormone Ratios for Men

DHEA/cortisol (Chapter 2)	15–25
Progesterone/estrogen (Chapter 3)	15–20
Total testosterone/estrogen (Chapter 3)	80–120
Estradiol/free testosterone (Chapter 3)	Less than 1.0

results fit together into a logical picture? Do the test results match with what I see in my clinical evaluation and with what you, as the patient, are feeling? If a reading doesn't make sense in terms of the whole picture, I look for explanations.

Medical testing is extremely precise, measuring elements in thousandths or millionths of a gram. With such precise measurements and concrete numbers, it's tempting to think of lab tests as infallible. But, of course, they are not. There are many factors that can affect the accuracy of your tests, including the methodology and quality control of the laboratory.

Sometimes a test result is inaccurate due to a problem with the blood draw or a laboratory error. Sometimes a test result is just an anomaly—a temporary spike or dip in your blood chemistry. The time of day, the phase of a woman's menstrual cycle, the timing of any hormones or other medications, even how much water you have had to drink—all of these factors can affect the results.

This is one of the many reasons that you want to be working with a qualified anti-aging specialist. An experienced practitioner will recognize when a particular test needs to be disregarded or repeated.

When the Numbers Don't Add Up

A couple of years ago, I ordered a set of hormone blood tests for a new 60-year-old patient of mine. Barry, who looked more or less his age, had never taken any hormone replacement or other anti-aging therapies. Most of his blood test results were about what I expected to see. His cortisol and estrogen levels were slightly elevated, as is common for someone his age. His DHEA and progesterone levels were quite low—all very typical. But his testosterone levels were off the charts. According to his testosterone readings, Barry should have been a 20-year-old bodybuilder! It didn't make sense.

I questioned Barry again about any medications or dietary habits that might explain his high testosterone levels but found nothing that would account for the reading. So we repeated the test. Sure enough, the subsequent test showed a different picture—a low to moderate testosterone level that matched the overall picture. Something had obviously gone wrong in the first test. Based on the first test results alone, I never would have recommended testosterone therapy for Barry. But in fact, Barry was in need of some testosterone replacement.

The point is that testing provides invaluable information, but it doesn't replace the need for expert guidance.

Alternative Testing Methods

In my practice, I rely primarily on blood testing for hormones. I find them to be the most reliable. The methodology for blood testing is well established and well documented. Because it has been in widespread use, blood testing has better established standards. Most of the research on hormones has used blood testing to measure and report on hormone levels. But other methods, such as saliva and urine tests, also have their advocates.

One advantage of saliva testing is that it does not require any needles. The saliva is simply collected on cotton swabs, sealed into plastic bags, and shipped to the laboratory. Saliva testing can even be ordered by mail.

While doubtless convenient, there is a far greater margin for error in the saliva collection process than in a traditional blood draw. For example, even a small amount of blood in the mouth at the time of saliva collection (such as bleeding from the gums following brushing or flossing) would render the test highly inaccurate.

Proponents of saliva testing argue that it is also more accurate than blood testing. They point out that the amount of hormone present in the saliva more closely reflects the amount of hormone that is active in the body's tissues ("free" or "unbound" hormone), as opposed to the amount being carried around in the bloodstream. After all, hormones do their actual work in the tissues of the body. The blood is simply the way they commute to work. Measuring blood levels of a hormone indicates the amount of *available* hormone but not necessarily the amount of *active* hormone.

Urine testing for hormones also has its proponents. Because hormones are secreted by the glands in pulses, hormone levels in the body fluctuate throughout the day. A blood test (or saliva test) measures the amount of hormones at a single moment in time. But hormones are also present in the urine. By collecting the urine output for twenty-four hours, the surges and dips in hormone levels can be averaged out. Instead of a single snapshot, you get the whole moving picture.

Obviously, a twenty-four-hour urine collection is a bit of an inconvenience. Another problem is that urine tests measure only hormone metabolites that have been excreted from the body. Hormones that have been excreted as waste products may not reflect a true picture of circulating hormone levels.

I grant that saliva testing and urine testing may offer certain advantages. Some measurements might even be more specific or accurate than we can get with a blood test. The problem comes with the interpretation of the information. What exactly are we measuring, and what is its significance? Both saliva and urine testing are still relatively new. There are no widespread standards or references for how the results can be interpreted. There is also no way to correlate the results of saliva testing to the more established standards of blood testing. No matter how accurate or specific they are, until we know more about what these results mean, their usefulness is somewhat limited.

With blood testing, the values are better established and referenced, and the collection and transport methods are far better controlled. A single blood draw can also suffice for hormone testing, risk factors, and any other blood chemistry work that is necessary. The fact that most labs require a doctor's prescription to order and receive test results is, to me, not a disadvantage. For now, I find blood testing to be the best method for hormone testing.

II.
TESTING FOR REVERSIBLE RISK FACTORS

In addition to hormone testing, we also use medical testing to identify correctable risk factors for disease. As we discussed in Part II, disease often begins with subtle biochemical imbalances or cellular dysfunction. Through testing, invisible conditions such as systemic inflammation or elevated homocysteine can be caught early and treated before full-blown disease has had a chance to develop. The following table summarizes the recommended risk factor screening tests.

Inflammation

As we discussed in Chapter 7, I recommend that your medical testing include tests for C-reactive protein (CRP) and fibrinogen, both of which can indicate the presence of dangerous systemic inflammation. Systemic inflammation may be completely without symptoms. But untreated inflammation can increase your risk of heart attack, cancer, and Alzheimer's disease.

RISK FACTOR PROFILE

Test	Standard range	Optimal
C-reactive protein (CRP)	Less than 4.9 mg/L	Less than 0.5 mg/L (men) Less than 1.3 mg/L (women)
Fibrinogen	200–400 mg/L	200–300 mg/L
Homocysteine	5–15 mcmol/L	Less than 8 mcmol/L
Cholesterol (total)	100–199 mg/dL	160–180 mg/dL
HDL	35–150 mg/dL	50–120 mg/dL
LDL	Less than 129 mg/dL	Less than 100 mg/dL
Triglycerides (TG)	Less than 199 mg/dL	40–100 mg/dL
Lp(a)	Less than 30 mg/dL	Less than 20 mg/dL
Total/HDL ratio		3–4 (men) 2–3 (women)
LDL/HDL ratio		Less than 2
TG/HDL ratio		Less than 2

I recommend testing for both of these inflammation markers because each measures a different by-product of the inflammation process. I find CRP to be highly significant (if elevated) but fibrinogen to be more sensitive. When CRP is elevated, it is a very reliable indicator that a serious inflammatory process is under way. Fibrinogen is more likely to detect subtle inflammation that might not cause an elevation in CRP. Elevated fibrinogen also suggests an elevated immune response as well as a degradation of the blood's flowing characteristics.

Once again, there is a critical difference between the standard reference range given by the laboratory and the optimal range for anti-aging and disease prevention. The standard reference range for CRP, for example, is anything less than 4.9 mg/L. And yet as CRP levels climb, so does your risk of heart attack. A CRP reading of 3.8, while well within the standard reference range, nonetheless correlates to a substantially elevated risk of future heart attack. Even if it is considered normal, why should you accept an increased risk of disease? If either of your inflammation markers is elevated, please refer to the anti-inflammatory nutrient protocols outlined in Chapter 7.

Methylation

In Chapter 8, we discussed the importance of maintaining adequate methylation. The most dangerous symptom of poor methylation is an accumulation of homocysteine in the blood. This toxic by-product can damage blood vessels and cell function and increase your risk of heart disease and Alzheimer's disease. Homocysteine testing is critical.

As with the inflammation markers, the safe range for homocysteine levels is considerably lower than the standard reference range given by most laboratories. While the standard allows for a homocysteine level up to 15 mmol/L, levels this high are associated with a 400 percent increase in coronary artery disease. Ideally, your homocysteine levels should be under 8 mmol/L. If they are not, please refer to Chapter 8 for nutrient protocols to lower homocysteine.

Blood Lipids

As discussed in detail in Chapter 8, cholesterol is not your enemy. It provides the essential building blocks for the steroid hormones and for healthy cells. Although it does play a secondary role, cholesterol does not cause heart disease and is not a reliable indicator of your heart disease risk.

The amount of total cholesterol in your blood is not nearly as important as the breakdown of the different types. Low-density lipoprotein (LDL) is the so-called bad cholesterol, which can accumulate in damaged blood vessels and is prone to oxidation. High-density lipoprotein

(HDL) is the good cholesterol, which protects the heart against the effects of high LDL.

The higher the percentage of HDL and the lower the percentage of LDL, the better. This ratio is a much more accurate predictor of your heart disease risk than the total cholesterol level. If you have a history of heart disease or have risk factors such as a cholesterol imbalance, I also recommend that you test for lipoprotein (a) and triglycerides. Lipoprotein (a) or Lp(a) is a modified form of LDL that is highly damaging to the arteries. Triglycerides (TG) are another type of blood fat associated with elevated heart disease risk. Both are important indicators of cardiovascular health and/or risk.

Abnormal levels or imbalances in any of the blood lipids are warning signs that must be taken seriously, although not necessarily with pharmaceutical therapies. Chapter 8 includes nutrient protocols for rebalancing cholesterol and triglycerides.

See also the LEF Disease Treatment and Prevention database under the heading "Cardiovascular Disease."

III.
BLOOD CHEMISTRY

In addition to the hormone and risk factor testing, your blood tests should include a basic blood chemistry workup. The table on pages 252–253 provides a guide to the function and interpretation of the basic blood chemistry tests.

See also the LEF Disease Prevention and Treatment database under the heading "Medical Testing."

The standard laboratory reference ranges are given below, along with the values that I consider to be optimal. If any of your values fall outside of the normal ranges, your doctor will most likely follow up with additional tests. But don't worry if some of your values are slightly outside of the optimal ranges indicated below. The optimal ranges represent an ideal. As you get further into your anti-aging program, you

Blood Chemistry

Blood component	Function	Reference range	Optimal range
White blood cell (WBC)	Low WBC indicates depressed immune function, commonly associated with viral infections. Elevated WBC is usually associated with bacterial infections.	4,000–10,800/mm^3	6,000–8,000/mm^3
Hematocrit (Hct)	Percentage of red blood cells. Low Hct indicates anemia. High Hct indicates thickened blood.	34–48 percent	40–48 percent
Mean corpuscular volume (MCV)	Mean size of red blood cells. Low MCV indicates iron deficiency anemia. High MCV indicates deficiency of folic acid or vitamin B$_{12}$.	80–99/mm^3	90–94/mm^3
Fasting blood sugar (FBS)	Nothing to eat or drink except water for at least ten hours before test. Levels above 100 indicate a predisposition toward diabetes. Levels above 125 indicate diabetes. Very low levels indicate hypoglycemia.	60–125 mg/dL	85–95 mg/dL
Fasting insulin	Nothing to eat or drink except water for at least ten hours before test. Elevated insulin is associated with hypertension, blood lipid disorders (such as high cholesterol), cardiovascular disease, obesity, or diabetes.	5–30 mU/L	5–8 mU/L
Albumin	Albumin is the most abundant protein in the body. Low albumin (below 4.0) suggests disease or malnutrition or accelerated aging.	3.5–5.0 g/dL	4.4–5 g/dL
Globulin	A protein associated with immune function. Elevated globulin may indicate infectious disease.	1.4–3.9 g/dL	2.5–3.0 g/dL
Albumin/globulin (A/G) ratio	A high A/G ratio indicates a strong immune system without current viral or bacterial challenge. Also used to check for renal (kidney) disease.	0.9–3.6	1.8–2.5

Blood Chemistry, cont.

Blood component	Function	Reference range	Optimal range
Sodium	Measure of fluid and electrolyte balance. High sodium produces high blood pressure.	125–150 mEq/L	138–145 mEq/L
Potassium	Indicates electrolyte balance and is especially important for those with heart disease. Low values are associated with fatigue.	3.4–5.3 mEq/L	4.4–4.8 mEq/L
Blood urea nitrogen (BUN)	Measures kidney and liver function. Dehydration can falsely elevate BUN.	6–24 mg/dL	12–20 mg/dL
Creatinine	Measures kidney function. High levels indicate kidney disease.	0.7–1.5 mg/dL	0.8–1.2 mg/dL
Iron	Low iron indicates iron deficiency anemia. Excess iron can damage blood vessels and contribute to heart disease.	32–168 mg/dL	60–100 mg/dL
Ferritin	Indicator of iron stores in the body. An accumulation of iron can raise risk of heart disease.	22–322 ng/mL	Less than 100 ng/mL
Bilirubin	Measures liver function.	0.1–1.2 mg/dL	0.1–1.2 mg/dL
Uric acid	High uric acid may lead to joint pain or gout. Low uric acid may reflect low folic acid levels.	2.6 – 7.2 mg/dL	3–5 mg/dL
Calcium	Calcium regulates muscle function, including that of the heart. But high blood calcium may damage blood vessels and lead to heart disease. Dietary calcium intake affects bone stores of calcium but not blood calcium levels. High blood calcium suggests a deficiency of vitamin K. (See also Chapter 11.)	8.4–10.4 mg/dL	9–10 mg/dL

will most likely see your blood chemistry values move closer and closer to these ideals. As you see this happening, it is confirmation that you are moving in the right direction.

WHEN TO DO YOUR TESTING

Medical testing comes into play during three important phases of your program. First, we will use testing to establish a baseline—a picture of where you are now. Second, medical testing during the implementation phase will allow us to fine-tune the protocols. Last, I recommend annual testing to monitor your long-term status.

Baseline Testing

I recommend that you schedule your initial medical testing during the first few weeks of your program. In the next two chapters, you will be starting a nutritional supplement program and implementing some anti-aging lifestyle changes. Both will have significant beneficial effects on your health, to the extent that they may already begin to reverse certain risk factors or hormone imbalances.

You may want to allow three to four weeks for the positive benefits of the basic program to take effect before scheduling your first round of testing. This will give the most accurate picture of what aspects of your health may require further intervention.

Fine-tuning

When working with hormones especially, the goal is to use the smallest amount needed to get optimal results. This is not a time to overshoot the target. The best way to do this, as I've said before, is to "start low and go slow." When I administer hormones, I start with a low dose and increase the amount gradually, using additional testing and your symptoms as a guide. If you are taking several different hormones, it's often necessary to adjust dosages up or down to find the "recipe" that works for you. Throughout this fine-tuning phase, I like to monitor hormone levels every six to eight weeks.

It's also critical to do follow-up testing on any abnormal risk factors, such as high homocysteine or inflammation markers. It is not enough to simply increase your intake of anti-inflammatory nutrients, for example, and hope for the best. You must be sure that the steps you have taken have been aggressive enough to handle the problem. Frequently, the starting dosages need to be increased in order to achieve target zones. Repeated testing is the only way to ensure that you are getting adequate protection.

Maintenance

Once you and your doctor arrive at your effective regimen, testing should be repeated annually. Although your anti-aging program will slow the aging process, your body is still a dynamic organism that will change over time. As you change, so will your hormone and nutrient requirements. Annual medical testing will allow you to monitor your evolution and progress, catch any new developments, and update your regimen as needed.

CHAPTER 11

Designing Your Anti-Aging Supplement Program

We turn not older with years, but newer every day.
—EMILY DICKINSON

A<small>N AGGRESSIVE PROGRAM OF</small> nutritional supplementation is a cornerstone of my approach to anti-aging and life extension. In the next chapter, we will be discussing the importance of the anti-aging diet. The foods you eat (as well as those you avoid) will have a profound impact on your health, both now and in the future. However, diet alone is not enough to counter the environmental, genetic, and metabolic forces that lead to premature aging and disease.

The reality is that virtually no one eats a nutritionally perfect diet, or anything even close to it. But even if you *were* to eat a precisely balanced diet, composed only of highly nutritious foods (and no empty calories), it would still be impossible to get the amount of nutrients needed for optimal health and function.

With dietary supplements, we can respond proactively to environmental, metabolic, and genetic factors that increase our risk of disease. We can compensate for the genetically programmed changes in cell and organ function that lead to biological aging. With the information gleaned from medical testing (as discussed in Chapter 10), we can customize a program of nutrients and hormone replacement based on individual risk factors, nutrient needs, and the rate at which your body is aging.

This is such an important point that it bears further emphasis. If the supplement program outlined in this chapter seems daunting, take a moment to consider what it is we are trying to accomplish. We are giving you the tools to avoid age-related and degenerative diseases such as heart disease, arthritis, diabetes, Alzheimer's disease, and macular degeneration. We are attempting nothing less than to forestall the aging process itself—to grow older without aging.

These are ambitious, even audacious goals. Success will require a conscious and committed effort, including aggressive nutritional intervention. I can promise you, however, that the investment is more than worthwhile.

STEP ONE: STARTING WITH THE BASICS

The first step is to implement a basic comprehensive regimen of vitamins, minerals, and essential fatty acids. I like to see this foundational level firmly established before we go on to add other more specialized supplements.

I start with a high-potency multivitamin and mineral formula, which is a convenient way to cover a lot of bases in one formula. But I'm not talking about the once-a-day type formulation that is available in groceries and drugstores, even those that are labeled as "high potency." *None comes close* to offering the level of nutritional support that I recommend.

The following table shows the nutrient values for several leading once-a-day multivitamins. As you can see, these formulas offer 100 percent of the Daily Value for many nutrients, sometimes more. But 100 percent of the government's recommendation for daily intake falls far short of the amount needed for optimal health and anti-aging. In many cases, you actually need up to ten times more than the Daily Value in order to promote truly optimal health.

Typical Multivitamin Formulas

Nutrient	Centrum	% DV	Thera M	% DV	One A Day	% DV
Vitamin A	3,500 IU	70	5,500 IU	110	5,000 IU	100
Vitamin C	60 mg	100	120 mg	200	90 mg	150
Vitamin D	400 IU	100	400 IU	100	400 IU	100
Vitamin E	30 IU	100	30 IU	100	45 IU	150
Vitamin K	25 mcg	31	—	—	—	—
Thiamine (vitamin B_1)	1.5 mg	100	3 mg	200	2.25 mg	150
Riboflavin (vitamin B_2)	1.7 mg	100	3.4 mg	200	2.55 mg	150
Niacin	20 mg	100	30 mg	150	20 mg	100
Vitamin B_6	2 mg	100	3 mg	150	3 mg	150
Folic acid	400 mcg	100	400 mcg	100	400 mcg	100
Vitamin B_{12}	6 mcg	100	9 mcg	150	9 mcg	150
Biotin	30 mcg	10	15 mcg	5	—	—
Pantothenic acid	10 mg	100	10 mg	100	10 mg	100
Calcium	162 mg	16	—	—	—	—
Iron	18 mg	100	18 mg	100	—	—
Phosphorus	109 mg	11	—	—	—	—
Iodine	150 mcg	100	150 mcg	100	—	—
Magnesium	100 mg	25	100 mg	25	100 mg	25
Zinc	15 mg	100	15 mg	100	15 mg	100

Typical Multivitamin Formulas, cont.

Nutrient	Centrum	% DV	Thera M	% DV	One A Day	% DV
Selenium	20 mcg	29	10 mcg	15	87.5 mcg	125
Copper	2 mg	100	2 mg	100	2 mg	100
Manganese	2 mg	100	5 mg	250	3.5 mg	175
Chromium	120 mcg	100	—	—	150 mcg	125
Molyb-denum	75 mcg	100	—	—	75 mcg	100
Chloride	72 mg	2	—	—	34 mg	1
Potassium	80 mg	2	—	—	37.5 mg	1
Boron	150 mg	*	—	—	—	—
Nickel	5 mcg	*	—	—	—	—
Silicon	2 mg	*	—	—	—	—
Tin	10 mcg	*	—	—	—	—
Vanadium	10 mcg	*	—	—	—	—
Lutein	250 mcg	*	—	—	—	—
Lycopene	300 mcg	*	—	—	—	—

*No DV established for this nutrient.

The Government's Recommendations Are Inadequate

Historically, the government's nutrient recommendations have been based on the amount of nutrients needed to avoid deficiency diseases such as scurvy, rickets, and pellagra. Once again, this reflects the disease-based approach to medicine that seems to pervade our society.

Instead of trying to determine what amount of nutrients will *maximize* health, the government instead has determined the *minimal* level of nutrition required to prevent overt disease. Only very recently has the FDA begun to acknowledge that nutrients can also protect against diseases such as heart disease, cataracts, cancer, and neurological disease.

Very slowly, some of the government's recommendations are now being nudged upward to reflect the growing evidence that higher levels of nutrients provide better protection against these diseases. In 2000, for example, the RDA of vitamin C was increased from 60 mg to 75 mg per day for women and to 90 mg per day for men.

But the newer recommendations still stop far short of the levels needed to preserve *optimal* health, which is our goal. In releasing the new recommendations for vitamin C, for example, the government ignored recommendations from their own researchers that the level be increased to 200 mg or more. While vitamin E is now universally recommended at dosages of 200 IU per day or more, the government's newest recommendations are just 30 IU. Despite mounting evidence of their ability to prevent disease, the government has yet to establish recommended intakes for phytochemicals such as lycopene and lutein.

It is shocking how unwilling the government is to respond to scientific advances in our understanding of nutrition and disease. The National Academy of Sciences (the body of scientists that sets the government's nutritional recommendations) appears to have a distinct bias against nutritional supplements. They rarely recommend nutrient intakes that exceed the amount that can be gotten through food sources alone.

Not only have they ignored the overwhelming evidence supporting higher nutrient recommendations, but they arbitrarily declare higher doses to be risky. Despite studies that repeatedly show that dosages of up to 4,000 mg of vitamin C per day are well tolerated, for example, the National Academy of Sciences has declared intakes over 2,000 mg a day to be unsafe.

Ironically, government scientists do acknowledge that those in poor health may benefit from increased levels of nutrients. As we saw throughout Part II, however, disease starts at the cellular level long before the first symptom is apparent. It is precisely at this cellular level that nutrient therapies can be of most benefit. Why wait until we are sick to give our bodies the nutrition they need? It is a backward, disease-oriented approach to health. In respect to nutrient guidelines, the government has failed in its self-appointed role as the referee of good science and good sense.

DECODING RDAS, RDIS, DVS, AND DRI

The government uses an alphabet soup of confusing and overlapping terms to express its extremely conservative ideas about nutrition.

RDA/RDI. The Recommended Dietary Allowance (or Recommended Dietary Intake) is the amount of proteins, vitamins, and minerals that the government considers adequate to meet the needs of most healthy adults.

DRV. The Daily Reference Values reflect the government's recommendations for nutrients, such as fat and fiber, that do not have an RDA but are considered to be important for health.

DV. Daily Values are the values developed by the FDA for use on food labels. They include both RDI and DRV.

DRI. The Daily Reference Intake is a collaborative effort between the United States and Canada that will eventually revise and replace the current U.S. RDA.

What "High Potency" Really Means

The chart below shows the nutrient values of the multivitamin formula (made by AMNI) that I use in my practice. You can see that many of the nutrients are included in amounts that are ten to fifty times the government's inadequate recommendations. Nonetheless, these amounts are not excessive. These are the nutrient amounts that promote healthy, youthful function and prevent disease and disability. (Formulations of this type are available in health and nutrition stores and by mail order. The Life Extension Foundation has formulated a high-potency daily nutritional supplement for its members, available by mail order.)

There is simply no way to fit the nutrients you need into one capsule or tablet. The multivitamin formula shown below, for example, requires six tablets per day. You might be wondering if you could simply take a handful of once-a-day vitamins to accomplish the same thing, but this is not a good idea. In order to get adequate levels of antioxidants and B vitamins, you would be getting unhealthy excesses of certain nutrients, such as iron or copper. In addition, the once-a-day type formulas are far more likely to use cheaper, synthetic vitamins or mineral salts that are poorly absorbed.

Multivitamin and Mineral Complex, six tablets per day

Nutrient	Amount	% DV	Functions
Vitamin A	5,000 IU	400%	Antioxidant, promotes immune function, tissue repair, eye health
Beta-carotene	15,000 IU		Precursor for vitamin A
Vitamin D	400 IU	100%	Assists in the use of calcium and phosphorus, needed for healthy bones, teeth, and muscle function
Vitamin E	400 IU	1,333%	Antioxidant, improves flowing characteristics of blood
Vitamin C	1,000 mg	1,666%	Antioxidant, increases resistance to infection, needed for collagen production, promotes healthy skin, hair, joints
Vitamin K	60 mcg	75%	Needed to make blood clotting factors, helps build bone and maintain healthy blood vessels
Thiamine (vitamin B_1)	100 mg	6,666%	Assists with carbohydrate digestion, promotes healthy function of heart and nervous system
Riboflavin (vitamin B_2)	50 mg	2,941%	Involved in energy production, promotes healthy skin and eyes
Niacin	50 mg	250%	Helps in conversion of carbohydrates to energy

Multivitamin and Mineral Complex, six tablets per day, cont.

Nutrient	Amount	% DV	Functions
Niacinamide	150 mg	750%	Helps in conversion of carbohydrates to energy
Pantothenic acid	400 mg	4,000%	Plays a central role in energy metabolism
Vitamin B_6	50 mg	2,500%	Promotes healthy nervous system, needed to form red blood cells, detoxifies homocysteine
Folic acid	800 mcg	200%	Helps in production of new blood cells and proteins, prevents birth defects, aids methylation and reduces homocysteine levels
Vitamin B_{12}	100 mcg	1,666%	Needed for nervous system function, aids methylation, and reduces homocysteine levels
Biotin	300 mcg	100%	Required for the manufacture of lipids and energy production, helps regulate metabolism of sugar
Choline	150 mg	*	Precursor to acetylcholine and phosphatidyl choline, needed for manufacture of neurotransmitters, promotes healthy brain function
Calcium	500 mg	50%	Builds stronger bones, joints, and teeth; regulates heart rhythm
Magnesium	500 mg	125%	Promotes nerve and muscle function, helps convert glucose into energy, aids in utilization of calcium
Potassium	99 mg	3%	Helps regulate blood pressure by controlling body's water balance, normalizes heart rhythm, prevents fatigue

Multivitamin and Mineral Complex, six tablets per day, cont.

Nutrient	Amount	% DV	Functions
Copper	2 mg	100%	Aids in transport of oxygen, needed for manufacture of cellular antioxidants
Manganese	20 mg	1,000%	Helps control blood sugar, energy metabolism, and hormone function; can increase cellular antioxidant activity; improves bone strength
Zinc	20 mg	133%	Supports immune function, promotes wound healing, regulates sex hormone activity, promotes prostate and breast health
Iodine	150 mcg	100%	Promotes healthy hair, nails, skin, and teeth; needed for proper thyroid function
Iron**	20 mg	100%	Needed for hemoglobin production, prevents anemia, promotes resistance to disease, may prevent hair loss in women
Chromium	200 mcg	166%	Helps the body utilize glucose for energy and regulate blood sugar
Selenium	200 mcg	285%	Antioxidant cofactor, protects heart, prostate; critical for glutathione synthesis and thyroid function
Molybdenum	150 mcg	200%	Cofactor for enzymes, aids in metabolism of amino acids
Boron	2 mg	*	Aids in calcium and magnesium use, essential to protect against bone loss
PABA	50 mg	*	Aids in utilization of pantothenic acid, helps in the breakdown and use of proteins

Multivitamin and Mineral Complex, six tablets per day, cont.

Nutrient	Amount	% DV	Functions
Inositol	50 mg	*	Helps to regulate cholesterol levels and support production of neurotransmitters

* No DV established.

** While critical to health, iron tends to build up in the body and can promote free radical damage, especially to the heart. Menstruating women, who lose iron each month, are frequently deficient in iron and should supplement. Adult men and postmenopausal women, however, should not take supplemental iron unless an iron deficiency is diagnosed. Most vitamin formulas are available with and without iron.

Additional Nutrients

A high-potency multivitamin and mineral supplement covers a lot of bases. But to complete the nutritional foundation, a few additional supplements are necessary.

Antioxidants

As discussed in Chapter 6, antioxidants are a key to the prevention of free-radical-associated diseases. Even with a high-potency formulation, additional vitamin C and vitamin E are usually needed to bring the total intake up to the levels recommended in Chapter 6 for antioxidant protection. A mixed carotenoid supplement supports and balances the vitamin A and beta-carotene included in the multivitamin. Coenzyme Q_{10} and alpha-lipoic acid are needed to support levels of cellular antioxidants. Additional zinc promotes the activity of the antioxidant enzymes. (See the table below for specific dosages.)

Essential Fatty Acids

In Chapter 7, we saw how hidden inflammation can invisibly drive disease processes from heart disease and cancer to Alzheimer's and arthritis. A fish oil supplement provides omega-3 fatty acids, which the body converts to active compounds called prostaglandins, which fight in-flammation. Omega-3 fatty acids provide the lipids needed to maintain healthy cell membranes, which are particularly important to the health and function of the brain, heart, and blood vessels. Fish oil also helps to condition the blood, improving its flowing characteristics (rheology).

Most Westerners are extremely deficient in these essential fatty acids, and adding fish oil supplements to the diet can bring about as-tonishing improvements in conditions such as arthritis and joint pain, asthma, allergies, and skin disorders (all of which are inflammatory conditions). Simply stated, fish oils are magic.

Increasing your consumption of these fatty acids too suddenly, how-ever, can lead to stomach upset and/or diarrhea. To avoid this, I advise you to begin with one capsule per day (1,000 mg) and increase gradu-ally to the recommended dose of 3,000 to 5,000 mg per day.

Omega-3 fatty acids are also found in vegetable sources, primarily flaxseed and flaxseed oil. However, the fatty acids in flax must be con-verted into the active compounds EPA and DHA before they are bio-logically active. The advantage of fish oils is that they already contain EPA and DHA. No conversion needs to happen in the body. For this reason, they are frequently more effective.

Antiglycation

The aging effects of glycation were discussed in detail in Chapter 9. Glycation-related damage to tissues and organs can be irreversible. To minimize the aging and disease-promoting consequences of glycation, add 1,000 mg of carnosine to your daily regimen.

Bone-Building Nutrients

Both men and women need to be concerned about preserving bone strength and mass as they age. Osteoporosis is not only a women's dis-ease. Men also lose bone mass—they just lose it more gradually. Because women tend to lose bone mass very rapidly following menopause, os-teopenia (weakened bones) and osteoporosis (porous bones) manifest earlier in life. But by the time men reach 75 or 80 they have completely "caught up" with their female counterparts and suffer from osteoporosis at the same rate as women.

To protect against bone loss, both men and women need to be concerned about calcium intake throughout their adult life. The government's recommendation for calcium is 1,000 mg per day. As the exception that proves the rule, this level is adequate. Magnesium (at half the calcium dosage, or 500 mg) aids in the utilization of calcium. Both nutrients are found in most multivitamins, but rarely at sufficient dosages. Supplement your multi with extra calcium and magnesium as needed to bring the total intake up to these levels.

The Overlooked Nutrient

Vitamin K is a nutrient that you may not have heard too much about unless you have ever been on anticoagulation therapies, such as Coumadin. In that case, you were probably instructed to avoid foods containing vitamin K (these include kale, brussels sprouts, spinach, and broccoli) because they would interfere with the effects of the anticoagulation therapy.

For a long time, vitamin K (phylloquinone) had only one known function in the body—to regulate coagulation factors in the blood. More recently, it has been discovered that vitamin K also plays a critical role in your body's management of its calcium stores.

It turns out that preventing osteoporosis is not just a matter of supplying the body with sufficient calcium. You must also ensure that the calcium is going where it is needed. Frequently, those who don't have enough calcium in their bones have too much calcium in their blood vessel walls. This leads to hardening of the arteries, which can cause heart attack and stroke.

This may explain why those with osteoporosis also have a much higher incidence of stroke and heart disease. It appears that these two diseases are, at least in part, two faces of a single problem: a dysfunction in the regulation of calcium.

Vitamin K helps to direct the body's calcium supplies into the bones, where it is needed to prevent osteoporosis. At the same time, it helps to keep calcium from being deposited in blood vessel walls and other organs. In this way, vitamin K is a critical part of the body's defense against both osteoporosis and cardiovascular disease.

The Life Extension Foundation has played an important role in bring-ing the little-known benefits of vitamin K to light. Most people do not get sufficient amounts of vitamin K from their diet, and few multivitamins contain this important nutrient. The formula I use is one of the few that does, although in relatively low amounts. The Life Extension Foundation recommends 5 to 10 mg per day for optimal health and longevity.

Filling in the Gaps

Even with a good, high-potency multivitamin, you will usually need to take some extra vitamin C, vitamin E, zinc, and calcium to bring your daily intake to the recommended levels. A few additional nutrients (mixed carotenoids, CoQ_{10}, alpha-lipoic acid, vitamin K, fish oil, and carnosine) round out the basic program.

Various multivitamin formulas will differ in the amounts of individual nutrients they contain. Begin with the most complete high-potency multi you can find, using the table above as a reference point. Then supple-ment as needed with individual nutrients to reach the recommended totals shown in the table on page 269.

How to Implement Your Basic Program

I recommend that you divide your daily supplements into three or four dosages. This allows your body to absorb the nutrients over the course of the day, and also minimizes any digestive upset from taking too many pills at once. Generally, my patients find it most convenient to take their nutrients with breakfast, lunch, and dinner, and before bed.

Vitamins, which are generally stimulating, are taken at breakfast and lunch. Fat-soluble vitamins such as CoQ_{10} are taken with fatty acids that aid in their absorption. Additional minerals are better absorbed when taken separately, and also can have a calming effect. These are taken at dinner and before bed. A pill sorter is an invaluable tool.

When first beginning a nutrient program, I suggest that you start slowly and allow your body a chance to adjust to a very dramatic differ-ence in nutrient levels. On pages 271 and 272 is a two-week implemen-tation schedule that works well for my patients.

Additional Nutrients

Mixed carotenoids	5,000 IU if not included in multi
Vitamin C	As needed to bring daily intake to 2,000–4,000 mg
Vitamin E (mixed tocopherols/ tocotrienols)	As needed to bring daily intake to 800–1,200 IU
Zinc	As needed to bring daily intake to 30–50 mg
Calcium	As needed to bring daily intake to 1,000 mg
Vitamin K	As needed to bring daily intake to 5–10 mg
Coenzyme Q_{10}	50–200 mg if not included in multi
Alpha-lipoic acid	250–500 mg if not included in multi
Fish oil (containing EPA and DHA)	3,000–5,000 mg
Carnosine	1,000 mg

The sample program below uses:

➢ BP-5 (by AMNI) high-potency multivitamin formula with chelated minerals (1 serving equals 6 tablets)
➢ Vitamin C, 1,000 mg tablets
➢ Vitamin E (mixed tocopherols and tocotrienols), 400 IU gel caps
➢ Mixed carotenoids, high-potency gel caps
➢ Coenzyme Q_{10}, 50–100 mg capsules
➢ Calcium, 500 mg tablets

- Max EPA/DHA fish oil, 1,000 mg gel caps
- Zinc, 15 mg tablets
- Alpha-lipoic acid, 100 mg capsules
- Vitamin K, 5 mg tablets
- Carnosine, 500 mg capsules

The Most Important Thing

The most important thing about this program, by far, is that you take your supplements, not that you take them exactly on time or in exactly the right order. If you find that trying to take supplements four times a day is simply not manageable, for example, it is perfectly all right to combine the morning and lunch supplements into one group and the dinner and evening supplements into another group. If you need to, you can increase the amounts more slowly, stretching your implementation phase out over several weeks.

For Men Only

In Chapter 3, we discussed nutrients that promote healthy prostate function and help to protect against prostate disease. Many of these, including selenium, zinc, and lycopene (a carotenoid), are already incorporated into the basic nutrient program. In addition, men may wish to add 120 to 250 mg of nettle extract and/or 50 to 100 mg of pygeum extract. Please also see Chapter 3.

Nutrients for Prostate Health	
Nettle extract	120–250 mg
Pygeum extract	50–100 mg

Taking It to the Next Level

After the two-week implementation phase, your body may be better nourished than it ever has been. You will probably feel a big difference

Week One

Time	Day 1	Day 2	Day 3	Day 4	Day 5	Day 6	Day 7
Breakfast	1 multi tab Carotenoids	1 multi tab Carotenoids Fish oil CoQ_{10}	1 multi tab Carotenoids Fish oil CoQ_{10}	1 multi tab Vitamin E Carotenoids Fish oil CoQ_{10}	2 multi tabs Vitamin E Carotenoids Fish oil CoQ_{10}	2 multi tabs Vitamin E Vitamin C Carotenoids Fish oil CoQ_{10}	3 multi tabs Vitamin E Vitamin C Carotenoids Fish oil CoQ_{10}
Lunch	1 multi tab	1 multi tab	2 multi tabs Alpha-lipoic acid	2 multi tabs Fish oil Alpha-lipoic acid	2 multi tabs Fish oil Alpha-lipoic acid	3 multi tabs Fish oil Alpha-lipoic acid	3 multi tabs Fish oil Alpha-lipoic acid
Dinner	Vitamin E Vitamin C Carnosine	Vitamin E Vitamin C Carnosine	Vitamin E Vitamin C Carnosine	Vitamin E Vitamin C Carnosine	Vitamin E Vitamin C Carnosine	Vitamin E Vitamin C Carnosine	Vitamin E Vitamin C Fish oil Carnosine
Bedtime	Calcium Zinc Vitamin K	Calcium Zinc Vitamin K	Calcium Zinc Vitamin K	Calcium Zinc Vitamin K	Calcium Zinc Vitamin K	Calcium Alpha-lipoic acid Zinc Vitamin K	Calcium Alpha-lipoic acid Zinc Vitamin K

Week Two, All Days

Breakfast	Lunch	Dinner	Bedtime
3 multi tabs	3 multi tabs	Vitamin C	Calcium
Vitamin E	Fish oil	Vitamin E	Alpha-lipoic acid
Vitamin C	Alpha-lipoic acid	Fish oil	Zinc
Mixed carotenoids		Carnosine	Vitamin K
Fish oil			
Coenzyme Q_{10}			
Carnosine			

in your energy levels, see improvements in your skin and nails, and notice clearer, more focused thinking. You may also experience reduced joint pain, greater stamina for exercise, and improved sleep. All of these are common responses to a high-caliber nutrient program.

After the first two weeks, you may be ready to declare your experience with anti-aging medicine to have been an unqualified success. But there is so much more to come. One of the fun things for me about anti-aging medicine is that each layer of the program brings you to a higher level of wellness and enthusiasm for life.

As we continue to move into higher levels of the program, you will begin to see that anti-aging is a never-ending upward spiral of increasing health, vitality, and well-being. What a contrast to the conventional view of aging as an unavoidable slide into increasing disability and dysfunction!

STEP TWO: ENHANCING BRAINPOWER

In weeks three and four, we will begin adding nutrients that enhance mental clarity, focus, and protect against age-related decline in brain function. You may already have noticed some signs of brain aging—a slight slowing of your reflexes, a foggy or unfocused feeling, increasing forgetfulness, or difficulty recalling words or names. Feeding the brain nutrients that enhance its activity and function will help to restore your mental sharpness, focus, and flexibility.

The basic nutrient program outlined above already includes many of the brainpower nutrients discussed in Chapter 5. **Coenzyme Q$_{10}$** helps to protect the brain cells from free radical damage and promotes energy production in the mitochondria. **B vitamins** aid in the production of neurotransmitters, which carry signals from cell to cell. **Essential fatty acids,** especially those found in fish oil, improve cell-to-cell communication by keeping the brain cell membranes supple and healthy. Fish oil also helps keep the blood free-flowing, which enhances the transport of oxygen to the hungry brain cells.

Having implemented your basic program, you will probably already feel a positive difference in your alertness and mood. Now we take that to the next level with additional brainpower nutrients. Beginning in week three, add the nutrients shown in the table below to your regimen. Supplement formulas that specifically target brain function will include many of these nutrients in one capsule. Take your brainpower nutrients in two divided doses, in the morning and before bed.

As we discussed in Chapter 5, you've also got to exercise your body and your brain to keep it in peak form. And for those who want to take a more aggressive approach, see Chapter 5 for more on "smart drugs."

Brainpower Nutrients

Ginkgo biloba	60–120 mg	Improves alertness by enhancing blood and oxygen flow to the brain
Acetyl-L-carnitine	1,000–2,000 mg	Improves mood, memory, and cognitive function by enhancing mitochondrial function
Phosphatidylcholine (PC)	3,000–6,000 mg	Enhances acetylcholine levels to enhance memory and recall
Phosphatidylserine (PS)	100–300 mg	Improves cell-to-cell communication and preserves the integrity and vitality of brain cell membranes
DMAE	100–300 mg	Enhances memory and cognitive function, raises levels of acetylcholine, and stabilizes brain cell membranes

STEP THREE:
RESTORING HORMONE BALANCE

At this point in your anti-aging program, we start to work with hormone levels. As we saw in Chapter 1, age-related changes in hormone levels are part of what drives the aging process. As hormone production sags, the body begins to slow down in its rejuvenation and repair of tissues and organs. Resistance to disease begins to weaken. Aging accelerates. In fact, the level of hormones in your body is one of the most telling biomarkers of aging.

By restoring these hormones to optimal, youthful levels, the body can be rejuvenated inside and out. Your body's production of hormones is greatly influenced by your nutritional status. Frequently, sagging hormone levels rebound somewhat as a result of optimizing nutrition. In particular, I have observed that adding essential fatty acids and carotenoids to the diet seems to pump up hormone production, especially in men.

As discussed in Chapter 10, I recommend that you have your levels of DHEA, cortisol, testosterone, estrogen(s), progesterone, thyroid hormone, and growth hormone evaluated. I prefer to test these hormone levels after the initial phase of the nutrition program has already been implemented. This allows the effects of the nutritional program to register. But at that point, additional hormone replacement may be required to bring your hormone profiles into optimal balance and your body into prime youthful function. For this, you will need to work with a qualified anti-aging specialist.

Please also refer to Part I for detailed information of on target levels, ratios, and dosage guidelines for the various hormones. Chapter 2 discusses the anti-aging effects of the adrenal hormone DHEA. Chapter 3 outlines the protocols for enhancing and balancing sex hormones in both men and women. Chapter 4 covers the master metabolic hormones produced in the thyroid and pituitary and how they can be supported with replacement hormones.

Working with a physician, all of these hormones can be restored to their optimal, youthful levels. Although the anti-aging benefits of hormone replacement are usually rapid and dramatic, it can take several weeks or even months of fine-tuning to optimize and stabilize your hormone profiles. Once you have reached target levels, I recommend that you have your doctor retest your hormones annually and adjust your program as needed.

STEP FOUR:
CORRECTING REVERSIBLE RISK FACTORS

The final step in your supplement program is to address any risk factors that may have turned up in your recommended testing. As discussed in Chapter 10, I recommend that you have your inflammation markers (CRP and fibrinogen) and homocysteine levels checked. These markers and their significance are discussed in detail in Chapters 7 and 8.

The basic program outlined above already includes nutrients that address many of these risk factors. Vitamins B_6 and B_{12} and folic acid lower homocysteine levels. Fish oil, ginkgo, and vitamin K help to reduce inflammation. So, as with the hormone testing, it makes sense to wait until after the basic nutrition protocol has been implemented before testing for these risk factors.

Elevated Homocysteine

If after implementing the basic nutrition protocol, homocysteine levels remain elevated (above 8 mcmol/L), additional homocysteine-lowering nutrients should be added to the regimen. The addition of 750 mg of trimethylglycine (TMG) will often be enough to lower homocysteine to safe levels. If needed, folic acid, vitamin B_6, and vitamin B_{12} can also be increased to the dosages shown on page 277. (Please also see Chapter 8 for more intensive protocols for stubbornly high homocysteine levels.)

Nutrients to Lower Homocysteine

TMG	750 mg
Vitamin B$_6$ or P5P	100 mg
Vitamin B$_{12}$	500–1,000 mcg
Folic acid	800–1,600 mcg

Elevated Inflammation Markers

Similarly, if your tests show indications of systemic inflammation despite the inflammation-reducing nutrients in the basic protocol, additional anti-inflammatory nutrients should be added. (C-reactive protein should be less than 0.5 mg/L and fibrinogen less than 300 mg/L.) Please also see Chapter 7.

Nutrients to Reduce Inflammation

Nettle leaf extract	900 mg
Bromelain	2,000 mg
Ginger	900 mg
Curcumin	1,200 mg

Elevated Cholesterol

In Chapter 8, I discussed nutritional regimens to balance cholesterol without prescription drugs. One natural cholesterol-lowering nutrient (the tocotrienol form of vitamin E) is already included in the basic protocol. If needed, additional tocotrienols can be added, up to 100 mg per day. Please also see Chapter 8 for more information on the use of high-dose niacin to reduce elevated cholesterol.

Nutrients to Reduce Cholesterol	
Vitamin E (as tocotrienols)	50–100 mg
Niacin	500–2,000 mg

GETTING TO THE PAYOFF

Now that you've customized your supplement program, you are probably looking at a fairly extensive list of supplements that you will be taking on a daily basis. As I noted at the beginning of this chapter, an aggressive program of supplementation such as this one may be a bit daunting at first. But before you make up your mind whether or not you can commit to the program long-term, I encourage you to try it for a minimum of six to eight weeks. I predict that you will find the results so rewarding that you will want to continue.

Darlene was a 51-year-old college professor who consulted me about an anti-aging program a few years ago. Since going through menopause the year before, she was feeling "old and worn out." Darlene desperately wanted to rejuvenate her body. But she told me flat out that she didn't think she'd be able to follow through with the supplement part of the program. "I'll make all the dietary and lifestyle changes," she told me, "but I've never been good about taking supplements. I find swallowing the pills very unpleasant. Vitamins and herbs upset my stomach. Usually, I just 'forget' to take them during the day."

If Darlene had followed all of the anti-aging diet and lifestyle recommendations outlined in the next chapter and done nothing else, I have no doubt she would have felt better and been healthier. But I knew that without the anti-aging supplement program, she was unlikely to get the dramatic results she was hoping for. I convinced her to make a provisional commitment to follow the supplement program for six weeks, no matter what.

We worked out a schedule that allowed her to begin with just a few basic supplements a day, increasing the number of supplements very gradually over a period of a month. Through experimentation, Darlene found that taking supplements with milk or juice worked better than taking them with water alone, and that eating a small piece of fruit immediately afterward helped to settle her stomach. But even so, it took quite a bit of discipline for Darlene to remember to take her supplements every day.

"I've tried to take supplements in the past," she told me, "but I always give up after a few days or a week at most." This time was different. She was surprised to find that it got easier and easier to swallow the capsules. It is definitely something that gets easier with practice. And by sticking with it, Darlene started to feel the payoff.

After three or four weeks, Darlene noticed she was waking up a few minutes before the alarm clock went off, feeling totally energized and alert. She had more energy throughout the day, enough to stop at the gym for a quick workout on the way home from work. Her skin looked clearer. Her libido perked up. The flu that was going around campus completely passed her by. By the time the six weeks were up, Darlene was absolutely committed to her supplement program—to the extent that she took all her supplements along on a weeklong skiing trip. "This is absolutely amazing," she said. "I wouldn't dream of going back to the way I used to feel."

If you are not used to taking supplements or you find it a bit challenging, take it slowly. Give yourself time to adjust to this new habit. You will find it gets easier and easier. At the same time, your payoff will get richer and richer.

CHAPTER 12

The Anti-Aging Lifestyle

The trick is to grow up without growing old.
—CASEY STENGEL

S A SOCIETY, WE tend to place a great deal of faith in the power of pills. Judging from the pharmaceutical commercials that now run constantly on television, pills can do a lot more than just lower your cholesterol, alleviate depression, and prevent heartburn. They also appear to improve your social life, your golf score, and the weather in your hometown. Of course, that's just marketing. But the reason this marketing is so effective is that we do, as a society, tend to believe that pills have an almost magical power to cure us without our having to change anything else about our lifestyle.

This attitude often carries over into the realm of nutritional medicine as well. When I develop anti-aging programs for my patients, I've noticed that they frequently think of the nutrient supplements as the "main" part of the program, with the dietary and lifestyle components being somehow secondary.

In the last chapter, I told you about my patient Darlene, who was not sure she could take a lot of supplements. As I pointed out to Darlene, it is not enough just to eat well and live a healthy lifestyle. To get the profound anti-aging benefits that I've described throughout this book, nutritional supplementation is a must. But the reverse is also true. The supplement program outlined in the previous chapter is not an antidote to bad habits or a substitute for a healthy lifestyle. In order to get the maximum results, you absolutely need both. The lifestyle program outlined in this chapter works with your anti-aging supplement program to counter the effects of aging and prevent disease.

There is simply no way to put all the benefits of a healthy diet, exercise, and lifestyle into a pill. The foods you eat, the amount and quality of exercise and rest you get, and even your mental attitude about life make an enormous difference in your health and vitality. More to the point, they all affect the rate at which your body is aging.

Chronic lack of sleep, for example, not only makes you feel tired and foggy but also increases the levels of stress hormones in your body. As we saw in Chapter 2, these hormones accelerate aging and promote disease. On the other hand, getting enough exercise not only keeps you trim and toned but also enhances the secretion of growth hormone, which can slow the rate at which your body is aging.

This chapter will outline my recommendations for diet, exercise, sleep, and stress reduction. Of course, any one of these topics could fill an entire book. Here, we'll focus specifically on the ways in which each of these aspects of your lifestyle can help you slow the aging process and prevent disease.

The recommendations in this chapter are not complicated. Some may differ from what you have read about diet and exercise in the past. Other aspects of the anti-aging lifestyle may simply be different from what you are used to. But nothing I'm asking you to do is difficult. And remember that none of us can be 100 percent on target 100 percent of the time. As long as you are moving in the right direction, every step you take gets you closer to your goal.

PARTNER UP

Occasionally, I have patients who come to me as a couple, interested in pursuing anti-aging as a team. Beth and William are a couple in their fifties who decided to make anti-aging a priority in their lives after they happened to see an interview that I did on television. Happily married for over twenty-five years, Beth and William hoped for many more years together. Obviously, neither wanted the other saddled with the burden of a sick or infirm spouse, but they had never considered what steps they might take to prevent that from happening.

After seeing the interview, they arranged a consultation with me and ultimately made a commitment to pursue an anti-aging program together. It was a rather dramatic change from the lifestyle they were used to, but the fact that they embarked on the journey together made the adjustment far easier. They both started taking anti-aging supplements, often calling during the day to remind each other to take their midday nutrients. William, who loved to cook, found that he enjoyed the challenge of adapting his favorite recipes to fit the anti-aging dietary guidelines. Beth kept a computer log of their medical test results. The two found that scheduling time for exercise and rest together became quality couple time that they looked forward to.

Together, Beth and William developed new habits and patterns and supported each other in making the necessary changes. And they appreciated the changes that they began to observe in their energy level, their moods, and even the appearance of their bodies. In my experience, this is one of the most effective scenarios for successful anti-aging.

Making the transition into a new lifestyle can be challenging, especially if you share a household with someone who has not made the same commitment to change. Lifestyle changes are easier to implement and more fun when you can share both the challenges and the benefits with a friend or partner. In reading this book, you have already indicated your interest in slowing down the aging process. If you have a partner or a close friend who might share your interest in anti-aging, I encourage you to recruit him or her to join you in your quest. It can be a tremendous advantage for both of you.

THE ANTI-AGING DIET

The anti-aging diet is quite different from the dietary recommendations handed down by the federal government. The most obvious difference is that the anti-aging diet is far higher in protein—containing at least twice as much protein as the government's guidelines. As a result, the anti-aging diet is much lower in carbohydrates than the government's recommendations.

Although they may be the foundation of the government's food pyramid, starches do *not* form the basis of a healthy diet, for reasons that are discussed below. At the same time, I am not advocating an Atkins-style diet of unlimited bacon cheeseburgers, hold the buns. For anti-aging and disease prevention, you need a balance of protein, carbohydrates, and fats. Even more critical, however, is the *quality* of protein, carbohydrates, and fats in the diet.

The ideal anti-aging diet is made up of roughly equal parts lean protein, complex carbohydrates, and healthful fats. For the average person, consuming about 2,000 calories per day, this works out to about 700 calories of each per day. Because fat has more than twice as many calories per gram than carbohydrates and protein, this means about 175 grams each of protein and carbohydrates and about 75 grams of fat per day.

Having gone through the math, I want you to forget about it. I find that diets that ask you to count calories or carbohydrate or fat grams are difficult if not impossible to follow in the real world. Unless you are willing to carry a food scale and calorie counter around with you everywhere you go, it is simply not realistic. Perhaps you would be able to keep that up for a few weeks, at best. But the anti-aging diet is not a short-term regimen. It is, quite literally, a diet for *life*.

There's a simpler way to optimize your diet without being a slave to your calculator. The anti-aging diet can be summed up in just four basic principles:

1. Cut out sugar and refined carbohydrates.

2. Eat more lean protein.

3. Replace unhealthy fats with healthful fats.

4. Consume the widest possible variety of produce and plenty of it.

Following these principles consistently is far more important than concentrating on the mathematical precision of your diet. In fact, if you simply follow these guidelines, you will find that you will effortlessly approach the goals of the ideal anti-aging diet without counting every calorie or gram of fat.

Dietary Principle #1:
Reduce the Sugar

The excess consumption of sugar and refined carbohydrates is by far the most dangerous and damaging dietary habit of our modern culture. Sugar and refined carbohydrates (things made with white flour) are very quickly digested and absorbed, causing a sudden rise in blood sugar. This triggers the release of insulin from the pancreas to clear the sugar out of the blood and into cells.

The more sugar and refined carbohydrates you eat, the more insulin is pumped through your system. Insulin causes excess sugar to be converted into fat for storage in the body. In fact, a diet high in sugar and refined carbohydrates leads to obesity much more directly and much more quickly than a diet high in fat.

Over time, insulin has a corrosive effect on blood vessels, increasing your risk of heart disease. And after a while, the body begins to lose its sensitivity to insulin, meaning that it takes more and more insulin to regulate your blood sugar. This resistance to insulin often leads to full-blown diabetes.

As we have seen in previous chapters, high blood sugar also promotes the damaging processes of inflammation and glycation, impairs the immune response, and promotes disease. Eating sugar and refined carbohydrates further speeds the aging process by suppressing the release of growth hormone.

In addition to these toxic effects on your body's biochemistry, refined carbohydrates offer virtually no nutritional benefits and frequently displace other, more healthful foods from the diet. Those who eat the most sugar consume more calories overall, and at the same time have a far lower intake of important nutrients.

For all of these reasons, I consider the drastic reduction of sugars and refined carbohydrates to be the most important dietary change you can make. It is also one of the most challenging. Sugar can be a hard habit to break. The intake of sugar has increased steadily over the last hundred years, right along with the incidence of related diseases such as obesity, diabetes, and cancer. Today, the average American consumes a staggering 20 teaspoons of sugar per day, or about 64 pounds per year.

Finding Hidden Sugar

To reduce the amount of sugar in the diet, you need to learn where it lurks. Sweet foods such as candy, pastries, cookies, and cakes are all obvious sources of sugar and should be reduced or, better yet, eliminated. But sugar also hides in many processed foods, such as condiments, salad dressings, frozen entrees, crackers, and snack foods that you might not think of as sweet.

To reduce sugar, reduce the amount of processed and prepared foods you consume. Also take the time to read and compare labels, noting the presence of sugar (or any of its many aliases) in the first few ingredients. Corn syrup, glucose, dextrose, fructose, maltose, malt syrup, and rice syrup are all forms of sugar commonly found in processed foods. (Low-fat and fat-free foods are particularly likely to be high in sugar.)

"Natural" sugars such as honey, maple syrup, and fruit juice sweeteners may be less refined than white sugar, but they have the same effect on the body and also need to be used in moderation.

One-fifth of the sugar consumed in this country is in the form of soft drinks, fruit drinks, and other sweetened beverages. So-called vitamin waters, performance drinks, and fruit juices may seem like healthy choices but are little more than sugar-water and should be avoided.

Remember that alcohol is metabolized by the body as a sugar. Reducing alcoholic intake is frequently the key to an improved sense of well-being and enhanced mental clarity.

Replace Refined Flours with Whole Grains

To avoid the consequences of chronically high blood sugar, you must also avoid foods made with refined white flour. This includes most breads, pasta, couscous, tortillas, and crackers. Although they may not taste sweet, these refined carbohydrates are converted quickly to sugar in the body, producing the same damaging effects as sugary foods.

Whole-grain breads, crackers, and pasta are healthier than products made with white flour. Because they contain more fiber, they are converted into sugars much more slowly than their refined counterparts and offer sustained energy without causing unhealthy spikes in blood sugar. Whole grains (wheat berries, brown rice, quinoa, millet, etc.) or rolled grains (oats, spelt, kamut, etc.) are also excellent sources of lower-sugar, complex carbohydrates.

When reading package labels, be aware that "wheat flour" and "unbleached wheat flour" are both names for white flour. Even products labeled "whole-grain" or "whole-wheat" are often made with white flour as the main ingredient. Look for products that specify "100 percent whole grain" or "100 percent whole wheat."

Your intake of grain products (even whole grains) should be limited to about five servings a day. A serving is 1 slice of whole-grain bread or ½ cup of cooked whole grains (such as rice), or 1 cup of cooked rolled grains (such as oats).

Dietary Principle #2:
Eat Healthy Fats

The anti-aging diet is not a low-fat diet. In fact, you will be getting about a third of your daily calories from fat. The key is that the anti-aging diet emphasizes healthy monounsaturated fats and essential fatty acids while reducing unhealthy saturated and trans fatty acids.

There is no doubt that a high intake of saturated fats (the fats found in meat and dairy products) promotes the development of heart disease and increases the incidence of obesity, diabetes, and cancer.

Even more damaging are trans fatty acids. Trans fatty acids are unsaturated oils that are treated with hydrogen (hydrogenated) to create an artificially saturated fat. Trans fats act just like saturated fats, only worse.

In addition to raising bad LDL cholesterol, they also lower protective HDL cholesterol and interfere with the detoxifying actions of the liver. Those with the highest intake of trans fats have a higher risk of cancer.

But fat is not the enemy! Without enough fat in the diet, your body cannot absorb fat-soluble vitamins such as vitamins A, D, and E. Deficiencies of these nutrients will compromise the health of your eyes, bones, heart, brain, and other organs. You also need essential fatty acids in order for your cells to function properly. A deficiency of EFAs can quickly lead to health problems, including skin disorders, hair loss, joint pain, inflammation, and circulatory disorders and heart problems.

The vital importance of healthy dietary fats became painfully obvious following the emergence of the Pritikin Diet for heart patients. This extremely low-fat diet did succeed in lowering cholesterol and reducing arterial damage in cardiac patients. However, those following this restrictive diet quickly began to show symptoms of fatty acid and fat-soluble vitamin deficiency. They suffered from dry, itchy skin, joint pain, allergies, constipation, and other maladies. Although the diet reversed heart disease, these patients were still in poor health.

The ability of the Pritikin Diet to reverse heart disease was clearly due to the elimination of unhealthy fats from the diet. Pritikin's error, however, was to throw the baby out with the bathwater. A very low-fat diet is also very low in monounsaturated fats and essential fatty acids. These are the fats that maintain cell function, lower LDL cholesterol, prevent oxidation of cholesterol in the body, and reduce inflammation. You do not want to take these fats out of your diet.

Replacing Unhealthy Fats with Healthy Fats

Cultures such as the Japanese and Greeks eat a diet that is slightly higher in fat than the typical American diet, yet these cultures have much lower rates of obesity, heart disease, arthritis, and other ailments than their American counterpart. This suggests that the total percentage of fat in the diet is not the critical factor. Rather, it is the type of fat that is being consumed.

The Japanese, for example, get most of their fat from deep-sea fish, which is rich in anti-inflammatory omega-3 fatty acids. I recommend the same to you. Because all of the fat it contains is extremely beneficial, you can consume salmon in abundance, without concern over the fat or mercury content.

In addition to fresh fish, the Mediterranean diet also features lots of olives, olive oil, avocados, and nuts, all of which are rich in healthy monounsaturated fats. These are precisely the types of fats that are emphasized in the anti-aging diet. The more you can shift your diet away from saturated fats and toward these healthy fats, the better.

For the purposes of anti-aging and disease prevention, no amount of trans fatty acids is acceptable. All foods containing hydrogenated or partially hydrogenated oils should be avoided. This includes most shortening, crackers, microwave popcorn, margarines, mayonnaise, cookies, commercial peanut butters (as opposed to "natural, nothing added" brands), cereals, cake mixes, muffins, and so on.

As the dangers of trans fats have become more apparent, the government is now moving to require that manufacturers list the amount of trans fats on the food information label, along with the amount of saturated fat. The new labeling requirements will go into effect by 2006. In response to consumer demand, more manufacturers are also starting to produce products made with nonhydrogenated oils, so it is becoming a bit easier to avoid these damaging fats.

USING HEALTHY FATS

> Use olive oil or canola oil instead of butter, margarine, or shortening.
> Dress salads with olive oil, walnut oil, or flaxseed oil instead of bottled salad dressings.
> Enjoy heart-healthy nuts, olives, and avocados in moderation, instead of cheese, chips, and other fatty snacks, which are high in saturated or trans fatty acids.
> Choose very lean cuts of meat and low-fat or nonfat dairy products to reduce your intake of saturated fat.
> Do not eat fried foods or reuse heated oils. Heating oil to a high temperature creates trans fats. Instead, sauté, poach, bake, or steam foods.

Eat Fat to Lose Weight

Millions of Americans have learned the hard way that a low-fat diet is not an effective strategy for losing weight. Low-fat diets trigger a famine response in which the body actually increases its production of body fat to compensate for the shortage in dietary fat. To make things even worse, when people reduce the fat in their diets, they tend to replace it with refined carbohydrates. The low-fat foods that crowd the grocery store shelves are, on average, far higher in sugar than the regular foods they replace. And, as we have seen above, refined carbohydrates promote fat storage, not fat loss. The fact is that low-fat, high-carbohydrate diets are counterproductive to weight loss.

Eating healthy fats such as those outlined here will actually help to tune your fat-burning metabolism. Reducing refined carbohydrates and increasing your protein intake will also promote weight loss.

Dietary Principle #3:
Pump Up the Protein

An anti-aging diet must be high in protein. One of the characteristics of a youthful body is its ability to rebuild, regenerate, and repair itself. In order to rebuild cells, tissues, and organs, your body needs high-quality protein and lots of it.

My recommendation is for you to eat at least one-third of your calories as high-quality, lean protein. For the average person, this translates into about six servings of protein foods per day, plus a protein powder supplement that I'll discuss in a moment. Keep in mind, however, that a serving is equivalent to about 3 ounces of meat, which is approximately the size of a deck of cards. In other words, a restaurant-sized serving of meat or fish is likely to be two or three servings.

In addition to six servings of protein foods, I recommend a daily protein shake made with 2 scoops of whey protein powder. Whey protein powder (available in health food and nutrition stores) is an ideal protein source that also enhances the level of glutathione, an important cellular antioxidant. (See also Chapter 6.) The powder tastes best when blended with milk, fruit, or yogurt. A handheld blender or old-fashioned milkshake mixer is very handy for this.

Not only is it critical that you consume enough protein, but the source of protein is also extremely important. For long-term health and anti-aging benefits, you need to emphasize sources of protein which are low in saturated fats. Here is a list of various sources of protein, from the most healthful to the least desirable.

> Fish should be eaten at least three times a week. Wild Pacific salmon is your healthiest choice. (To minimize mercury exposure, avoid swordfish, king mackerel, and tilefish, and limit your consuption of tuna and bluefish to two servings per month.)

> Eggs and egg whites are an inexpensive, high-quality source of complete proteins. Contrary to popular notion, eating eggs does not raise your cholesterol levels, although the yolks do contain saturated fats. Some growers are now using feed that enhances the omega-3 fatty acid content of eggs, which improves their nutrient value.

> Lean chicken, turkey, or Cornish game hens (white meat only, no skin) from organically raised animals. Wild game birds (pheasant, grouse, etc.) contain less saturated fat and more healthy fats than livestock animals.

> Lean cuts of beef or pork from organically raised animals. Meat from venison, buffalo, and other game animals contains less saturated fat and more healthy fats than meat from livestock animals.

> Low-fat, organic dairy foods (milk, yogurt, kefir, cottage cheese, and cheeses made with skim milk) are a moderately good source of protein and also provide calcium. Limit your intake of cheeses that are high in saturated fat, however. This includes hard cheeses such as cheddar and soft cheeses such as Brie.

> Beans and legumes are good-quality protein but have less protein per ounce than meats. You would have to eat an awful lot of beans

and legumes to get the recommended amount of protein if these were your only source. I recommend that you enjoy beans and legumes in place of carbohydrates, rather than in place of protein foods.

> Not recommended: smoked meats, bacon, ham, sausages, and cold cuts. These should be eliminated from your diet. Most are quite high in saturated fat and contain harmful nitrites and nitrates. Try to avoid meats cooked at very high temperatures (barbecued, grilled, or fried). Cooking meats at high temperatures creates harmful compounds that promote inflammation and accelerate aging in the tissues of the body.

A Word About Vegetarianism

People embrace vegetarianism for a number of reasons, which may include moral, ethical, religious, and environmental issues. But when a patient tells me that he or she is vegetarian for health reasons, I feel compelled to point out that a strict vegetarian (vegan) diet may not be the healthiest diet for humans and is not ideal for an anti-aging regimen.

Animal protein sources contain specific nutrients that our bodies need in order to function optimally, including B vitamins, and important amino acids such as carnosine, methionine, taurine, and carnitine, all of which are scarce in vegetable sources.

Although it is possible to compensate for most of these nutrients in a vegetarian diet, it takes careful planning and effort. Many vegetarians are, in fact, deficient in protein, B vitamins, calcium, selenium, essential fatty acids, and other nutrients, *even when they take nutritional supplements.*

Lacto-ovo-vegetarians, who consume eggs and dairy products, are much more likely to get adequate protein and B vitamins. Those who include fish as well as eggs and dairy products in their diet will also get valuable omega-3 fatty acids.

292 Individualizing Your Anti-Aging Program

Dietary Principle #4:
Eat More Red, Yellow, and Green Foods

In its "Five a Day" campaign, the government has recognized that the incidence of many of today's most deadly diseases would be slashed if Americans would eat more fruits and vegetables. Fruits and vegetables offer a disease-fighting triple whammy. They are high in antioxidants, fiber, and disease-fighting phytochemicals. All of these nutrients are known to offer powerful protection against disease.

Calorie for calorie, fresh vegetables contain more nutrients than any other kind of food. The incredible variety of produce available today presents a bounty of colorful, flavorful choices that offer something for every palate. But Americans are still only managing to eat a measly three servings a day, and most of those are in the form of high-fat french-fried potatoes.

My personal prescription is for you to eat at least six servings of fresh (not fried) vegetables each and every day. This may seem like a daunting task, but remember that a serving of vegetables is only ½ cup of hard vegetables (carrots, squash, etc.) or 1 cup of leafy greens. A good-sized mixed green salad, for example, can provide three servings at a single sitting.

In addition, eat two or three servings of whole fruit (not fruit juice) each and every day. Whole fruits are preferable to fruit juices because the fiber in the fruit serves to slow the absorption of sugar into the bloodstream. Combining fruits with foods that contain protein and/or healthy fats also helps keep blood sugar steadier by slowing the absorption of the natural sugars in fruits. Apples, for example, can be combined with peanut butter or low-fat cottage cheese. You'll find that you stay satisfied for longer because the increase in blood sugar will be more gradual and sustained.

PRODUCE PICKS

➤ As a rule of thumb, the more brightly colored the vegetables, the more valuable they are nutritionally. Spinach, for example, contains more nutrients than iceberg lettuce, and pink grapefruit is higher in phytonutrients than white grapefruit.

➤ To ensure the most comprehensive intake of beneficial phytochemicals, eat the widest possible variety of fruits and vegetables. In particular, try to be sure that all the "stoplight" colors are represented in your diet: red (tomatoes, red peppers, strawberries, watermelon), yellow (mango, pineapple, carrots, squash, cantaloupe, grapefruit), and green (spinach, broccoli, cabbage, kale, beans).

➤ Avoid white potatoes, which are converted into sugar very quickly. In fact, a boiled red potato will cause a rise in blood sugar similar to the effects of straight table sugar. Sweet potatoes, despite their name, do not raise blood sugar as quickly, and also contain far more beta-carotene.

➤ Choose seasonal, local produce, and buy organic whenever possible. Organically grown vegetables not only are higher in nutrients but also reduce your exposure to pesticides, fungicides, artificial fertilizers, and other toxic chemicals used in conventional agriculture.

➤ When fresh produce is not available, frozen vegetables, which generally contain more nutrients than canned, are the next best choice. Canned tomatoes are a notable exception. In fact, the cancer-fighting compound in tomatoes (lycopene) is actually enhanced through the cooking process, especially when cooked in oil.

➤ Don't forget fresh herbs as a valuable and delicious source of antioxidants and other nutrients. Oregano, thyme, sage, and rosemary are all known for their antioxidant activity. Turmeric and ginger contain natural anti-inflammatory compounds. Chives, onions, leeks, and garlic all contain valuable sulfur-containing phytochemicals that fight free radical activity and protect against cancer, especially of the stomach.

Anti-Aging Diet Recommendations at a Glance

Food type	Daily servings	One serving equals:
Protein	6	3 ounces fish (fatty fish such as salmon and tuna also provide 1 serving of healthy fat) 3 ounces meat or chicken 1 large egg 1 cup low-fat milk, yogurt, kefir, or buttermilk ½ cup low-fat cottage cheese or skim ricotta ¼ cup skim mozzarella or string cheese 1 cup beans or legumes
Whole grains, legumes	5	1 cup cooked oats or whole-grain cereal 1 cup beans or legumes ½ cup cooked brown rice 1 slice whole-grain bread or ½ large whole-wheat pita pocket ½ cup whole-wheat pasta
Vegetables	6	½ cup carrots, beans, peppers, tomatoes, broccoli, etc. 1 cup raw spinach, lettuce, or mesclun mix 1 cup cooked kale or collard greens ½ cup sweet potato or baked winter squash
Fruits	2	1 orange, apple, banana, or pear 1 cup berries, cherries, or grapes 1 cup melon, pineapple, or mango
Healthy fats	4–5	1 tablespoon olive, canola, walnut, or flaxseed oil ½ small avocado ¼ cup nuts 2 tablespoons peanut butter or other nut butter ¼ cup sunflower or pumpkin seeds 3 ounces salmon or other fatty fish (also counts as 1 serving of protein)

Putting It All Together

As you make the transition to the anti-aging diet, you will probably need to do a bit of label reading to guard against excess sugar, saturated fat, and trans fats. But you don't have to weigh and measure every mouthful of food. You can transform your diet into the ideal anti-aging diet without a lot of muss and fuss, simply by following the four dietary principles and the serving guidelines listed on page 294.

Below is an example of what a typical day on the anti-aging diet might include. But don't feel limited to the suggestions here. The guidelines are flexible enough to accommodate every lifestyle, region, and palate. Your menu can be as simple or as gourmet as you choose. Be creative and enjoy yourself.

Remember that every step you take toward the goal is a valuable and beneficial step in the right direction. Also keep in mind that a small change that you stick with for the long term can make a bigger difference than a big change that lasts only a day or two.

Breakfast
  Large bowl oatmeal
  ½ grapefruit
  1 soft-boiled egg

Morning Snack
  Protein shake with 2 scoops whey powder, 1 cup yogurt, and 1 cup
    berries

Lunch
  1 large mixed salad with tomatoes, peppers, etc., topped with
    3 ounces chicken breast and dressed with olive oil and vinegar
  ½ whole-wheat pita

Afternoon Snack
  Guacamole made with ½ mashed avocado and ¼ cup salsa
  Baked corn tortilla chips

Dinner
   Large piece of salmon baked with lemon and chives
   Steamed brown rice
   Spinach sautéed in olive oil and garlic

Evening Snack
   ½ cup baby carrots with 2 tablespoons natural peanut butter or
   ¼ cup hummus

If You Are Overweight

If you are overweight, you already know that it is very important to achieve a healthy weight. Excess weight promotes disease and aging and is fast becoming one of the leading causes of death and disability in this country. But chances are good that you have tried to lose weight, probably more than once.

The good news is that the anti-aging diet outlined here, along with the entire anti-aging program (exercise, supplements, hormone balancing, etc.), will naturally promote fat loss and weight loss, if needed. The different elements of the program work together synergistically to optimize your health and your weight. Enhanced nutrition will increase your physical and mental sense of well-being. Elevated mood and energy levels will enable a more active lifestyle. More youthful hormone profiles will shift your metabolism away from fat storage and toward building lean muscle tissue, and so on.

Most of my patients lose 5 to 10 pounds of excess fat simply by implementing the anti-aging program. It is not at all uncommon for people following this program to lose 25 or 30 pounds over the course of a year, without any attempt to diet or lose weight.

If, however, you still have weight to lose, you may need to reduce your intake of food by 15 to 20 percent until you reach a healthy weight. Follow the guidelines and maintain the proportions of the anti-aging diet (one-third lean protein, one-third complex carbohydrate, and one-third healthy fat). Simply cut out one serving per day of grains, proteins, and healthy fats. There is no need to reduce the amount of fruits and vegetables. Eliminate all alcoholic beverages and add more activity to your life (see Exercise, below.)

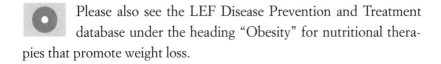 Please also see the LEF Disease Prevention and Treatment database under the heading "Obesity" for nutritional therapies that promote weight loss.

EXERCISE SMARTER, NOT HARDER

I can't overemphasize how important regular exercise is to the success of your anti-aging program. Some of the benefits of exercise, such as the improvement in heart and lung function, simply cannot be achieved in any other way. Exercise also greatly enhances the benefits of hormone replacement and other supplements—and vice versa. The combination of exercise and anti-aging supplements is far more effective in reducing body fat, increasing muscle tone, and creating a more youthful appearance than either approach alone.

One of the many benefits of exercise is that it tends to increase libido and sexual function in both men and women. There is no reason for sexual desire or activity to decline with age. In fact, researchers have documented that those who continue to have active sex lives as they get older are consistently healthier and younger-looking than those who do not. Simply stated, sex is anti-aging, and those who exercise more tend to have more active sexual lives.

The number one reason people give for not exercising is that they don't have enough time. It is best to exercise on a daily or near daily basis, but you don't have to sweat for an hour at a time in order to get the anti-aging benefits of exercise. In fact, exercising too hard or for too long is counterproductive. Not only is it time-consuming and injury-promoting, but extended endurance training is not the best way to build up your strength or stamina. (Surprisingly, it's also not the best way to burn fat.)

Symptoms of Aging	Benefits of Exercise
• Decline in heart function	• Improved heart function
• Decline in lung function	• Improved lung function
• Loss of bone density	• Increased bone density
• Increase in body fat	• Reduced body fat
• Decreased flexibility	• Decreased joint pain
• Loss of muscle mass	• Improved muscle strength and tone
• Decline in glucose tolerance (risk for diabetes)	• Improved glucose tolerance
• Decline in sex drive and performance	• Improved libido and sexual function
Decline in growth hormone Slow metabolism	Reduced blood pressure Reduced cholesterol Reduced anxiety, stress

The Efficiency Trap

The body is a highly adaptive piece of machinery. When it is repeatedly presented with the same challenge, it will adapt to allow it to meet the challenge with less effort. This is what I call the efficiency trap. Because of the body's adaptive responses, long-duration exercise, such as long-distance running or biking, actually works against the goals of an anti-aging exercise program.

Over time, exercise sessions that involve intense and sustained effort for periods longer than forty-five minutes will actually encourage your heart, lungs, and muscles to become smaller. This allows them to expend less energy during long bouts of activity. So instead of burning more calories, the body becomes more efficient and burns fewer. And while they might be able to go for hours using relatively little energy, a smaller heart and lungs have less reserve capacity. This means they are less able to respond to a sudden extraordinary demand for effort.

And instead of reducing excess fat deposits, long-duration exercise actually causes the body to increase the production and storage of fat. This may sound paradoxical, but it's true. Your body will do exactly what you train it to do. And long-duration exercise trains your body to store fat. Here's why.

When you exert yourself, your body initially uses carbohydrates to fuel your muscles. But after about fifteen minutes of strenuous activity, that energy supply is depleted. At that point, the body will be forced to tap into its energy stores, converting fat into fuel for the duration of the activity.

Ironically, although burning fat may be your goal, your body does not necessarily see this as a good thing. The body is programmed to hoard energy (fat) as a hedge against starvation. No matter how much fat you may have in storage, whenever your body is forced to tap into these energy stores, it sounds the alarm that famine may be at hand.

So if you exercise for long periods of time on a daily basis, your body will step up the production and storage of body fat to compensate for the amount of fat being burned through repeated, long-duration exercise—regardless of how much excess fat you may have to burn.

But marathon runners are awfully thin, you might be thinking. It's true, people who exercise intensely for many hours every day burn an enormous amount of calories. As a result, they may be quite thin. They are not necessarily lean, however. For one thing, as we have just seen, their bodies are working hard to replace all of the fat that they burn. Second, after forty-five minutes of hard exercise, the body actually begins to cannibalize its own muscle tissue as an energy source, instead of fat. And so, although they may be very thin, long-distance runners may actually have a higher percentage of body fat (and lower percentage of lean muscle) than people who use interval and resistance training.

More to the point, few of us have the time or inclination to exercise for hours a day. In truth, the vast majority of Americans find it difficult to find time for any exercise at all. That's why it's imperative that an exercise program deliver maximal strengthening and fat-burning benefits in the least amount of time.

The Power of Interval Training

Interval training is a way of working around the body's adaptive response to sustained exercise. By avoiding the efficiency trap, interval training maximizes your calorie and fat burn. It is a more effective way to increase the strength and aerobic capacity of your heart and lungs. Best of all, it takes only twenty to thirty minutes a day.

Instead of exercising for long periods of time, you will alternate short bursts of intense effort with short periods of recovery. Your body will, of course, adapt to this challenge as well. But interval training causes the body to adapt in a much more beneficial way. Instead of creating smaller and more efficient organs, interval training develops the capacity of the heart and lungs to work harder and more powerfully.

Over the long term, interval training also promotes fat burning instead of fat storage. A brief session of interval training uses the carbohydrates available in the muscle for energy instead of tapping into fat stores. This means you will actually burn less fat *during* exercise than you would if you exercised for longer. However, you will also avoid triggering your body's fat-hoarding survival instinct.

Instead, interval training steps up your fat-burning metabolism in the hours *following* exercise. Instead of storing more fat as a response to endurance training, you will continue to burn fat and calories at a higher rate for up to sixteen hours following an interval training session. In fact, studies have shown that those who use interval training burn *up to nine times more fat* than those who burn the same number of calories doing sustained moderate-intensity exercise.

How to Do Interval Training

Tennis and racquetball are ideal interval training sports because they alternate short bursts of activity with recovery periods. Walking, running, biking, swimming, and other endurance sports can all be easily adapted to interval training. You will need a stopwatch or sports watch until you get the feel for the intervals.

Begin by warming up at a moderate pace for five minutes to bring blood into the heart and muscles and to lubricate the joints. When you feel warm and your heartbeat and breathing are slightly accelerated, you are ready to begin your intervals.

The technique is to alternate two-minute sprints with one to two minutes of recovery. The sprint intervals should be at about 80 to 90 percent of your maximum possible exertion. In other words, you will walk, jog, run, swim, row, or bike just about as hard or fast as you can, but just for two short minutes. Then you will back off the pace and recover for one to two minutes. Your recovery intervals should be at 40 to 50 percent of maximum possible exertion. In other words, you want to slow down enough to catch your breath, but keep moving. By the end of your recovery interval, you should be ready for another sprint.

Simply alternate sprint and recovery intervals for a total of twenty minutes. Your workout will be finished before you even realize you have broken a sweat. Many treadmills, stationary bikes, stair steppers, and other types of fitness equipment have a preprogrammed interval training option which automatically changes the speed, resistance, or incline of the machine in order to increase and decrease the intensity during the workout. Done on a daily basis, twenty minutes of interval training is all it takes to get fit and turn up your fat-burning metabolism. In addition to being very time-efficient, interval training also reduces the risk of exercise-related injuries.

Anyone, at any level of fitness or stamina, can effectively use interval training because the exertion level is completely relative. Whether your sprint pace is a five-minute mile or a fast walk, as long as you are pushing yourself close to *your* maximum exertion during your sprint intervals, you will reap the benefits.

If you are someone who really enjoys long-distance running, biking, or other endurance sports, this doesn't mean that you necessarily need to stop doing these activities. But you can and should still use interval training as a part of your daily training. Instead of maintaining a steady pace for the entire distance, build some sprint and recovery intervals

IS ARTHRITIS OR JOINT PAIN
PREVENTING YOU FROM EXERCISING?

Many people find it difficult to exercise because of pain or stiffness in their knees, hips, shoulders, and back due to osteoarthritis. Ironically, exercise is one of the most effective ways to relieve and prevent pain and loss of flexibility from osteoarthritis. Many arthritis sufferers find that swimming or water aerobics allow them to exercise without pain. Regular exercise of this sort may even allow you to "graduate" to other forms of pain-free exercise.

Strength training (discussed below) also helps to strengthen the muscles, tendons, and ligaments that support joints, thereby reducing pain. Be sure as well to stretch regularly (discussed below) to increase and maintain your flexibility and range of motion.

Finally, nutritional supplementation can help reduce joint pain and inflammation. In addition to the anti-inflammatory nutrients discussed in Chapter 7, consider taking joint-supportive nutrients such as glucosamine, chondroitin, and/or methylsulfonylmethane (MSM) in the following amounts:

Glucosamine sulfate: 1,000–1,500 mg per day

Chondroitin sulfate: 800–1,200 mg per day

MSM: 3–10 g per day, as tolerated

These nutrients help to stimulate the production of fresh cartilage in the joint, relieving pain. Keep in mind that it may take up to twelve weeks to see the maximum benefit from this protocol.

 Please see also the LEF Disease Prevention and Treatment database under the heading of "Arthritis."

into your workouts. This will help you to build a larger, stronger, and more resilient heart and lungs. It will also help you increase your overall speed and power by building larger muscles.

The Importance of Strength Training

Interval training will help strengthen your heart and lungs, improve your circulation and blood chemistry, and release feel-good endorphins. But in addition to the aerobic conditioning you get from interval training, you also need to do some sort of strength or resistance training to build and maintain muscle strength.

Strength training not only makes you stronger, it will also make you leaner. Because muscle tissue burns far more calories at rest than other types of tissue, strength training is one of the most effective ways to increase your calorie- and fat-burning metabolism.

Strength training also offers a host of anti-aging benefits.

> Strength training increases the production of testosterone in the body. At the same time, the fat-reducing benefits of strength training can reduce the amount of circulating estrogen in the body. (Fat cells store and manufacture estrogen in both men and women.) The net result is a more favorable testosterone/estrogen balance, which, as discussed in Chapter 3, is important for men and women alike.

> Exercise can also reduce cortisol levels, which enhances the ratio of anti-aging DHEA to cortisol (see Chapter 2 for details on why this is so important).

> Exercise helps to lower blood sugar by using the blood glucose as fuel for the muscles. Strength training also helps to improve your body's sensitivity to insulin by increasing the number of insulin receptors in the muscle tissue.

> Strength training helps to maintain bone density and mass, which helps to decrease the risk of osteoporosis later in life.

> By strengthening the ligaments, tendons, and muscles that support the joints, strength training can decrease or prevent joint pain and preserve flexibility.

How to Do Strength Training Effectively

Strength or resistance training can be done with free weights or machines, or any other form of resistance, such as weighted cuffs, rubber resistance bands, or tubes. You can even use the weight of your own body, as with push-ups, chin-ups, lunges, and dips. But in order to be effective, you must use enough weight or resistance to fatigue the muscle.

There are a lot of misconceptions about strength training. Women, in particular, often fear that working with weights will cause them to bulk up. Many believe that using very light weights and doing a lot of repetitions will "tone" without building muscle. Not only is this approach very time-consuming, but it accomplishes almost nothing.

As any skinny adolescent boy can attest, the fact is that bulking up is very difficult to do. Men or women who want to be bodybuilders have to spend many hours a week lifting very heavy weights, following rigid diets, and (usually) enhancing the effects with amino acids and other body-building supplements. Big muscles are simply not something that happens by accident.

When done correctly, strength training will tighten and sculpt the muscles of your body and burn away excess body fat. But contrary to popular misconceptions, strength training makes most people *smaller,* not bigger. This is because a pound of muscle takes up only one-fifth the space taken up by a pound of fat.

Train to Fatigue

In order to get the many benefits of strength training, you have to challenge your muscles in a very specific way. If you can repeat any strength training exercise more than twelve times, you are not using enough resistance or weight. Increase the resistance until you find that the ninth or tenth repetition is difficult to complete. To increase the difficulty without increasing the resistance, you can also increase the time your muscles spend under tension by slowing your movements down and not allowing the muscles to relax in between repetitions.

The good news is that when you use enough resistance to fatigue the muscle, one set of eight to ten repetitions is all you need to do. You can easily work all the major muscles in the body in about twenty minutes.

And while aerobic interval training should be done five or six days a week, you can get the benefits of resistance training in only two sessions a week. (Take at least one day off between sessions.)

You can do strength training in a health club or in your home, with an instructor, with a videotape, or on your own if you are more experienced. Pilates classes also focus on building strength, using external resistance or just the weight of your body to build muscle tone. If you have never done strength training, I highly recommend that you invest in a few sessions with a personal trainer to learn how to do strength training correctly. The better your form, the better your results will be and the lower your risk of injury.

Ironically, when you use good form, you will probably need less weight to fatigue the muscle, because proper form will more effectively isolate the muscle you are trying to train. But you will get far more benefit from lifting slightly less weight with good form than you will from lifting more weight with poor form. Ultimately, the amount of resistance doesn't matter. What matters is that the (correct) muscle is fatigued when you finish your set. As you become more experienced, books or fitness magazines can be an excellent resource for expanding your repertoire of training routines and techniques.

Keep It Challenging

As we have seen, exercise is an adaptive activity. The body changes in response to the demands of exercise. Therefore, the same activity will become less and less challenging over time. As exercise becomes less challenging, it also becomes less effective. Therefore, it's important to continue to challenge yourself in order to continue to reap benefits from the time you spend exercising.

For interval training, this means that both your sprint and recovery speeds should increase as you become more fit. You may cover more distance in the same amount of time as you get stronger. You do not, however, have to increase the total amount of time you spend exercising.

When engaging in strength training, continue to increase the resistance whenever the current level ceases to fatigue the muscle after eight to twelve repetitions. Increasing the number of repetitions will not be nearly as effective as increasing the resistance.

Maintain Flexibility

Flexibility is a use-it-or-lose-it sort of thing. Unless you make an effort to maintain your flexibility, you will become less and less flexible as you get older. This greatly increases your risk of injury and discomfort and makes it increasingly difficult to exercise and do other things you enjoy.

You can maintain your flexibility by doing simple stretches on a daily basis. Contrary to what you may have heard in the past, the best time to stretch is at the *end* of your daily exercise routine, when your muscles, tendons, and ligaments are warm and lubricated. Stretching can help to relax your body and your muscles after a workout and also facilitates muscle recovery and development. If you also like to stretch before your workout, be sure you first warm up your body with five to ten minutes of moderate activity, such as brisk walking. Stretching when the muscles are cold can lead to muscle pulls and tears.

When the muscles are warm, stretch your legs, arms, shoulders, torso, and spine, using gentle reaching, bending, and twisting movements. Extend each stretch until you feel a light resistance and then hold without bouncing. Breathe deeply and try to deepen your stretch slightly on each exhalation. After fifteen to twenty seconds, release the stretch and rest in a neutral position before continuing with the next stretch.

Yoga tapes or classes are a wonderful way to increase your strength and flexibility. As an added benefit, yoga frequently incorporates physical and mental relaxation exercises that help to reduce the aging effects of stress hormones. Some types of yoga, often called power yoga, can also provide a terrific aerobic workout as well.

The following table shows an example of how the various components of an anti-aging exercise program can all be incorporated into a varied weekly routine. You can, of course, freely substitute your own favorite activities for the ones listed here, as long as you are getting twenty minutes of interval training, involving some high-intensity intervals, on most days of the week, along with regular strength training and daily stretching for flexibility.

A SEVEN-DAY EXERCISE PLAN

Monday	1. Warm up with 5 minutes of brisk walking. 2. Speed-walk, jog, or run through the neighborhood or on a track for 20 minutes, alternating between sprint and recovery intervals. Make sure your sprint pace is intense enough that you are fatigued by the end of each sprint. 3. Stretch for 5 to 10 minutes.
Tuesday	1. Warm up on a treadmill or stationary bike for 5 minutes at low- to medium-intensity effort. 2. Use a stationary bike or stair stepper for 20 minutes, using the interval training program. Be sure the intensity is high enough that you are fatigued at the end of each high-intensity interval. 3. Do 10 minutes of weight training focusing on arms, back, and shoulders. Use enough weight to fatigue the muscles. 4. Finish with stretching exercises for 5 to 10 minutes.
Wednesday	1. Warm up with 5 minutes of light jogging. 2. Play 45 minutes of basketball, soccer, tennis, or racquetball. Play hard! Run for the ball. 3. Do stretching exercises for 5 to 10 minutes.
Thursday	1. Warm up with 5 minutes of light- to moderate-intensity activity. 2. Swim laps for 20 minutes, alternating intervals of high- and low-intensity effort. Push yourself as hard as you can during the sprint intervals. 3. Do 15 minutes of resistance exercise using water weights, focusing on legs, buttocks, and abdomen. Use enough resistance to fatigue the muscles. 4. Finish with stretching exercises for 5 to 10 minutes.
Friday	Take the day off! Enjoy a leisurely walk and some gentle stretching before bed.
Saturday	1. Warm up with 5 minutes of light activity. 2. Take a 20- to 30-minute bike ride on hilly terrain. Try not to slow down on the hills. If it's very flat where you live, build in intervals by alternating high-speed sprints with moderate-speed recovery intervals. 3. Do a 30-minute yoga tape.
Sunday	1. Warm up with 5 minutes of low to moderate activity. 2. Canoe, kayak, or row for 30 minutes. Be sure to alternate intervals of very intense effort with intervals of moderate effort. 3. Complete the workout with stretching exercises for 5 to 10 minutes.

It may take you a while to work up to this amount of exercise, and that is perfectly all right. If you are already exercising two or three days a week, you can probably work up to my exercise recommendations within a few weeks or months. If you don't exercise at all, it may take you six months or more to gradually build up your stamina and enthusiasm for regular exercise. Take it gradually and try to keep it fun.

Remember that shorter, more frequent exercise is much more beneficial (and easier to fit in to your life) than longer, infrequent sessions. Start by trying to engage in some sort of vigorous activity at least six days a week, even if it is only for five or ten minutes. Once you are in the habit of exercising daily, you can more easily increase the intensity and duration of your sessions until you reach the goals I have set for you.

Even committed exercisers occasionally go through periods of time when they are simply too busy to fit it all in. When this happens to you, try not to fall off the wagon entirely. Again, remember that short, frequent sessions, even ten minutes a day, are far more beneficial than a weekly (or monthly) blow-out and make it easier to get back into your regular schedule when the crunch is over.

TIPS FOR GETTING THE MOST OUT OF EXERCISE

1. Exercise on an empty stomach (no food two hours prior) to support the exercise-induced release of growth hormone.
2. For a very efficient workout that combines interval training with strength training, alternate two-minute bursts of intense aerobic activity (jumping rope or stationary biking, for example) with two minutes of strength training exercises, using these as your recovery intervals.
3. Doing a variety of different kinds of exercise (cross-training) will reduce injury and boredom and will increase your strength and stamina. Try different workouts on different days, alternating biking and swimming, for example.
4. Recreational activities such as hiking, canoeing, volleyball,

dancing, or even vigorous gardening (raking, hoeing) can be counted toward your weekly exercise goal of six aerobic workouts, as long as the activity incorporates brief intervals of intense exertion. Just as you want your muscles to be fatigued after strength training, you want your body to be fatigued by the end of each sprint interval.

! Some discomfort while exercising is normal, particularly if you have not been exercising regularly. Pain is not normal and, contrary to popular notions, does not lead to improvement. If something hurts, or you feel dizzy or very short of breath, slow down or stop. If you have chronic or serious medical conditions, check with your physician before beginning any new program of exercise.

COUNTERING THE AGING EFFECTS OF STRESS

In Chapter 2, we discussed in great detail the aging and disease-promoting effects that stress can have on the body. Supplemental DHEA can do a lot to compensate for the negative effects of stress on the body. But using DHEA as an antidote to a stressful life is not enough. As I emphasized in the opening of this chapter, to effectively combat aging, we can't just throw pills at the problem. We must combine supplementation and hormone replacement with meaningful changes in lifestyle and habits. In this case, that means making stress reduction and relaxation a priority in your life.

Many people consider the time they spend watching television to be their "relaxation" time. And judging by the number of hours the average American spends in front of the television, we ought to be the most relaxed nation on earth. But watching television has no beneficial effects on stress hormones, and some research indicates that it may have negative effects on brain function and hormone levels. Sleep, while it has restorative effects (discussed below), is also not the equivalent of relaxation.

The type of relaxation that has beneficial effects on the body is usually achieved through a focused and intentional practice such as meditation, yoga, or breathing exercises. A relaxation practice does not need to be lengthy, difficult, or complex to be effective. A wide variety of mind-body disciplines, including various forms of yoga, meditation, prayer, and tai chi, have been shown in medical studies to reduce the effects of stress on our bodies. Artistic and creative endeavors, including writing, drawing, painting, music, and dancing, are also effective stress reduction tools.

Specifically, studies have demonstrated that meditation and yoga can lower cortisol and raise DHEA levels. Relaxation and stress reduction techniques have also been shown to improve immune response, decrease pain, alleviate depression, and lower blood pressure.

Some stress reduction techniques are purely physical and/or mental, but many incorporate a spiritual aspect as well. If you have a spiritual practice that is meaningful to you, chances are that you came to it for reasons other than its anti-aging benefits. But a daily spiritual practice can pay additional dividends in terms of its strictly physiological effects on your body. Stress researchers working under Dr. Herbert Benson at Harvard University have found that heartfelt prayer (regardless of the spiritual or religious orientation of the subject) is one of the most effective methods of reversing the effects of stress on the body.

There are research centers around the country that have focused on documenting the medical and hormonal effects of stress reduction programs. Some of these offer on-site programs as well as a variety of instructional books and tapes (see box). As they have become more and more popular, yoga, meditation, tai chi, and other classes can now be found in virtually every locality. Any one of these practices can vastly increase your quality of life. Check with local health clubs, hospitals, wellness centers, dance and movement studios, and yoga centers for offerings.

Try several disciplines, if necessary, to find one that suits your personality and lifestyle. The goal is to find something that you can fit into your life on a daily basis. Even a few minutes of focused stress reduction every day is a powerful way to slow the aging process and prevent disease. It can also offer personal and spiritual benefits that extend far beyond the specific realm of stress-related illness.

RESEARCH CENTERS AND
STRESS REDUCTION PROGRAMS

Center for Mindfulness in Medicine, Health Care, and Society
55 Lake Avenue
North Worcester, MA 01605
Phone: 508-856-2000
E-mail: mindfulness@umassmed.edu
Web site: www.umassmed.edu/cfm/

Now part of the University of Massachusetts Medical School, the Center for Mindfulness is an outgrowth of the original Stress Reduction Clinic founded by Jon Kabat-Zinn and featured on Bill Moyers's PBS series *Healing and the Mind*. The center sponsors research and also offers retreats and other stress reduction programs. You can purchase stress reduction tapes and books through the site as well.

The Mind/Body Medical Institute
824 Boylston Street
Chestnut Hill, MA 02467
Phone: 617-991-0102
Toll free: 866-509-0732
E-mail: MBMI@caregroup.harvard.edu
Web site: www.mbmi.org

Founded by Herbert Benson, M.D., the Mind/Body Medical Institute is affiliated with Harvard University Medical School. The Institute sponsors and publishes research, and it also provides outpatient medical services, training for health professionals, and corporate and school-based programs. The Web site includes extensive re-search and references as well as an online store of books, audio-, and videotapes.

The Institute of HeartMath
14700 West Park Avenue
Boulder Creek, CA 95006
Phone: 831-338-8500
E-mail: info@heartmath.org
Web site: www.heartmath.org

The Institute of HeartMath has researched and developed several novel techniques for managing the biological stress response. Published research demonstrated substantial reductions of cortisol and increases in DHEA in subjects employing a HeartMath technique called Cut-Thru. The institute offers a variety of programs and re-treats for individuals, families, and corporate groups. The Web site details their research and techniques and offers a variety of programs by audio- and videotape.

SLEEP AND AGING

A couple of years ago, researchers at the University of Chicago took a group of healthy, college-age men and kept them up until one o'clock in the morning every night for six nights, waking them up each morning at five. After just six nights of sleep deprivation (sleeping only four hours a night), these young men, all in their early 20s, had cortisol levels typical of men in their 60s.

In other words, your body perceives the lack of sleep as stress and responds by producing stress chemicals. With an understanding of the relationship between cortisol and aging, discussed in Chapter 2, you can fully appreciate the significance of these findings. The development of cortisol-driven diseases (high blood pressure, diabetes, obesity, memory loss, etc.) can be significantly hastened by chronic sleep loss.

A very large study of over seventy thousand nurses, for example, found that nurses who slept from five to seven hours per night had more heart attacks than their colleagues who averaged eight hours.

Chronic stress—and this includes inadequate sleep—is aging and disease promoting. You may feel that you can fit more into every day by sleeping less. But ultimately you will fit more into your life by living longer. If you are serious about an anti-aging and life-extension program, getting sufficient sleep is a priority.

If you have difficulty waking up when the alarm goes off, or find yourself fighting sleepiness in the middle of the day or early evening, this is a sign that you are under-rested. You may need to go to bed earlier each night in order to be fully rested by the time you have to get up.

Steps to Better Sleep

If you are setting aside enough time for sleep but are not able to sleep, you are not alone. Here are some of the things I've found to be most helpful for my patients who have difficulties with occasional or chronic insomnia.

1. In general, vitamins tend to be stimulating, while minerals are lightly sedating. Take your vitamins in the morning and any additional mineral supplements at night.

2. Baths with Epsom salts can also help to promote sleep. The salts contain high amounts of magnesium, which is absorbed through the skin. Use several handfuls of Epsom salts in a bath of warm water and soak for fifteen to twenty minutes.

3. Exercising in the evening can create a surge of stimulating hormones that makes it difficult to fall asleep. If possible, exercise in the morning or afternoon.

4. If your hormone regimen calls for progesterone, take this hormone in the evening, as it tends to be sedating.

5. Melatonin is a hormone produced by the pineal gland that can help to induce sleep. The pineal gland regulates the body's circadian rhythms (the synchronization of our sleep/wake cycles with day and night). In cases of insomnia due to jet lag, melatonin can help by resynchronizing the sleep cycle. Published studies have found that melatonin increases the speed of falling asleep, the duration of sleep, and the quality of sleep. As a safe and effective sleeping aid, take 3 mg of melatonin at bedtime.

MAKING IT STICK

If you've ever failed to keep a New Year's resolution past the first few weeks of January, you know that deciding to make a change for the better is fairly easy, but making those changes permanent is often difficult. Embarking on a serious anti-aging and life extension program can present the same challenge. No doubt you are feeling quite enthusiastic about the prospect of living longer and looking and feeling more youthful. You are probably very motivated to start your anti-aging program and begin reaping the benefits.

It's not uncommon for people to begin an anti-aging program with great enthusiasm, only to find that six months later, they've all but reverted to their previous habits. The program we've outlined here is ambitious and may involve some fairly big changes in your daily routines. Being prepared for lapses in focus and motivation can help you to overcome them.

Start Low, Go Slow

My advice to you is to incorporate the program gradually, instead of in one mighty burst of enthusiasm that may fade once the novelty wears off. The weekend warrior who packs a year's worth of exercise into a few weekend outings does not get the same physiological benefits as those who exercise more moderately but regularly. (The warrior is also far more prone to serious injury.) Likewise, the things you do day in and day out will have a greater impact on your long-term health than the occasional superhero effort (or lapse).

The recommendations outlined in this chapter represent your goals, not necessarily your starting point. If your current lifestyle is not that different from the guidelines in this chapter, that's terrific. But if embracing an anti-aging lifestyle will require a significant reorientation, take it slow. Resist the temptation to decide that starting tomorrow, you will begin meditating thirty minutes a day, eliminate all sugar from your diet, exercise every afternoon, and be in bed two hours earlier than usual. A dramatic transformation that lasts only a week or two will have almost no enduring effects.

Instead, resolve simply to increase your consumption of vegetables this week, or to reduce your sugar consumption by one-third. Set aside five minutes each morning before breakfast to do some breathing exercises. Plan to walk the dog for twenty minutes in the evening instead of the usual five-minute to-the-corner-and-back. Every small change that becomes a lasting habit makes a big difference.

As each small change slowly becomes habitual, raise the bar for yourself. Break up your twenty-minute walk with two-minute intervals of jogging. Add another serving of vegetables to each meal and reduce your sugar intake by another third. Enroll in a weekly yoga class. And so on . . .

This gradual but powerful renovation of your lifestyle parallels my approach to hormone replacement and nutrient supplementation: start low and go slow. Allow yourself time to adjust, mentally, physically, and logistically to the changes you are making.

As your nutrient status, hormone balance, and biochemistry gradually improve, you will feel profound changes in your energy, mood, and sense of well-being. As risk factors decline and function improves, you will begin to look and feel noticeably more youthful. The program becomes self-perpetuating. Your results will provide all the motivation you need to continue what you are doing, and to take the next steps.

PART IV

THE FUTURE OF
LIFE EXTENSION SCIENCE

The Life Extension Foundation has many missions. One is to inform and educate consumers and professionals about the state of life extension and anti-aging science. Another is to fight against anticonsumer legislation that blocks access to information and therapies. A third is to fund the most promising anti-aging and life extension research.

Part IV gives you a glimpse into the future, with an update on the most cutting-edge research, much of which is actively funded by LEF, and a preview of the therapies that we believe will revolutionize the practice of medicine within our lifetimes.

CHAPTER 13

Extending Human Life Span

If I'd known I was going to live this long,
I would have taken better care of myself.
—EUBIE BLAKE

CENTURIES AGO, THE AVERAGE person didn't live much past the age of 35. Of course, some lived well past the average life expectancy, to the "old" age of 60 or even 65. And a very small percentage of individuals lived to be extremely old. But no one, not even the oldest of the old, survived past 120 years of age.

Today, the average life expectancy for a human being born in an industrialized nation is close to 80 years. With anti-aging and disease prevention therapies, one can hope to live well beyond the average life expectancy in good health. But it is still the case that no one, not even the oldest of the old, survives much past 120 years of age.

Despite all the medical and scientific advances of the last century, the maximum human life span remains a fixed threshold that has yet to be crossed. The search is on for therapies and technologies that will allow us to step across that threshold. We already have extensive research on a very simple approach that can significantly extend the maximum life span of other mammalian species. It is calorie restriction, or CR.

EATING LESS, LIVING LONGER

Animals who spend their lives on a very restricted (but highly nutritious) diet live longer—much longer—than animals who are allowed to eat as much as they want. This is true in every species in which it has been tested: mice, rats, dogs, and monkeys. On average, calorie restriction extends the life expectancy of an animal by about one-third.

Not only does it increase *average* life expectancy, but calorie restriction also shatters the *maximum* life span of species. The maximum life span of mice and rats is normally about 3 years. Calorie-restricted mice, however, can live to be 4 or 5 years old—an astonishing 40 to 60 percent increase in maximum life span. When translated into human terms, this would be a maximum life span of more than 160 years.

Most important, calorie restriction significantly retards aging and the onset of disease. This means that the additional years that calorie restriction adds to life are healthy and active years, not additional years of geriatric frailty. Very old CR mice are remarkably physically active and mentally alert, comparable to their much younger counterparts. They tend to remain disease-free until the very end of their long lives.

A Preemptive Strike Against Aging

In the comprehensive anti-aging program outlined in Part III, we have implemented nutritional and hormonal therapies that compensate for genetic changes that drive the aging "program." Because our cells become less able to defend themselves against free radicals as we age, for example, we have added an aggressive program of antioxidant nutrition. Because the production of hormones tends to decline as we age, we support declining hormone levels with bioidentical hormone replacement, and so on.

You will notice that the anti-aging effects of calorie restriction in mice (see box) parallel the goals of your anti-aging program. CR mice have more youthful hormone profiles, lower blood fats, decreased oxidative damage, reduced inflammation, and increased insulin sensitivity.

But calorie restriction does not *compensate* for age-related changes in cell and organ function. It appears to operate on a genetic level to *prevent* these age-related changes from happening in the first place. This represents a quantum leap forward in the fight against aging.

EFFECTS OF CALORIE RESTRICTION ON BIOMARKERS OF AGING AND DISEASE IN MICE

> Improves DNA repair
> Reduces free radical activity and oxidative damage
> Lowers body temperature
> Lowers cholesterol and triglycerides
> Lowers blood sugar and insulin levels
> Prevents insulin resistance (protective against diabetes and cardiovascular disease)
> Maintains fertility into advanced age
> Protects against glycation (accumulation of damaged proteins)
> Inhibits inflammatory processes
> Protects against degeneration of neurons (protective against cognitive decline and brain disease)
> Prevents age-related decline of DHEA
> Prevents age-related immune dysfunction
> Reduces incidence of cancer
> Increases resistance to stress

Better Late Than Never

Whenever it is introduced, calorie restriction appears to extend the *remaining* life span of an animal by about 40 percent. The earlier in life it is introduced, the greater the remaining life span and the greater the total gain in life span. However, research demonstrates that calorie restriction can extend life span even in older animals.

In one experiment, mice were allowed to eat freely until they were a year old, which, for a mouse, is considered middle age. The researchers then reduced their caloric intake for the rest of their lives. Even when the regimen was not introduced until middle age, the mice lived longer, healthier lives than they otherwise would. They did not live quite as long as mice that had followed CR throughout their entire lives, but they lived significantly longer than mice who ate normally throughout life. Recent findings at the University of California at Riverside indicate that CR can extend life span in mice even when it is not introduced until late in life, when the mice are already "old."

These findings have profound significance. They suggest that CR may do more than just slow or delay the aging process. It may actually be able to reverse some of the genetic changes of aging, effectively rejuvenating the elderly. Obviously, the burning question for scientists is whether the life-prolonging and rejuvenating effects of calorie restriction extend to other species, including humans.

Calorie Restriction in Primates

In the late 1980s, researchers at the University of Wisconsin launched a multidecade study to test the effects of calorie restriction on rhesus monkeys, which have a maximum life span of about 30 years. Similar experiments are under way at the National Institute on Aging.

The effects of CR on the biomarkers of aging in monkeys were quickly evident. Like the mice, CR monkeys show physiological signs of retarded aging. Researchers at the University of Wisconsin note that the calorie-restricted monkeys are leaner and healthier, with lower blood sugar and blood insulin levels than the control monkeys.

As the monkeys in these experiments have begun to reach "old age," it is also clear that the incidence of age-related diseases such as cancer and diabetes is much lower in the CR monkeys. At the National Institute on Aging, the control animals are dying of disease at roughly twice the rate of the calorie-restricted animals.

It is already clear that CR will extend the average life span of monkeys by preventing the onset of age-related disease. But it is still too soon to know whether CR will extend the maximum life span of these animals. Although researchers fully expect that to be the case, the results will not be in until the oldest of the animals die, somewhere around the year 2010 or later.

Calorie Restriction in Humans

In order to determine whether CR can extend the maximum human life span, researchers would have to find a group of people willing to dramatically decrease their intake of food under rigidly controlled conditions. Even so, a life span study on humans would obviously take many decades to complete, probably outlasting the researchers involved.

But we do have data on the shorter-term effects of calorie restriction, and the preliminary information is quite promising. In the early 1990s, eight adults were sealed into the Biosphere in the Arizona desert for a two-year experiment intended to simulate life in a space colony. Among the participants was scientist Roy Walford, who has been involved with calorie restriction research for decades.

After a few months inside the colony, it became clear that the environment inside the Biosphere was not capable of producing enough food to feed the inhabitants the number of calories they needed. For twenty-one of the twenty-four months they spent in the Biosphere, all eight of the crew members were forced to follow a calorie-restricted regimen, consuming about 30 percent fewer calories than normal. They were, however, very careful to get sufficient protein, vitamins, minerals, and fatty acids to prevent nutrient deficiencies or malnourishment.

For the first six months of the calorie restriction regimen, all of the participants lost weight, even though none was overweight at the beginning of the experiment. Weight loss averaged 27 pounds for the men and 15 pounds for the women, rendering all of the participants "underweight" for their height. After six to eight months, however, the weight loss tapered off as the participants' metabolisms adjusted to the lower calorie intake.

But weight loss was not the only effect of calorie restriction. The participants saw a dramatic decrease in average cholesterol (from 191 to 123), a drop in fasting blood sugar (from 92 to 74), and a 25 percent drop in blood pressure. In a research paper published afterward, Walford noted that the biological changes in the Biosphere subjects paralleled the changes seen in CR mice and monkeys. Walford also observed that "despite the selective restriction in calories and marked weight loss, all crew members remained in excellent health and sustained a high level of physical and mental activity throughout the entire two years."

The Secret of Okinawa

There is more tantalizing evidence that calorie restriction may indeed slow aging and extend life span in humans. Inhabitants of Okinawa, a group of forty islands at the southern edge of the Japanese islands, live longer on average than any other culture in the world. According to data compiled by the World Health Organization and the Japanese Ministry of Health and Welfare, natives of these South Pacific Islands live to an average age of almost 82 years, about 7 percent longer than the average life expectancy for Americans.

The inhabitants of Okinawa also eat about 40 percent fewer calories than Americans and about one-fifth fewer calories than other Japanese. The traditional, native diet of the Okinawans, which is heavy on fruits and vegetables and light on red meat and dairy products, is naturally low in calories. But there is a cultural component as well. Traditional island wisdom dictates that one should stop eating when one is only about four-fifths full. Even though Okinawans eat much less from childhood on throughout life, they are not malnourished, due to a highly nutritious diet. But they are much healthier.

Rates of disease and disability due to aging in the Okinawan population are much lower than in other populations and strikingly consistent with the results of calorie restriction in animals. Elderly Okinawans are 75 percent more likely to retain their cognitive ability, are 80 percent less likely to suffer from breast and prostate cancers, and have 80 percent fewer heart attacks than Americans.

Although these population-based data are not the same as a placebo-controlled trial, they are nonetheless extremely compelling. Additional studies to research the effects of CR in human beings are in the planning stages at the Pennington Biomedical Research Center in Baton Rouge, Louisiana, as well as at Tufts University School of Medicine in Boston. But for some, the evidence that calorie restriction can improve health, prevent disease, and may even extend human life span is already compelling enough to embrace calorie restriction as an anti-aging therapy.

IS CALORIE RESTRICTION FOR YOU?

Calorie restriction is, to say the least, not for everyone. The inhabitants of the Biosphere were quick to point out that they spent most of the two years feeling uncomfortably hungry. Those who choose to follow a CR lifestyle must be motivated enough to withstand a near constant state of hunger. They also need to be extremely disciplined about how they spend the limited number of calories they have each day.

Calorie restriction involves reducing calories by 30 to 40 percent of the amount that would maintain a healthy weight. For most healthy adults, this would mean an intake of 1,200 to 1,400 calories per day. But with calories this low, it is imperative that every single calorie count nutritionally. There is no room for empty calories. Malnutrition is neither healthy nor anti-aging.

The Biosphere inhabitants, for example, consumed an extremely nutrient-dense diet of vegetables, fruits, nuts, grains, and legumes, with small amounts of dairy, eggs, and meat.

If you are interested in exploring calorie restriction as a way to increase your longevity, there are organizations that can provide information and serve as support. One such group is the Calorie Restriction Society, 1827 West 145th Street, Suite 205, Gardena, CA 90249 (www.calorierestriction.org).

For the vast majority of people, however, going hungry every day is simply not a realistic option. But there are clues that suggest that fasting every other day may be as effective or even more effective than continuous calorie restriction.

Modified Calorie Restriction

Researchers have found that mice that are allowed to eat as much as they want—but only every other day—show benefits similar to those seen in mice on continuous calorie restriction diets. Even when their weekly calorie intake is the same as a normally fed mouse, mice who fast every other day age more slowly and live longer than mice with no type of calorie restriction. They have lower blood glucose and insulin levels than mice who eat a normal diet every day. They also have more youthful brain chemistry and are less susceptible to stress and shock.

These are very exciting findings. It suggests that even after short periods of food deprivation, the body appears to adjust its metabolism in ways that are anti-aging and longevity-enhancing. And for many people, fasting for twenty-four hours at a time, even several times a week, is far more realistic than radically reducing the amount of food they eat every day.

Controlled studies on the effects of fasting in older people are currently being planned by the National Institute on Aging. In the meantime, you may wish to consider intermittent fasting as a form of modified calorie restriction. Most healthy people can safely fast for twenty-four to thirty-six hours at a time without difficulty or danger.

 No calorie restriction or fasting should be undertaken without your physician's clearance.

To make fasting more comfortable, you can drink clear low-salt broth, a small amount of diluted fruit or vegetable juices, and herbal teas. Also drink plenty of water during your fast.

If you need to lose weight, fasting every other day will probably result in significant weight loss, providing you do not increase your food intake on other days. If you do not need to lose weight, these studies suggest that you can safely increase your intake of healthful foods on days when you are eating, without interfering with the anti-aging benefits of the fasts.

With a calorie restriction regimen, excellent nutrition is an imperative. When the quantity of food is reduced, the quality of what you eat becomes even more important. On days when you are not fasting, scrupulously follow the dietary guidelines in Chapter 12, which maximize nutrition and regulate blood sugar.

Among my own patients who fast, most do not take vitamins, minerals, antioxidants, and fatty acids on fast days, but continue to take hormones and any brainpower supplements. On days when they are eating, they take the maximal recommended levels of nutrients. (Please also see Chapter 11.) Discuss your supplement regimen (and any drugs you may be taking) with your physician before beginning a fasting regimen to determine which supplements should be reduced or eliminated on fast days.

Although intermittent fasting may be less daunting than ongoing calorie restriction, it still requires a degree of motivation and discipline. Not everyone will be comfortable or happy with this degree of restriction. If fasting is not for you, be assured that the anti-aging diet and supplement program outlined in Chapters 11 and 12 is a powerful approach that will slow premature aging and prevent disease.

And if scientists can understand more about how calorie restriction works, it may be possible to develop drug therapies that would mimic the effects of calorie restriction without the ascetic lifestyle.

CAN WE REWRITE THE GENETIC PROGRAM FOR AGING?

Aging is controlled in large part by our genetic programming. We are not yet at the point where we can overwrite the genetic program. But we are getting closer every day. One branch of genetic research focuses on figuring out which genes cause which effects. With that knowledge, dysfunctional or undesirable genes could theoretically be removed, modified, or replaced with other genes. In other words, we might one day be able to remove or modify genes that cause brown hair and replace them with genes that cause blond hair. But the genetics of aging and disease are not just a matter of which genes you have or don't have. It has quite a bit to do with how and when the genes that you have express themselves.

At the moment of conception, you already have all the genes you will ever have in your lifetime. But these genes do not all "speak" at once. For example, your hair color may change throughout your lifetime, turning darker as you grow from a child to an adult, and then turning gray or white (or falling out) as you age. In this case, the gene that triggers hair to turn gray may be silent until you are in your 50s, at which point it begins to express itself.

Epigenetics is a fairly new branch of genetics that focuses on the factors affecting genetic expression. For example, it might be possible to simply silence the gene that causes your hair to turn gray. In order to do that, we would need to know which environmental or biological cues trigger that particular gene to begin to express itself.

Many things affect how and when a gene "speaks up" or turns itself off. Nutrition and stress are two factors that have been discussed in detail in previous chapters. Both can affect the behavior of genes in ways that determine our susceptibility to disease.

Calorie restriction appears to alter the expression of genes that are key to aging and longevity more profoundly than any other therapy yet identified. A better understanding of how calorie restriction affects genetic expression will bring us closer to authentic anti-aging therapies.

High Technology Speeds the Search for Anti-Aging Therapies

A new research technology called the gene chip has greatly accelerated the pace at which scientists can research aging and anti-aging therapies such as calorie restriction. Gene chip technology can analyze the genetic expression of thousands of genes at once. For example, with gene chip technology, researchers at the University of Wisconsin compared genetic expression in old and young mice. With the power to analyze many thousands of genes at once, the researchers were able to create a very detailed but also very broad genetic map of aging.

With gene chip technology, anti-aging therapies can be evaluated on a genetic level. Scientists used gene chip technology to map out the impact of calorie restriction on over twelve thousand different genes from laboratory mice. They confirmed that the genetic profile of elderly CR mice was similar to the genetic profile of youthful mice. In other words, CR prevented many of the genetic changes seen in aging mice. The gene chip analysis also allowed scientists to document exactly which genes were affected by calorie restriction.

GENES AFFECTED BY CALORIE RESTRICTION

Calorie restriction triggers changes in the expression of genes involved in:

> ➤ Metabolism of carbohydrates (sugars) for energy
> ➤ Breakdown and synthesis of proteins
> ➤ Synthesis and metabolism of lipids such as cholesterol and triglycerides
> ➤ Signal transduction controlling the life cycle of cells: cell growth, proliferation, and programmed death (apoptosis)
> ➤ Production of insulin, growth hormone, and IGF-1
> ➤ Cellular protection against free radical damage
> ➤ Cellular mechanisms of inflammation
> ➤ Detoxification of foreign chemicals and toxins

The Search for Mimetics

Although calorie restriction is the most effective anti-aging and life extension therapy yet discovered in mammals, most people are not willing to make the necessary sacrifices. And so the search is on for therapies that might be able to mimic the effects of calorie restriction, without the hardship. If a drug or natural substance can be found that closely mimics the genetic effects of CR, the drug might also have the potential to extend the maximal human life span.

The exciting thing about gene chip technology is that it will greatly accelerate this research, putting lifesaving and life-extending therapies into your hands much more quickly. Earlier, we saw that calorie restriction is effective even when it is begun late in life. Now, gene chip technology suggests why this is the case. After just four weeks, mice on a calorie-restricted diet already display 70 percent of the genetic changes that are evident in mice that have been on calorie restriction for two years.

This discovery is great news for the researchers searching for calorie restriction mimetics. Instead of the years required for a longevity study, a potential anti-aging drug or nutrient can now be screened in a matter of weeks.

Focusing the Search: Is Insulin the Key?

Even with the dramatic acceleration of research made possible by gene chip technology, researchers must still start somewhere. Given a virtually unlimited number of possible drugs and compounds that could be screened, they are focusing their research on substances that are most likely to mimic the effects of calorie restriction. What is it about calorie restriction that makes animals live so much longer? A good number of genes appear to be affected. But is there a primary genetic shift (or a few key shifts) that gives rise to all the other changes that have been observed?

Of all of the changes that calorie restriction brings about, one of the most striking is the reduction of fasting blood sugar and insulin. Calorie restriction has a dramatic effect on blood sugar regulation, reducing the amount of insulin needed by the body. This has been seen consistently in mice, in monkeys, and even in the Biosphere inhabitants.

Some researchers now believe that the genes that regulate insulin sensitivity may be at the heart of aging and longevity. In species ranging from microscopic worms to rodents, a single mutation in the gene that regulates insulin is enough to significantly extend life span. These key insulin-regulating genes appear to affect the behavior of multitudes of genes further "downstream."

This suggests the possibility that the complex of changes associated with aging may be triggered by just a few primary genes (such as those governing insulin control). In that case, we could, in one stroke, forestall hundreds of other genetic changes associated with aging simply by modulating the expression of these key aging genes. Instead of stamping out brush fires all over the aging body, we might be able simply to take the matches out of the forest.

Accordingly, researchers searching for calorie restriction mimetics have begun by screening glucoregulatory drugs, those known to affect blood sugar and insulin sensitivity. Using gene chip technology, researchers have evaluated the effects of several of these drugs on the genetic expression of aging. So far, the most promising results have been with the insulin-sensitizing drug metformin (brand name Glucophage), which was originally developed for diabetics. In mice, the administration of metformin gave rise to many of the same changes in genetic expression that are seen with calorie restriction.

Further research is needed to determine whether metformin might have the ability to extend life span in humans, but metformin clearly has anti-aging benefits. In addition to its ability to increase insulin sensitivity and lower blood sugar and insulin levels, metformin reduces appetite, body weight, and body fat in both diabetics and nondiabetics. It also protects against glycation and the formation of advanced glycation end products (or AGEs), the importance of which was discussed in Chapter 9.

Metformin lowers cholesterol and blood pressure and helps keep the blood thin and "unsticky," protecting against the development of cardiovascular disease. Cardiovascular disease is responsible for four in ten deaths in the United States. Among type 2 diabetics however, three-quarters die from cardiovascular disease or its complications. By preventing damage to the arteries, metformin also protects against damage to the eyes, kidneys, and nerves.

Many physicians have begun to prescribe metformin for patients who they feel are at increased risk of diabetes or cardiovascular disease. And many researchers have expressed interest in metformin as an anti-aging drug for the general population. As the recent gene chip analysis reveals, metformin mimics some of the effects of calorie restriction on gene expression.

Like most drugs, however, metformin is not without risks and toxicities.

 Metformin is not recommended for anyone with a history of liver or kidney problems or those with a history of alcohol abuse. When used over the long term, metformin can interfere with the absorption of vitamin B_{12}, which can lead to a toxic buildup of homo-cysteine. (See Chapter 8.) Some people experience nausea, stomach pain, gas pain, and/or diarrhea when they take metformin, side effects that may disappear over time.

AUTHENTIC ANTI-AGING THERAPIES ARE ON THE HORIZON

The ideal anti-aging therapy will be something that is safe and nontoxic and can be taken over the long term without concern. Metformin is an exciting step in the right direction, because it illuminates the key role of insulin regulation in aging. This insight, along with the acceleration of this research through gene chip technology, brings us significantly closer to finding or developing even safer and more effective anti-aging therapies.

I am quite confident that we will have effective calorie restriction mimetics in the near future, making the life-extending benefits of calorie restriction widely available.

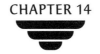

CHAPTER 14

The Cellular Time Machine

I don't want to achieve immortality through my work.
I want to achieve it by not dying.
—WOODY ALLEN

CALORIE RESTRICTION (OR A drug that would mimic the effects of calorie restriction) has the potential to dramatically extend the human life span by slowing aging and delaying the onset of age-related diseases. Used in conjunction with an anti-aging program such as that described in Part III, this approach could add thirty to forty healthy years to the maximum human life span.

But there is another exciting approach to the treatment of aging and age-related diseases that has enormous promise.

Imagine a future in which aging, diseased, or damaged body parts—heart, liver, kidney, pancreas—could be replaced by fresh new organs grown from your very own cells. There would be no anguished waiting for an available organ and no risk of rejection, no need for a lifetime of toxic drugs to suppress your immune system.

And what if the same technology could be used to infuse aging skin with pristine new skin cells, identical to the skin cells that you had when you were born? Spinal cord injuries or stroke damage could be repaired with new neurons. A cancer patient's blood could be reseeded with youthful new blood cells to recharge a failing immune system. Healthy new bone cells could knit together frail, porous bones. New heart muscle cells could repair the damage from a heart attack. These healthy new cells, tissues, and organs would all be created from your very cells, with your own unique genetic identity intact, through a process called "nuclear transfer."

Nuclear transfer is a scientific breakthrough that could eventually provide each person with a limitless supply of perfectly matched cells, tissues, and organs to replace worn-out, diseased, or damaged parts as needed. The successful development of this technology would move life extension to a whole new level. With the ability to replace or repair virtually any tissue in the body, this discovery has the potential to extend human life span indefinitely.

The Cellular Time Machine

Nuclear transfer allows your individual cells to travel back through time. An aging skin cell taken from your arm, for example, could be returned back to a time so early in your development that you did not yet have skin cells, much less aging ones. Nuclear transfer technology can transform a mature cell into a very special and powerful type of cell called an embryonic stem cell, or ESC. ESCs normally exist for only a few weeks during the very earliest embryonic stages of life before being transformed into specialized cells. But with nuclear transfer, we may soon be able to re-create ESCs from an adult cell.

These embryonic stem cells have two essential properties that make them very different from any of the cells in your body right now. For one thing, they are immortal. When we say that a cell is immortal, it doesn't mean that the cell never dies. If its environment gets too hot, or too salty, or too dry, an embryonic stem cell will certainly die. The immortality feature has to do with the fact that unlike normal cells, which can divide only a limited number of times before they get old and die, embryonic stem cells can continue to divide indefinitely, creating an unlimited number of generations.

Embryonic stem cells are also pluripotent, meaning that they have the potential to develop into any type of cell in the body. Although they have this potential, embryonic stem cells are themselves completely undifferentiated. They are not yet skin cells, or muscle cells, or blood cells, or brain cells. They are waiting for the chemical and electrical signals that will tell them when and how to develop into an ear or a heart or a liver.

These two unique properties—immortality and pluripotency—are what make ESCs so potentially useful. They are ageless, able to produce billions of cells without wearing out or getting old. And, in principle, they can be used to produce every type of cell needed in the body.

The opportunity to research and work with embryonic stem cells makes it possible to learn exactly what triggers these cells to differentiate into all of the different cell types and body parts. The nuclear transfer technology that allows us to produce these cells from an adult cell may someday empower us to fix almost anything that can go wrong with the human body.

Eminent scientists including Nobel laureates, as well as organizations such as the National Academy of Sciences (the body of scientists that advises Congress), the National Institutes of Health, and the American Medical Association, are emphatic that research on embryonic stem cells must continue. It is our best and brightest hope for cures for today's incurable diseases and conditions (including aging).

Unfortunately, the future of this research is threatened because of a highly emotional and political debate over the ethics and morality of human cloning. *Nuclear transfer* is, you see, another term for *cloning*.

THERAPEUTIC CLONING VERSUS REPRODUCTIVE CLONING

For many people, the word *cloning* summons up nightmarish visions of a Huxley-esque brave new world in which babies are engineered "to order" on embryo farms. The fear that nuclear transfer will lead to baby farms or engineered superhumans is misplaced. The moral, ethical, and social problems with the reproductive cloning of human beings are obvious, and there is widespread scientific and popular support for regulations that would prohibit reproductive cloning of humans.

Therapeutic cloning, on the other hand, is not the cloning of a human being but the cloning of very early stage human cells. These cells have the potential to generate genetically and immunologically compatible cells and tissues, which could be used to save the life of the person from whom the cell was taken. There is no way that therapeutic cloning could ever accidentally result in the creation of a new human being, for reasons we'll explore in a moment. Along with most scientists, the majority of Americans support therapeutic cloning.

Although both scientists and laypeople can clearly distinguish between reproductive and therapeutic cloning, there have been repeated attempts in the United States Congress to enact legislation banning both types of research. So far, efforts to outlaw therapeutic cloning have failed, but the climate for stem cell research is generally not good. A federal funding ban prohibits research on cloning at any public research facility or any private institution that receives government funding.

Other ESC research has been sharply restricted as well. Much of the research on ESCs has been done using cells taken from frozen embryos created for fertility therapy. Once a couple completes fertility treatments, the unused embryos are routinely destroyed. Some couples have chosen to donate these embryos instead to medical research, in the hopes of finding treatments for today's incurable diseases. The ethics of using these embryonic cells for research has become the subject of another vigorous and emotional debate.

Restrictions now prohibit the use of federal funding for research on ESCs created or harvested after August 2001. This leaves only about two dozen government-approved, preexisting ESC lines available to researchers, and many of these are contaminated and of limited use for research.

The federal funding ban does not restrict privately funded research on new stem cell lines, which might be gathered from frozen embryos before they are destroyed (with the consent of the donors), or created through cloning techniques. But the ongoing political controversy has negatively affected all kinds of ESC research, including nuclear transfer technology. Biotechnology companies are understandably reluctant to invest heavily in research that may be banned or curtailed by future legislation. Although some research continues, scientists feel that their progress against incurable illnesses such as Parkinson's disease or Alzheimer's disease is greatly hampered by these limitations.

HOW ARE STEM CELLS OBTAINED?

> Frozen embryos that are created in the course of fertility therapy contain ESCs. When a couple no longer needs these embryos, they are destroyed. Before being destroyed, ESCs can be removed from the embryos. The federal research ban applies to any newly harvested ESCs from frozen embryos, but allows research on a limited number of preexisting cell lines.

> Nuclear transfer produces ESCs from the DNA of a donor but does not create a viable human embryo. These cells are genetically matched to the donor's cells. The federal research ban applies to any ESCs created through nuclear transfer.

> Adult stem cells (discussed below) are produced in bone marrow, brain, and other tissues in the body. They are multipotent, meaning they can develop into some types of cells, but not all types of cells. Adult stem cell research is not limited by the federal restrictions on ESC research, but its potential applications are more limited.

WHY DO WE NEED IMMORTAL CELLS?

Long before you are born, your immortal, pluripotent embryonic cells are gone forever. A few have been replaced by less versatile adult stem cells. Most, however, have been replaced by more mature cells—heart cells, brain cells, blood cells, immune cells, and so on. These cells are called *somatic* cells, from the Greek word for "body." The somatic cells are no longer immortal, nor are they pluripotent.

Somatic cells can only divide to create more cells of the same type. And, unlike embryonic stem cells, all somatic cells will eventually age and die. Even in the womb, these cells are already ticking off the countdown toward your mortality.

When grown in a tissue culture, somatic cells divide only a certain number times before they grow old and die. This limit, known as the Hayflick limit, after the scientist who first observed the phenomenon, is thought to act as a sort of firewall against DNA mutations. The more times a cell divides and copies its DNA, the more opportunities there are for errors. By limiting the number of times a cell can divide, the body lowers the chance of DNA mutations. This also ensures that any mutations that do occur will eventually die out.

The Hayflick limit is apparently regulated by telomeres, strings of nucleotides found at the end of each cell's chromosomes. Telomeres act as a sort of end cap to tie off the end of the chromosome strand and protect our DNA sequence from damage, much like a bumper prevents damage to the fender of a car. Telomeres are made out of the same material as DNA, but they don't contain any genetic instructions.

When a cell divides, it creates a complete copy of its DNA sequence, so each new cell has its own copy of the organism's genetic blueprint. But every time the cell divides and the chromosomes are copied, a tiny bit at the end gets cut off, and the telomere gets a bit shorter.

The more times a cell has divided, the shorter the telomere at the end of the chromosome. In this way, telomere length is a clock that indicates the age of the cell line. As their telomeres get shorter and shorter, the cells divide more and more slowly. When a telomere gets to a certain length, the cell stops dividing and dies.

Exceptions to the Hayflick Limit

Our bodies are made up mostly of somatic cells with a few very specialized exceptions. Our "germ" cells, egg and sperm cells, retain their immortality. This allows the species to continue to reproduce, creating new generations.

Another exception to the rule is more sinister. A cancer cell is a cell that has mutated in such a way as to override the Hayflick limit. With nothing to stop its division, it can replicate out of control, eventually overwhelming the body's systems. The thing that germ cells and cancer cells have in common is that they both produce an enzyme called telomerase, which rebuilds the telomere to its original length after each cell division. Because the telomere never gets shorter, the cell never reaches its Hayflick limit. It can continue to divide, with the potential to create an infinite number of new generations.

Are Telomeres the Key to Immortality?

Some writers have advanced the theory that telomeres determine our longevity. When we have gone through our allotted number of cell divisions and used up our telomere lengths, the theory goes, our cells stop dividing, and we die.

While it is certainly true for cells in petri dishes, it is an oversimplification to say that telomeres determine the longevity of an entire organism. Some cells, such as neurons in the brain, either do not divide or divide much more slowly than other cells, such as skin and intestinal cells. We also have a supply of adult stem cells that provide brand-new cells to replace cells that have become impaired or died. People who die in old age still have billions of cells that are capable of dividing, as well as other cells, such as neurons, that may not need to divide.

But there is no doubt that older cells behave differently than younger cells. These age-related differences in cellular behavior appear to be regulated in part by telomere length.

Location, Location, Location

Telomeres appear to affect the expression of genes through something known as the telomere positioning effect, or TPE. The position of a gene relative to the end of the telomere seems to affect when that gene is turned on or off.

For example, let's say that the gene that causes your hair to be brown is located close to one end of your chromosome. When you are young and your telomeres are still quite long, this gene expresses itself loud and clear. But as your cells age and your telomeres get shorter, this gene gets closer and closer to the end of the telomere. (Or, more accurately, the end of the telomere gets closer and closer to the gene.) At a certain point, when the distance between the gene and the end of the telomere is short enough, the brown hair gene falls silent, and a gene that causes your hair to turn gray begins to express itself.

Many of the factors known to accelerate aging have been shown to accelerate telomere loss, supporting the link between telomere length and aging. For example, you may recall a study I mentioned in Chapter 2, in which women who were under severe stress displayed genetic changes associated with accelerated aging. In that study, the researchers saw a dramatic shortening of telomere length in the DNA of women who were under chronic stress! Research also shows that oxidative damage, discussed in Chapter 6, causes excessive telomere loss. Homocysteine, discussed at length in Chapter 8, has also been shown to accelerate the aging of cells by increasing the amount of telomere loss with each division of the cell.

This suggests that therapies that slow the loss of telomeres or extend the length of telomeres might prevent the expression of genes that cause aging. Here too, the theory is supported by evidence that anti-aging therapies such as antioxidants also preserve telomere length. Calorie restriction, discussed in Chapter 13, also has a favorable effect on telomere length.

Therapeutic Implications for Telomere Research

Because telomerase is one of the distinguishing features of cancer cells, scientists have high hopes that telomere research may one day yield a very sensitive diagnostic tool to detect cancer. Scientists at Geron Corporation have already developed a very sensitive method of detecting the presence of telomerase in a cell. The TRAP assay was shown to be up to 98 percent accurate in identifying cancer cells, with no false positives (meaning that the test did not detect telomerase in any of the noncancerous tissues tested).

The company is now using TRAP technology to develop products that would allow doctors to detect telomerase in blood, urine, saliva, or

Pap smears. The availability of a very sensitive, very accurate, and universal cancer marker would obviously be a major breakthrough in the fight against cancer by allowing cancer to be detected earlier, when treatment is more successful. These tools are still in preclinical testing, however, and will have to complete the lengthy FDA approval process before coming on the market.

Even more promising is the possibility that an agent that blocks the action of telomerase might prove to be the universal cure for cancer, changing "immortal" cancer cells back into mortal cells, which would stop dividing and die after a certain number of divisions. This approach has been shown to be effective in test tubes. Again, a successful telomerase inhibitor could be a major step toward defeating cancer. But the development of telomerase blockers that would be safe and effective in human cancer patients will likely take several more years.

Researchers are also trying to figure out a way to use telomerase to fight aging and extend life span. If telomerase could be used to restore the telomere length in a somatic cell, it might suppress the expression of the genes that would normally begin to "speak up" as cells get old and telomeres get shorter. In the test tube, telomerase can successfully rejuvenate aging cells and extend their life span by restoring telomere length. It also appears that treating somatic cells with telomerase does not turn them into cancer cells.

How long before a telomerase-based anti-aging therapy might be in your hands? The development of telomerase as an anti-aging drug will take many years of research and testing in order to get FDA approval. Another option would be to induce the expression of telomerase in somatic cells by genetic engineering, but the genetic manipulation of telomerase is even trickier.

Even if scientists perfect a method to safely turn on the gene that expresses telomerase, we would still have to figure out how to get that gene into the body's cells (and be sure that we could turn it back off again). The anti-aging effects of telomerase therapy would also be largely limited to types of cells that divide quickly and therefore suffer from telomere loss. Cells such as neurons or heart muscle cells, which don't divide, would not benefit directly from telomerase therapy.

THE PROMISE OF THERAPEUTIC CLONING

Now that we have discussed the possible use of telomerase to rejuvenate old dividing cells, let's go back to the promise of embryonic stem cell research. First, let's see how nuclear transfer is achieved at labs such as Advanced Cell Technology (ACT), headed by Dr. Michael West, a leading advocate of research into ESCs. To execute the nuclear transfer, Dr. West's team used DNA taken from an aging somatic cell and a mature, unfertilized egg cell, harvested from an egg donor using a technique very similar to that used for in vitro fertilization. Working with small surgical instruments under a high-power microscope, scientists removed the nucleus from the egg cell, leaving only the shell and cytoplasm (somewhat like taking the yolk out of a chicken egg, leaving only the shell and the egg white).

Then the nucleus of the somatic cell, containing the DNA of its donor, was injected into the enucleated egg cell, and the shell was gently fused back together. By placing this egg cell into a bath of chemicals, the scientists stimulated the egg cell to begin dividing, much the way an egg that has been fertilized by a sperm would begin dividing. But unlike a fertilized egg, which contains genetic material from both the mother and the father, the cloned cell contained only the DNA of the somatic cell donor.

Harvesting Embryonic Stem Cells

Whether created through nuclear transfer (cloning) or fertilized through sexual reproduction, a newly dividing egg cell will eventually reach a stage called a blastocyst. This is a tiny ball of about one hundred undifferentiated cells, containing the magical embryonic stem cells.

Although each embryonic stem cell contains the complete genetic blueprint from which an entire human being can be formed, construction is not yet under way. It is as if the architectural plans for a new building have been filed with the building office, but no permit has been issued, no materials have been bought, and no workers have been hired. Many more things need to happen before any building can begin.

In order to begin developing into a human being, the blastocyst must implant itself in the lining of the uterus. Under normal conditions (sexual reproduction), about 80 percent of blastocysts fail to successfully implant in the lining of the uterus and therefore never develop past this primitive stage. For the lucky blastocyst that does achieve implantation, a new phase of construction begins. This is, in effect, the biological building permit that allows a blastocyst to develop further.

The chemical environment in the uterus cues the embryonic cells to differentiate into the different types of cells that make up a human body and to begin organizing themselves into human form. As the cells begin to differentiate, of course, they lose their immortality and their pluripotency.

If reproductive cloning were the goal, scientists would have to implant the cloned blastocyst into the uterus of a birth mother. Without this step, the blastocyst has absolutely no way of ever developing into a human.

But the goal of therapeutic cloning is not to create a human being but merely to create the blastocyst, from which embryonic stem cells can be harvested and used therapeutically. Once harvested, the ESCs could be induced to develop into mature, specialized cells that could then be used to treat the patient from whom the somatic cell was taken. By learning which chemical and environmental cues trigger differentiation, scientists could direct the development of some of the ESCs to create specific cells, tissues, or even organs. These could be reimplanted, infused, or transplanted back into the patient using a variety of methods.

New hearts could be grown for heart-disease patients, Parkinson's patients could be given new brain cells, diabetics could be given new insulin-producing cells. Because the cells would be an exact genetic match, there would be no chance of rejection of the new tissues. No one would have to die waiting for an organ donor to become available. Aging tissues could theoretically be rejuvenated with young new tissues indefinitely.

Embryonic cells also offer a new vehicle for genetic therapies to prevent and cure disease and aging. The genes of ESCs are easier to manipulate than those of somatic cells, and because they reproduce so quickly, the new genetic program could be quickly disseminated in the target cells or tissues. The possibilities for the treatment of genetically modulated diseases are virtually unlimited. It is no wonder that therapeutic cloning is supported by eminent scientists of every religious and philosophical background.

How Close Are We to Harvesting Embryonic Stem Cells for Therapeutic Uses?

Although Dr. West's team succeeded in creating a cloned egg cell that began to divide, the cells did not continue dividing long enough to reach the blastocyst stage. No ESCs were harvested from this first early attempt. Three years later, in 2004, a team of South Korean scientists reported that they had successfully grown cloned human cells to the blastocyst stage and were able to harvest ESCs from them.

Scientists have become adept at nuclear transfer (cloning) in animals, including sheep, mice, cats, and cows. Now they hope to use everything they have learned about cloning animals to speed the progress of human therapeutic cloning. But while cow eggs are readily available for nuclear transfer, the supply of human donor eggs is more limited and more precious.

Once we become more adept at nuclear transfer in human cells, there is still much work to be done to learn how to induce the growth of ESCs into the various cells needed for therapy. Once again, the research on animals is more advanced. Mouse ESCs have been successfully cultured into a variety of different cell types, including blood and immune cells, heart cells, insulin-secreting cells, and neural cells. Researchers have had success using neural cells from ESCs to repair spinal cord injuries in experimental animals.

Human ESC research, on the other hand, is still in its infancy. The first human ESCs were isolated (from noncloned human embryos) in 1998. Human ESCs have been successfully developed into neural precursor cells and other more mature types of brain cells. Researchers have begun to identify how to induce the growth of specific types of neurons with the use of various nutrients.

Some of these cells were transplanted into the brains of newborn mice. These mice all had suppressed immune systems that prevented them from rejecting the human ESCs as foreign. Weeks later, researchers found that these cells had migrated to various parts of the mice's brains, developing further into mature neurons. The goal of therapeutic cloning, of course, is to produce human ESCs that would be genetically identical to the patient, completely avoiding the issue of rejection.

ADULT STEM CELL RESEARCH

Federal funding restrictions have unfortunately slowed the progress of human ESC research in the United States. Many of the resources that would otherwise be poured into this research are, for now, being directed toward adult stem cell research. Unlike ESCs, adult stem cells can be harvested from adult human beings without cloning or the creation of an embryo. While adult stem cell research is less controversial, its applications are more limited.

Adult stem cells are a little different from embryonic stem cells. They are multipotent, meaning that they can give rise to a variety of different cell types. But they are not pluripotent—they cannot give rise to every type of cell. The stem cells in our bone marrow, for example, can produce various kinds of blood and immune cells. But they cannot produce heart muscle or liver cells. They also do not divide as quickly as embryonic stem cells and are more difficult to grow in cultures.

With the advance of therapeutic cloning and the increased availability of ESCs, adult stem cell therapies may, in the long run, become less important. But in the meantime, this more mature research is far closer to yielding new therapies for conditions such as heart disease and Parkinson's disease.

Scientists have already produced dramatic results by administering bone marrow stem cells to lethally irradiated mice. The transplanted stem cells created a new supply of living blood cells and then migrated to the heart, where they began to repair the damage to the heart muscle. Surgeons in Europe have gotten very promising results by transplanting stem cells into a human patient following a heart attack.

Stem cell therapy is also widely seen as the best hope for incurable neurological diseases such as Parkinson's disease, Hodgkin's disease, and amyotrophic lateral sclerosis (ALS). A Canadian research team has reported very promising results in the experimental use of stem cells for the treatment of Parkinson's disease in humans. Surgeons extracted stem cells from the brain of a Parkinson's patient and then grew them in a laboratory. The stem cells yielded millions of new dopamine-producing brain cells, which were then reinfused into the patient's brain. Within three months, tests showed a 55 percent improvement in dopamine uptake in his brain. A full year later, evaluations using a standardized rating scale showed an 83 percent improvement in his condition, with no Parkinson's medications.

The time and energy that are going into adult stem cell therapy will not go to waste. Many lives may be saved with adult stem cell therapies before ESC therapies are fully developed. And much of the research on adult stem cells will further the development of ESC therapies provided that ESC researchers are allowed and encouraged to continue their work.

FIGHTING FOR PROGRESS

Of course, if Congress outlaws therapeutic cloning, much of this very exciting research—work that has the potential to extend your life span almost indefinitely—will come to a halt. Funding restrictions on ESC and cloning research are already in place. Efforts to ban both reproductive and therapeutic cloning continue, over the loud objections of the Juvenile Diabetes Research Foundation, the American Liver Foundation, the Association of American Medical Colleges, the American Society of Cell Biologists, and the Alliance for Aging Research.

Despite the possibility of a federal ban on embryonic stem cell research and therapeutic cloning, California passed a referendum in 2004 authorizing 3 billion dollars in funding for stem cell research, much of it for ESC research. Similar efforts are under way in other states such as New York, New Jersey, and Massachusetts. ESC research is also being pursued aggressively in countries such as England, South Korea, China, and Russia.

How can we ban research that has the potential to save thousands of lives every day, offering hope to the millions of people who are suffering and dying from diseases for which we currently have no cure?

Some feel that therapeutic cloning will somehow open the door to reproductive cloning in the future. Others oppose therapeutic cloning on the basis that it violates the rights of the blastocyst, which has the potential to become a human being.

Advocates for therapeutic cloning argue that the rights of a primitive one-hundred-cell blastocyst, without organs, nerve cells, awareness, or sensation, cannot be placed above the rights of the millions of fully developed human beings whose lives could be saved through ESC-generated therapies, merely because that one-hundred-cell mass contains a complete copy of the donor's DNA.

If you feel strongly about therapeutic cloning and ESC research, you must join the debate. You can directly affect the future of this research by communicating your position on therapeutic cloning to your government representative, particularly your senators. You can access the Senate's Web site at www.senate.gov. You can also visit the Coalition for the Advancement of Medical Research Web site at www.camradvocacy.org for more information on this issue as well as sample letters that can be sent to government officials.

CHAPTER 15

A Bridge to the Future

Youth is not a time of life; it is a state of mind.
—SAMUEL ULLMAN

THE ANTI-AGING AND life extension technologies discussed in the previous chapters are experimental, but the research is progressing at astonishing speed. I can clearly envision a future in which healthy human life span may be measured in centuries rather than decades and when the diseases that kill us today will be footnotes in our medical history.

As close as these advances sometimes seem, however, it may still take years or decades before these experimental therapies and technologies are in our hands. One of the things that the anti-aging program outlined in Part III can do is buy time. By slowing down the speed at which your body is aging and taking steps to protect against degenerative disease, you can vastly increase your quality of life. At the same time, you increase the chances that you will live to experience and benefit from future advances in anti-aging and life extension technology.

Sadly, there are many people for whom these advances will not arrive quickly enough to make a difference. Millions of people are suffering from diseases or infirmities for which we do not yet have cures. Despite the best efforts of conventional and anti-aging medicine, they may die before these cures are found.

SUSPENDING TIME UNTIL
CURES CAN BE FOUND

In theory, cryonic suspension represents the ultimate time-buying strategy. This somewhat radical approach involves cooling the body after death to extremely low temperatures to prevent physical decay and storing it in the hopes that medical technology will someday advance to the point where the body can be successfully revived and healed of its ailments.

Although it may sound like pure science fiction, human cryonic suspension has actually been in practice since the 1960s. Although the methodology is constantly evolving, the basic procedure is to remove the blood and fluids from the body and replace them with solutions of cryopreservation agents, which protect the body against freezing damage. The body is then cooled to subzero temperatures (between -130 and -196 degrees Fahrenheit), arresting physical decay indefinitely.

In the early days of cryonics, scientists used chemicals such as glycerol and DMSO (dimethyl sulfoxide) as cryopreservants. These are similar to the naturally occurring chemicals that allow animals such as frogs, fish, insects, and reptiles to spend long periods of time with their bodies partially frozen. Today, improved cryopreservants and cooling technologies offer even greater protection against freezing, at lower, less toxic concentrations. The most advanced method is vitrification, which virtually eliminates the formation of ice crystals. A small number of private companies currently offer long-term cryonic preservation as an alternative to burial or cremation.

Despite decades of practice, cryonics still has not caught on in a big way. There are about 120 bodies currently being held in a state of cryopreservation, and about 1,000 other people have made arrangements for cryonic suspension following death. There are, of course, no guarantees that we will ever be able to successfully revive these patients. Right now, the decision to choose cryonic suspension involves a great deal of faith in future medical technology.

Scientists are probably fifty to a hundred years away from the successful animation and repair of any of today's cryonically preserved patients. There are at least four major scientific hurdles that still need to be overcome before this is possible.

1. **Rewarming technology.** Scientists are making great strides in materials and methods that minimize cellular and structural damage when cryopreserving organs and entire bodies. (These advances will be discussed in more detail below.) But as hard as it is to cryopreserve tissues without damage, it's even harder to warm them up without destroying them. Research is proceeding in this field.

2. **Tissue repair capability.** Second, because no technology is perfect, cryonically preserved patients cannot be revived until we have the ability to repair any damage to cells, tissues, or organs that may have occurred during either the cryopreservation or rewarming process. Patients who were suspended in the 1960s and 1970s were preserved using older technology and will probably require more repair, and therefore more advanced technology, to be successfully revived. Ironically, they may have to wait longer than those preserved more recently.

   The maturation of nanotechnology will most likely be the advance that will make successful reanimation of today's patients possible. Advances in nanotechnology could someday produce cell-size surgical robots, which could swim through the body repairing damage and restoring function at the cellular level.

3. **Medical advancement.** Third, doctors need to have the means to heal diseases or conditions that were present before death and which might threaten a patient's survival after revival. If a patient died of a disease (or symptoms of aging) that current medical technology cannot treat, that patient cannot be revived until we have a treatment or cure for the disease, as well as technology to repair any damage that accumulated before pronouncement of death. In other words, we may first need to have technology that allows us to grow healthy new organs, or a

therapy to stop cancer, or a gene therapy to reverse aging, before cryobiologists can proceed with reanimation.

4. **Neural preservation.** Perhaps the most difficult challenge facing cryobiologists is the preservation or regeneration of proper neural function. Other tissue and organs can be repaired or replaced, but the essence of individual personhood resides in the brain. Can a cryopreserved brain be revived with its complex and delicate neural programming intact? Even if normal neurological function were possible, how well might a cryonically suspended brain retain vital information such as memories, personality, and learning?

Hamsters cooled until more than 60 percent of the water in their brains was in the form of ice crystals have been revived with no observable neurological or behavioral impairment. The latest cryopreservation techniques allow the cooling of brain tissue to superlow temperatures with far less ice formation.

In addition to having some tolerance for ice formation, brain stem cells also appear to have extra resistance to oxygen deprivation. At the Salk Institute, brain stem cells harvested from the brains of cadavers that had been dead for more than twenty hours (but not cryopreserved) were found to be viable, able to divide and differentiate into various types of brain cells.

All of this is hopeful evidence that if cryobiologists can master techniques that can cool and then rewarm the brain without causing too much ice damage, the brain may be resilient enough to retain or recover complete neurological function.

BEYOND THE SCIENCE: IS IT ETHICAL?

Quite apart from the scientific challenges that remain to be solved, there are obviously some important social and philosophical issues involved in cryopreservation of human beings. From a legal point of view, you are free to choose cryopreservation following death, the way you might choose to have your remains cremated or buried. (Cryopreservation is an option only after a patient has been pronounced dead.)

There is a possibility that cryonically preserved patients may never be reanimated. In that case, the cryonic preservation was little more than a high-tech embalming procedure. But what if doctors of the future succeed in reviving us but cannot completely heal or repair us? What will our medical and legal rights be, both before and after revival, and who will protect them if we cannot? Who will bear the financial responsibility for our care, either before or after revival, if we cannot?

In choosing cryopreservation, one is, in effect, projecting oneself into an unknown future, the social, political, scientific, and environmental conditions of which we cannot begin to imagine. We are placing our trust in generations that have not yet been born, relying on them to provide ongoing care and trusting them to make decisions about our welfare. Are we asking too much of future generations or science?

These are questions that anyone seriously considering cryopreservation must think about very carefully. But ultimately, the ethical and philosophical considerations that surround the cryopreservation of humans may be only temporary ones. The same technology that would make reanimation possible might also make cryopreservation unnecessary for most people. The advances that would allow us to repair damaged tissues and organs and reverse disease and aging in cryopreserved patients could be applied to reverse damage and disease in the living, preventing death instead of repealing it.

In the final analysis, long-term cryopreservation may be only a temporary stopgap, a bridge that may allow a generation or two of pioneers to cross from the technologically limited shores of the present to the brighter beaches of a future in which disease and aging are no longer.

RESOURCES FOR CRYONICS
INFORMATION AND SERVICES

Alcor: 877-462-5267, www.alcor.org

American Cryonics Society: 800-523-2001, www.americancyronics.org

Cryonics Institute: 586-791-5961, www.cryonics.org

Cryonics Society of Canada: www.cryocdn.org

Suspended Animation, Inc: 561-997-4062

TransTime: 510-346-8846, www.transtime.com

TECHNOLOGY TO SAVE THE LIVING

The cryonic suspension of a body is the most sensational and controversial application of cryobiology, but there is much more to the science than cryopreservation of humans for future reanimation. Advances in cryopreservation will allow doctors to save millions of lives in ways that have nothing to do with the cryonic preservation of human bodies. It is very much a medical technology for the living.

Actually, some applications of cryopreservation are already quite routine. Human sperm are regularly cooled to liquid nitrogen temperatures for storage and then later used to create successful pregnancies. Cryonics also allows the preservation of blood cells and stem cells for long periods of time. Stem cells removed from human umbilical cords have been shown to be viable after up to fifteen years of cyropreservation. Once the therapeutic cloning techniques discussed in Chapter 14 have been mastered, this same technology will allow us to preserve those precious cells for future use.

Cells or small groups of cells can be successfully frozen because they can be cooled very quickly, minimizing the damage from the formation of ice crystals. More advanced techniques are needed in order to freeze large organs in such a way that ice crystallization is minimized and the vital cell-to-cell relationships within the organ are not compromised.

Scientists are very close to mastering the technology that would allow them to cool and store tissues and organs in such a way that they can be thawed, transplanted, and restored to proper function in the body. Recently, researchers achieved a major milestone toward this goal, preserving whole ovaries from rats and then successfully reimplanting them in rats. The frozen ovaries functioned completely normally after transplantation, even leading to pregnancies in the recipients.

Successful cryopreservation of organs will be a major advance in transplant medicine. Right now, patients routinely die waiting for an appropriate organ to become available from a donor. When hearts do become available, those that cannot be used within a few hours are wasted. With advances in cryopreservation, livers, kidneys, hearts, lungs, and corneas—whether harvested from donors or grown in the laboratory from embryonic stem cells—could be preserved indefinitely until needed, eliminating millions of tragic and needless deaths.

From Ice to Glass: Vitrification Is the Key

The successful cryopreservation of organs or even whole bodies depends on mastering a process called vitrification. The big problem with cooling organs to subzero temperatures is that the water contained in the cells and tissues forms ice crystals. These ice crystals squeeze, tear, and rearrange the cells, so the organ cannot function when rewarmed.

Vitrification is a technique that allows tissue to be transformed into a hard, glassy solid as it cools, with little or no ice crystal formation. Cellular structure can be almost perfectly preserved, greatly increasing the chances that the organ will function normally once it is rewarmed. "Vitrification," says leading cryophysicist Brian Wowk, "is a way of stopping biological time without disturbing the natural order inside living cells."

The problem is that the amount of cryopreservants that would have to be used to produce total vitrification of an organ (and no harmful ice crystals) would be chemically toxic to the cells. For decades, this problem has limited the success of cryopreservation of organs (as well as humans).

Dr. Wowk and his colleagues at 21st Century Medicine, a laboratory in southern California funded by the Life Extension Foundation, have been researching the vitrification problem from a number of angles. Dr. Gregory Fahy, the world's foremost cryopreservation expert, has developed methods that involve the gradual introduction of cryopreservants as the tissue reaches lower and lower temperatures. This can increase the effectiveness of the chemicals while reducing their toxicity. The researchers also have developed new vitrification solutions with novel chemicals that block the formation of ice and which are effective at less toxic concentrations.

These advances in vitrification may make the long-term preservation of viable human organs, including the brain, a medical and scientific reality in the foreseeable future.

Other Low-Temperature Technologies

Rapid cooling technologies may also buy valuable time for living patients. Researchers at the LEF-funded Critical Care Research Laboratory, also in southern California, have been working on an automated liquid ventilation system that could lower the whole-body temperature of a patient extremely rapidly by introducing a liquid perfluorocarbon solution into the lungs. Combined with other techniques, this allows a temporary slowdown of biological activity without lasting damage. Critical Care Research has also developed a battery of drugs that protect brain cells and other cells from the damage that would otherwise result from the lack of oxygen due to ischemia (reduced or no blood flow).

Ischemia is a major underlying cause of aging and degenerative disease and causes serious damage in severely injured patients. Critical Care's advanced cooling and resuscitation technologies will be able to save the lives of heart attack, stroke, and accident victims by temporarily reducing their metabolic activity.

ARE WE PLAYING GOD?

It used to be that once a person's heart had stopped, that person was considered to be legally, medically, and irretrievably dead. Now hundreds of thousands of such patients are routinely revived with the use of cardiopulmonary resuscitation technology. We no longer consider a patient dead just because the heart has stopped for a few minutes. And soon, the technologies developed through LEF-funded research may once again rewrite the definition of death.

One of the objections that has been raised over cryonic research is that scientists are attempting to "play God" by resurrecting the "dead." Doctors sometimes induce comas in patients to allow them to recover from radical heart surgeries. Cryonic suspension might be defined as a long-term coma that allows a patient to wait until technology can offer a cure. These are differences of degree, not of kind.

The goal of all of these technologies, from defibrillators to cryopreservation, is simply to offer people the opportunity to live longer, healthier lives. On what basis can we determine that one is acceptable and one is not? Throughout history, the line in the sand that has separated scientific advancement from "playing God" has been drawn and redrawn many times.

Now, some of the best minds in science are focused on overcoming the medical and technological challenges involved with cryopreservation. They are not indifferent to the ethical and philosophical issues. But they clearly see that whether it is used for fertility therapy, transplant medicine, or to buy time until a cure for aging or disease is found, cryotechnology will save and enhance lives.

THE NATURE OF PROGRESS

Science continues to expand our reach and our possibilities, to redefine the possible. The regeneration of damaged nerve tissue, the biological rejuvenation of aging cells, the nonsexual reproduction of a mammal, the extension of the maximal life span of a species—all of these were thought to be impossible only a short time ago.

Scientific advancement has always spawned controversy. Human flight, now an everyday occurrence, was once thought to be against the will of God. In vitro fertilization, once as controversial as therapeutic cloning, now fulfills the dreams of parents who would otherwise be unable to have children of their own.

Vast social and philosophical adjustments are sometimes required before a new technology can be accepted. The adjustment can be a painful process, but it is one we have little choice but to embrace. As history has demonstrated, scientific progress leads to longer, healthier, and more productive lives.

As we become more familiar with new technologies, we usually find that developments that at first seemed dangerous or unwise (air travel, smallpox vaccinations, organ transplants, the Internet) turn out to be technologies that we would not want to—or cannot—live without.

Afterword from
the Life Extension Foundation

Social scientists warn that if science succeeds in dramatically extending our life span, we could face grave social and economic crises due to world overpopulation and an increasing elderly (by which they mean "useless") population. They fail to grasp the true promise of the anti-aging and life extension movement.

Although the average age of the population will rise, medical costs will actually decrease as we eliminate the diseases that now cripple and eventually kill most of our citizens. Instead of overloading our elder care system with more invalids, we will extend the functional careers of talented, productive people. Those who enjoy the wisdom that comes with a lifetime of experience will have the energy and vitality to apply that knowledge to solving social and scientific problems.

The science of life extension gives rise to ethical, philosophical, social, and even theological questions. While LEF recognizes the significance of these issues and the need for debate and commentary, we believe that it is neither desirable nor possible to stop the great march of science and discovery. It appears to be our destiny to understand and solve the problem of aging, becoming the first species ever to consciously and directly participate in our evolutionary progress.

We invite you to be there, to participate in this exciting, challenging future. To speed the progress of life extension research, consider membership in the Life Extension Foundation. In addition to access to information about the latest scientific developments, your membership dollars will fund research into lifesaving and life-extending technologies.

For more information, contact the Life Extension Foundation at 877-877-9705 or online at www.lef.org.

Appendix
Finding an Anti-Aging Physician

The following organizations can refer you to members or board-certified anti-aging physicians in your area.

American Academy of Anti-Aging Medicine (A^{4}M)
1510 West Montana Street
Chicago, IL 60614
www.worldhealth.net

The American College for Advancement in Medicine (ACAM)
23121 Verdugo Drive, Suite 204
Laguna Hills, CA 92653
www.acam.org

American Association for Health Freedom (formerly the American Preventive Medical Association)
9912 Georgetown Pike, Suite D-2
Great Falls, VA 22066
www.healthfreedom.net
E-mail: aahf@healthfreedom.net

Life Extension Foundation
P.O. Box 229190
Hollywood, FL 33022
www.lef.org

References

CHAPTER 2: OVERCOMING THE AGING EFFECTS OF STRESS

Epel ES, Blackburn EH, et al. Accelerated telomere shortening in response to life stress. Proc Natl Acad Sci USA. 2004 Dec;101(49):17312–5.

Watson RR, Huls A, et al. Dehydroepiandrosterone and diseases of aging. Drugs Aging. 1996 Oct;9(4):274–91.

Brindley D, Rolland Y. Possible connections between stress, diabetes, obesity, hypertension. Clin Sci. 1989;77:453–61.

Cohen S, Tyrrell D. A psychological stress and susceptibility to the common cold. NEJM. 1991;325:606–12.

Ben-Eliyahu S, et al. Stress increases metastatic spread of a mammary tumor in rats. Brain Behav Immun. 1991;6:193–205.

Sapolsky R. Neuroendocrinology of stress and aging. Endocrine Rev. 1986; 7:284–301.

Uno H, Ross T. Hippocampal damage associated with prolonged and fetal stress in primates. J Neurosci. 1989;9:1705–11.

Kerr S, Campbell L. Chronic stress-induced acceleration of electrophysiologic and morphometric biomarkers of hippocampal aging. J Neurosci. 1991;11:1316–24.

Watanabe Y, Gould E. Stress induces atrophy of apical dendrites of hippocampal CA3 pyramidal neurons. Brain Res. 1992;588:341–45.

Villareal DT, et al. Effects of DHEA replacement on bone mineral density and body composition in elderly women and men. Clin Endocrinol. 2000; 53:561–68.

Lee KS, et al. Effects of DHEA on collagen and collagenase gene expression by skin fibroblasts in culture. J Dermatol Sci. 2000;23:103–10.

Baulieu EE, Thomas G, et al. DHEA and aging: contribution of the DHEAge Study to a sociobiomedical issue. Proc Natl Acad Sci USA. 2000 Apr 11; 97(8):4279–84.

de Pergola G. The adipose tissue metabolism: role of testosterone and DHEA. Int J Obes Relat Metab Disord. 2000;24 Suppl 2:S59–63.

Arlt W, Callies F, Allolio B. DHEA replacement in women with adrenal insufficiency—pharmacokinetics, bioconversion and clinical effects on well-being, sexuality and cognition. Endocr Res. 2000 Nov;26(4):505–11.

Reiter WJ, et al. DHEA in the treatment of erectile dysfunction: a prospective, double-blind, randomized, placebo-controlled study. Urology. 1999; 53:590–94.

Arlt W, Callies F, et al. Dehydroepiandrosterone replacement in women with adrenal insufficiency. N Engl J Med. 1999 Sep 30;341(14):1013–20.

Stomati M, et al. Six month oral DHEA supplementation in early and late postmenopause. Gynecol Endocrinol. 2000;14:342–63.

Khorram O, Vu L, Yen SS. Activation of immune function by dehydroepiandrosterone (DHEA) in age-advanced men. J Gerontol A Biol Sci Med Sci. 1997 Jan;52(1):M1–7.

Barret-Connor E, et al. Endogenous levels of DHEA-S but not other sex hormones are associated with depressed mood in older women: the Rancho Bernardo Study. J Am Geriatr Soc. 1999;47:685–91.

McCormick DL, Rao KV. Chemoprevention of hormone-dependent prostate cancer in the Wistar-Unilever rat. Eur Urol. 1999;35:464–67.

Barnhart KT, Freeman E, et al. The effect of dehydroepiandrosterone supplementation to symptomatic perimenopausal women on serum endocrine profiles, lipid parameters, and health-related quality of life. J Clin Endocrinol Metab. 1999 Nov;84(11):3896–902.

Khalil A, Fortin JP, LeHoux JG, Fulop T. Age-related decrease of dehydroepiandrosterone concentrations in low density lipoproteins and its role in the susceptibility of low density lipoproteins to lipid peroxidation. J Lipid Res. 2000 Oct;41(10):1552–61.

CHAPTER 3: TUNING THE SEX HORMONES

Shah SH, Alexander KP. Hormone replacement therapy for primary and secondary prevention of heart disease. Curr Treat Options Cardiovasc Med. 2003 Feb;5(1):25–33.

Heersche JN, Bellows CG, Ishida, Y. The decrease in bone mass associated with aging and menopause. J Prosthet Dent. 1998 Jan;79(1):14–16.

Chang KJ, Lee T, et al. Influences of percutaneous administration of estradiol and progesterone on human breast epithelial cell cycle in vivo. Fertil Steril. 1995 Apr;63(4):785–91.

Formby B, Wiley TS. Progesterone inhibits growth and induces apoptosis in breast cancer cells: inverse effects on Bcl-2 and p53. Ann Clin Lab Sci. 1998 Nov;28(6):360–69.

Leonetti H. Clinical study on the use of natural progesterone cream in the prevention of osteoporosis. 1998 (unpublished). Bethlehem, PA: Bethlehem Obstetrics Clinic.

Cowan LD, Gordis L, et al. Breast cancer incidence in women with a history of progesterone deficiency. Am J Epidemiol. 1981 Aug;114(2):209–17.

Cooper LS, Gillett CE, et al. Survival of premenopausal breast carcinoma patients in relation to menstrual cycle timing of surgery and estrogen receptor/progesterone receptor status of the primary tumor. Cancer 1999 Nov 15;86(10):2053–58.

Badwe RA, Mittra I, Havaldar R. Timing of surgery during the menstrual cycle and prognosis of breast cancer. J Biosci. 2000 Mar;25(1):113–20.

Macleod J, Fraser R, Horeczko N. Menses and breast cancer: does timing of mammographically directed core biopsy affect outcome? J Surg Oncol. 2000 Jul;74(3):232–36.

Mohr PE, Wang DY, et al. Serum progesterone and prognosis in operable breast cancer. Br J Cancer 1996 Jun;73(12):1552–55.

Lee J, Hopkins V. What Your Doctor May Not Tell You About Menopause. 1996. New York: Warner.

Head KA. Estriol: safety and efficacy. Altern Med Rev. 1998 Apr;3(2):101–13.

Takahashi K, Manabe A, et al. Efficacy and safety of oral estriol for managing postmenopausal symptoms. Maturitas. 2000 Feb 15;34(2):169–77.

Granberg S, Eurenius K, et al. The effects of oral estriol on the endometrium in postmenopausal women. Maturitas. 2002 Jun 25;42(2):149–56.

Lemon HM. Pathophysiologic considerations in the treatment of menopausal patients with oestrogens; the role of oestriol in the prevention of mammary carcinoma. Acta Endocrinol Suppl.1980;233:17–27.

Women's Health Initiative Investigators. Risks and benefits of estrogen plus progestin in healthy postmenopausal women. JAMA. 2002;288:321–33.

Colditz GA, Hankinson SE, et al. The use of estrogens and progestins and the risk of breast cancer in postmenopausal women. N Engl J Med. 1995 Jun 15;332(24):1589–93.

Smart CR, Byrne C, et al. Twenty-year follow-up of the breast cancers diagnosed during the Breast Cancer Detection Demonstration Project. CA Cancer J Clin. 1997 May-Jun;47(3):134–49.

Lauritzen C. Results of a 5-year prospective study of estriol succinate treatment in patients with climacteric complaints. Horm Metab Res. 1987 Nov; 19(11):579–84.

Vincent A, Fitzpatrick LA. Soy isoflavones: are they useful in menopause? Mayo Clin Proc. 2000 Nov;75(11):1174–84.

Castelo-Branco C, Figueras F, et al. Facial wrinkling in postmenopausal women. Effects of smoking status and hormone replacement therapy. Maturitas. 1998 May 20;29(1):75–86.

Tzingounis VA, Aksu MF, Greenblatt RB. Estriol in the management of the menopause. JAMA. 1978 Apr 21;239(16):1638–41.

Sherwin BB. Estrogenic effects on memory in women. Ann NY Acad. Sci. 1994 Nov 14;743:213–30; discussion, 230–31.

Jacobs DM, Tang MX, et al. Cognitive function in nondemented older women who took estrogen after menopause. Neurology. 1998 Feb;50(2):368–73.

Smetnik VP. [Principles of hormone replacement therapy in climacteric.] Vestn Ross Akad Med Nauk. 1997;2:34–38 (Russian).

Resnick SM, Metter EJ, Zonderman AB. Estrogen replacement therapy and longitudinal decline in visual memory. A possible protective effect? Neurology. 1997 Dec;49(6):1491–7.

DeGregorio MW, Taras TL. Hormone replacement therapy and breast cancer: revisiting the issues. J Am Pharm Assoc. 1998 Nov-Dec;38(6):738–44; quiz, 744–46.

Rossouw JE, Anderson GL, et al. Risks and benefits of estrogen plus progestin in healthy postmenopausal women: principal results from the Women's Health Initiative randomized controlled trial. JAMA. 2002 Jul 17;288(3): 321–33.

Liske E. Therapeutic efficacy and safety of *Cimicifuga racemosa* for gynecologic disorders. Adv Ther. 1998 Jan-Feb;15(1):45–53.

Warnecke G. Using phyto-treatment to influence menopause symptoms. Med Welt. 1985;36:871–74.

Lehmann-Willenbrock E, Riedel HH. Clinical and endocrinological examinations concerning therapy of climacteric symptoms following hysterectomy with remaining ovaries. Zentralbl Gynakol. 1988;110(10):611–18.

Stolze H. An alternative to treat menopausal complaints. Gynecology 1982; 3:14–16.

Duker EM, Kopanski L, et al. Effects of extracts from *Cimicifuga racemosa* on gonadotropin release in menopausal women and ovariectomized rats. Planta Med. 1991 Oct;57(5):420–24.

Rafi MM, Rosen RT, et al. Modulation of bcl-2 and cytotoxicity by licochalcone-A, a novel estrogenic flavonoid. Anticancer Res. 2000 Jul;20 (4):2653–8.

Tamir S, Eizenberg M, et al. Estrogenic and antiproliferative properties of glabridin from licorice in human breast cancer cells. Cancer Res. 2000 Oct 15; 60(20):5704–9.

Hardy ML. Herbs of special interest to women. J Am Pharm Assoc. 2000 Mar; 40(2):234–42.

Cassidy A, Bingham S, Setchell, KD. Biological effects of a diet of soy protein rich in isoflavones on the menstrual cycle of premenopausal women. Am J Clin Nutr. 1994 Sep;60(3):333–40.

Wagner JD, Cefalu WT, et al. Dietary soy protein and estrogen replacement therapy improve cardiovascular risk factors and decrease aortic cholesteryl ester content in ovariectomized cynomolgus monkeys. Metabolism. 1997 Jun;46(6):698–705.

St. Germain A, Peterson CT, et al. Isoflavone-rich or isoflavone-poor soy protein does not reduce menopausal symptoms during 24 weeks of treatment. Menopause. 2001 Jan-Feb;8(1):17–26.

Chang HC, Doerge DR. Dietary genistein inactivates rat thyroid peroxidase in vivo without an apparent hypothyroid effect. Toxicol Appl Pharmacol. 2000;168(3):244–52.

Duncan AM, et al. Modest hormonal effects of soy isoflavones in postmenopausal women. J Clin Endocrinol Metab. 1999;84(10):3479–84.

Persky VW, et al. Effect of soy protein on endogenous hormones in postmenopausal women. Am J Clin Nutr. 2002;75(1):145–53.

Jones KJ. Steroid hormones and neurotrophism: relationship to nerve injury. Metab Brain Dis. 1988 Mar;3(1):1–18.

Alexander GM, Swerdloff RS, et al. Androgen-behavior correlations in hypogonadal men and eugonadal men. II. Cognitive abilities. Horm Behav. 1998 Apr;33(2):85–94.

Gelfand MM, Wiita B. Androgen and estrogen-androgen hormone replacement therapy: a review of the safety literature, 1941 to 1996. Clin Ther. 1997 May-Jun;19(3):383–404.

Zgliczynski S, Ossowski M, et al. Effect of testosterone replacement therapy on lipids and lipoproteins in hypogonadal and elderly men. Atherosclerosis. 1996 Mar;121(1):35–43.

Wu SZ, Weng XZ. Therapeutic effects of an androgenic preparation on myocardial ischemia and cardiac function in 62 elderly male coronary heart disease patients. Chin Med J (Engl). 1993 Jun;106(6):415–18.

Wu S, Weng X. Regulation of atrial natriuretic peptide, thromboxane and prostaglandin production by androgen in elderly men with coronary heart disease. Chin Med Sci J. 1993 Dec;8(4):207–09.

Wu SZ, Weng XZ, Yao XX. [Antianginal and lipid lowering effects of oral androgenic preparation (Andriol) on elderly male patients with coronary heart disease] Zhonghua Nei Ke Za Zhi. 1993 Mar;32(4):235–38 (Chinese).

Anderson RA, Bancroft J, Wu FC. The effects of exogenous testosterone on sexuality and mood of normal men. J Clin Endocrinol Metab. 1992 Dec; 75(6):1503–7.

Keel BA, Abney TO. Effects of estradiol administration in vivo on testosterone production in two populations of rat Leydig cells. Biochem Biophys Res Commun. 1982 Aug 31;107(4):1340–48.

King DS, Sharp RL, Vukovich MD, Brown GA, Reifenrath TA, Uhl NL, Parsons KA. Effect of oral androstenedione on serum testosterone and adaptations to resistance training in young men: a randomized controlled trial. JAMA. 1999 Jun 2;281(21):2020–28.

Gann PH, Hennekens CH, et al. A prospective study of plasma hormone levels, nonhormonal factors, and development of benign prostatic hyperplasia. Prostate. 1995 Jan;26(1):40–49.

Donnelly BJ, Lakey WH, McBlain WA. Estrogen receptor in human benign prostatic hyperplasia. J Urol. 1983 Jul;130(1):183–87.

Andro MC, Riffaud JP. *Pygeum africanum* extract for the treatment of patients with benign prostatic hyperplasia: a review of 25 years of published experience. Curr Ther Res Clin Exp. 1995;56(8):796–817.

Gann PH, Ma J. Lower prostate cancer risk in men with elevated plasma lycopene levels: results of a prospective analysis. Cancer Res. 1999;59(6): 1225–30.

Leitzmann MF, Stampfer MJ. Zinc supplement use and risk of prostate cancer. J Natl Cancer Inst. 2003 Jul 2;95(13):1004–7.

Wilt TJ, Mulrow C, et al. Saw palmetto extracts for treatment of benign prostatic hyperplasia: a systematic review. JAMA. 1998 Nov 11;280(18): 1604–9.

Goldmann WH, Sharma AL. Saw palmetto berry extract inhibits cell growth and Cox-2 expression in prostatic cancer cells. Cell Biol Int. 2001;25(11): 1117–24.

CHAPTER 4: TAPPING THE POWER OF THYROID
AND GROWTH HORMONE

Vanderpump MP, Tunbridge WM, et al. The incidence of thyroid disorders in the community: a twenty-year follow-up of the Whickham Survey. Clin Endocrinol (Oxf). 1995 Jul;43(1):55–68.

Hak AE, Pols HA, et al. Subclinical hypothyroidism is an independent risk factor for atherosclerosis and myocardial infarction in elderly women: the Rotterdam Study. Ann Intern Med. 2000 Feb 15;132(4):270–78.

Michalopoulou G, Alevizaki M. High serum cholesterol levels in persons with "high-normal" TSH levels: should one extend the definition of subclinical hypothyroidism? Eur J Endocrinol. 1998 Feb;138(2):141–45.

Cararis GJ, Manowitz NR, et al. The Colorado Thyroid Disease Prevalence Study. Arch Intern Med. 2000;160:526–34.

Arvat E, Broglio F. Insulin-like growth factor 1: implications in aging. Drugs Aging. 2000 Jan;16(1):29–40.

Rudman D, Feller AG, et al. Effect of human growth hormone in men over 60 years old. N Engl J Med. 1990 Jul 5;323:1–6.

Jorgensen J, Thuesen L. Three years of growth hormone treatment in growth hormone-deficient adults: near normalization of body composition and physical performance. Eur J Endocrinol. 1994;130:224–28.

Blackman MR, et al. Growth hormone and sex steroid administration in healthy aged women and men. JAMA. 2002;288(18):2282–93.

Hoffman AR, Lieberman SA. Functional consequences of the somatopause and its treatment. Endocrine. 1997 Aug;7(1):73–76.

Ceda GP, Dall'Aglio E. The insulin-like growth factor axis and plasma lipid levels in the elderly. J Clin Endocrinol Metab. 1998 Feb;83(2):499–502.

Attanasio AF, Bates PC. Human growth hormone replacement in adult hypopituitary patients. J Clin Endocrinol Metab. 2002, Apr;87(4):1600–6.

Chromiak JA, Antonio J. Use of amino acids as growth hormone-releasing agents by athletes. Nutrition. 2002 Jul-Aug;18(7–8):657–61.

Corpas E, Blackman MR. Oral arginine-lysine does not increase growth hormone or insulin-like growth factor-I in old men. J Gerontol. 1993 Jul;48 (4):M128–33.

CHAPTER 5: MAXIMUM BRAINPOWER FOR LIFE

McDowell K, Kerick SE, et al. Aging, physical activity, and cognitive processing: an examination of P300. Neurobiol Aging. 2003 Jul-Aug;24(4): 597–606.

Kleijnen J, Knipschild P. Gingko biloba for cerebral insufficiency. Br J Clin Pharmacol. 1992 Oct; 34(4):352–58.

Solomon PR, Adams F. Ginkgo for memory enhancement: a randomized controlled trial. JAMA. 2002;288(7):835–40.

Subhan, H. The psychopharmacological effects of ginkgo in normal healthy volunteers. Int J Clin Pharmacol Res. 1984;4(2):89–93.

Carta A, Calvani M, et al. Acetyl-L-carnitine and Alzheimer's disease: pharmacological considerations beyond the cholinergic sphere. Ann NY Acad Sci. 1993;695:324–26.

Bossoni G, Carpi C. Effect of acetyl-L-carnitine on conditioned reflex learning rate and retention in laboratory animals. Drugs Exp Clin Res (Switzerland). 1986;12(11):911–16.

Valerio C, Clementi G, et al. The effects of acetyl-L-carnitine on experimental models of learning and memory deficits in the old rat. Funct Neurol (Italy). 1989;4(4):387–90.

Cipolli C, Chiari G. Effects of L-acetylcarnitine on mental deterioration in the aged: initial results. Clin Ter (Italy). 1990;132(6 Suppl):479–510.

Seidman MD, Khan MJ, et al. Biologic activity of mitochondrial metabolites on aging and age-related hearing loss. Am J Otol. 2000 Mar;21(2):161–67.

Matthews RT, Yang L, et al. Coenzyme Q_{10} administration increases brain mitochondrial concentrations and exerts neuroprotective effects. Proc Natl Acad Sci USA. 1998 Jul 21;95(15):8892–7.

Crook TH, Tinklenberg J, et al. Effects of phosphatidylserine in age-associated memory impairment. Neurology (United States). 1991 May;41(5):644–49.

Milanova D, Nikolov R, et al. Study on the anti-hypoxic effect of some drugs used in the pharmacotherapy of cerebrovascular disease. Methods Find Exp Clin Pharmacol (Spain). 1983 Nov;5(9):607–12.

Balestreri R, Fontana L. A double-blind placebo controlled evaluation of the safety and efficacy of vinpocetine in the treatment of patients with chronic vascular senile cerebral dysfunction. J Am Geriatr Soc. 1987 May;35(5): 425–30.

La Rue A, Koehler KM, et al. Nutritional status and cognitive functioning in a normally aging sample: a 6-y reassessment. Am J Clin Nutr. 1997 Jan;65(1): 20–29.

Ortega RM, Requejo AM, et al. Dietary intake and cognitive function in a group of elderly people. Am J Clin Nutr. 1997 Oct;66(4):803–09.

Deijen JB, van der Beek EJ, et al. Vitamin B_6 supplementation in elderly men: effects on mood, memory, performance and mental effort. Psychopharmacology (Berl). 1992;109(4):489–96.

Perrig WJ, Perrig P, Stahelin HB. The relation between antioxidants and memory performance in the old and very old. J Am Geriatr Soc. 1997 Jun; 45(6):718–24.

Dustman RE, Emmerson RY, et al. Age and fitness effects on EEG, ERPs, visual sensitivity, and cognition. Neurobiol Aging. 1990 May-Jun;11(3): 193–200.

Gomez-Pinilla F, So V, Kesslak JP. Spatial learning and physical activity contribute to the induction of fibroblast growth factor: neural substrates for increased cognition associated with exercise. Neuroscience. 1998 Jul;85 (1):53–61.

Rodriguez-Gomez JA, Venero JL, et al. Deprenyl prevents protein oxidation. Brain Res Mol Brain Res. 1997 Jun;46(1-2):31–38.

Yen TT, Knoll J, et al. Extension of lifespan in mice treated with dinh lang (Policias fruticosum L.) and (-)deprenyl. Acta Physiol Hung. 1992;79(2): 119–24.

Knoll J. Deprenyl medication: a strategy to modulate the age-related decline of the striatal dopaminergic system. J Am Geriatr Soc. 1992 Aug;40(8): 839–47.

Emmenegger H, Meier-Ruge W. The actions of hydergine on the brain: a histochemical, circulatory and neurophysiological study. Pharmacology. 1968;1(1):65–78.

Boismare F, Le Poncin M, Lefrancois J. Biochemical and behavioural effects of hypoxic hypoxia in rats: study of the protection afforded by ergot alkaloids. Gerontology. 1978;24 Suppl 1:6–13.

Sozmen EY, Kanit L, et al. Possible supportive effects of co-dergocrine mesylate on antioxidant enzyme systems in aged rat brain. Eur Neuropsychopharmacol. 1998 Feb;8(1):13–16.

Markstein R. Hydergine: interaction with the neurotransmitter systems in the central nervous system. J Pharmacol. 1985;16 Suppl 3:1–17.

Cahn J, Borzeix MG. [Cerebral blood flow and metabolism, and neurologic deficit in an experimental infarction: application to the study of an ergot derivative] Presse Med. 1983 Dec 29;12(48):3058–60 (French).

Cover CC, Poulin JE, et al. Posttranslational changes in band 3 in adult and aging brain following treatment with ergoloid mesylates, comparison to changes observed in Alzheimer's disease. Life Sci. 1996;58(8):655–64.

Ditch M, Kelly FJ, Resnick O. An ergot preparation (hydergine) in the treatment of cerebrovascular disorders in the geriatric patient: double-blind study. J Am Geriatr Soc. 1971 Mar;19(3):208–17.

Gallai V, Mazzotta G, et al. A clinical and neurophysiological trial on noötropic drugs in patients with mental decline. Acta Neurol (Napoli). 1991 Feb;13(1):1–12.

Canonico PL, Aronica E, et al. Repeated injections of piracetam improve spatial learning and increase the stimulation of inositol phospholipid hydrolysis by excitatory amino acids in aged rats. Funct Neurol. 1991 Apr-Jun; 6(2):107–11.

Bartus RT, et al. Profound effects of combining choline and piracetam on memory enhancement and cholinergic function in aged rats. Neurobiol Aging. 1981;2:105–11.

Ferris SH, et al. Combination of choline/piracetam in the treatment of senile dementia. Psychopharm Bull. 1982;18: 94–98.

Friedman E, et al. Clinical response to choline plus piracetam in senile dementia: relation to red-cell choline levels. N Engl J Med. 1981:304(24): 1490–91.

Buresova O, Bures J. Piracetam-induced facilitation of interhemispheric transfer of visual information in rats. Psychopharmacol (Berlin). 1976; 46:93–102.

Chase CH, et al. A new chemotherapeutic investigation: piracetam effects on dyslexia. Annals of Dyslexia. 1984;34:29–48.

De Deyn PP, Orgogozo JM, et al. Acute treatment of stroke. PASS group. Piracetam Acute Stroke Study. Lancet. 1998 Jul 25;352(9124):326.

Pilch H, et al. Piracetam elevates muscarinic cholinergic receptor density in the frontal cortex of aged but not of young mice. Psychopharmacol. 1988;94:74–78.

Paula-Barbosa MM, Brandao F, et al. The effects of piracetam on lipofuscin of the rat cerebellar and hippocampal neurons after long-term alcohol treatment and withdrawal: a quantitative study. Alcohol Clin Exp Res. 1991 Oct;15(5):834–38.

Jouvet M, Albarede JL, et al. Noradrenaline and cerebral aging. Encephale. 1991 May;17(3):187–95.

Saletu B, Frey R, et al. Differential effects of a new central adrenergic agonist— modafinil and d-amphetamine on sleep and early morning behaviour in elderly. Arzneimittelforschung. 1989 Oct;39(10):1268–73.

Laffont F, Mayer G, et al. Modafinil in diurnal sleepiness, a study of 123 patients. Expl Fonct Neuro CHU Paris France. Sleep. 1994 Dec;17(8):5113–15.

Billiard M, Besset A, et al. Modafinil, a double blind multicentric study. Sleep. 1994 Dec;17(8):5107–12.

Saletu B, Frey R, et al. Differential effects of a new central adrenergic agonist—modafinil and d-amphetamine on sleep and early morning behaviour in young healthy volunteers. Int J Clinical Pharm Res. 1989;9(3):183–85.

Lagarde D, Batejat D, et al. Interest of modafinil, a new psychostimulant during a sixty-hour sleep deprivation experiment. Fundam Clin Pharmacol. 1995;9(3):271–79.

Goldenberg F, Weil JS, Van Frenkeel R. Effects of modafinil on diurnal variation of objective sleepiness in normal subjects. 5th Int Cong Sleep Research. 1987(149).

CHAPTER 6: CURTAILING OXIDATION:
RUST-PROOFING YOUR CELLS

Harmon D. Free radical theory of aging: effect of free radical reaction inhibitors on the mortality rate of male LAF1 mice. J Gerontol. 1967:23:476.

Meydani SN, et al. Vitamin E supplementation and in vivo immune response in healthy subjects. JAMA. 1997;227:1380–86.

Bostick RM. Reduced risk of colon cancer with high intake of vitamin E: The Iowa Women's Health Study. Cancer Res. 1993;53:4230–37.

Jacobs EJ, Connell CJ. Vitamin C and vitamin E supplement use and colorectal cancer mortality in a large American Cancer Society cohort. Cancer Epidemiol Biomarkers Prev. 2001 Jan;10(1):17–23.

Fleischauer AT, Simonsen N, Arab L. Antioxidant supplements and risk of breast cancer recurrence and breast cancer-related mortality among postmenopausal women. Nutr Cancer. 2003;46(1):15–22.

Di Matteo V, Esposito E. Biochemical and therapeutic effects of antioxidants in the treatment of Alzheimer's disease, Parkinson's disease, and amyotrophic lateral sclerosis. Curr Drug Target CNS Neurol Disord. 2003 Apr; 2(2):95–107.

Martin A. Antioxidant vitamins E and C and risk of Alzheimer's disease. Nutr Rev. 2003 Feb;61(2):69–73.

Seddon M, et al. Dietary carotenoids, vitamins A, C, and E & age related macular degeneration. Eye Disease Case Control Study Group. JAMA. 1994; 272:1413–20.

Goodman GE, Schaffer S. The association between lung and prostate cancer risk, and serum micronutrients: results and lessons learned from beta-carotene and retinol efficacy trial. Cancer Epidemiol Biomarkers Prev. 2003 Jun;12(6):518–26.

Ito Y, Wakai K. Serum carotenoids and mortality from lung cancer: a case-control study nested in the Japan Collaborative Cohort (JACC) study. Cancer Sci. 2003 Jan;94(1):57–63.

Handelman GJ. The evolving role of carotenoids in human biochemistry. Nutrition. 2001 Oct;17(10):818–22.

Holick CN, Michaud DS. Dietary carotenoids, serum beta-carotene, and retinol and risk of lung cancer in the alpha-tocopherol, beta-carotene cohort study. Am J Epidemiol. 2002 Sep 15;156(6):536–47.

Yoshikawa K, et al. Study of prediagnosed selenium levels in toenails and the risk of advanced prostate cancer. J Natl Cancer Inst. 1998;90: 1219–24.

Givannucci E, et al. Intake of carotenoids and retinol in relation to risk of prostate cancer. J Nat Cancer Inst. 1995;87:1767–76.

Clark L, et al. Effects of selenium supplementation for cancer prevention in patients with carcinoma of the skin. JAMA. 1996;276:1957–63.

Russel T, et al. Coenzyme Q_{10} administration increases brain mitochondrial concentration and exerts neuroprotective effects. Proc Nat Acad Sci. 1998;95:8892–97.

Singh RB, et al. Randomized double blind placebo-controlled trial of coenzyme Q_{10} in patients with acute myocardial infarction. Cardiovasc Drugs Ther. 1998;12:347–53.

Johnston CS, Meyer CG, Srilakshmi JC. Vitamin C elevates red blood cell glutathione in healthy adults. Am J Clin Nutr. 1993;58:103–5.

Bunin AI, Filina AA, Erchev VP. A glutathione deficiency in open-angle glaucoma and the approaches to its correction. Vestn Oftalmol. 1992;108: 13–15.

Sen CK. Glutathione homeostasis in response to exercise training and nutritional supplements. Mol Cell Biochem. 1999 Jun;196(1-2):31–42.

Bounous G, Gervais F, Amer V, et al. The influence of dietary whey protein on tissue glutathione and the diseases of aging. Clin Invest Med. 1989;12: 343–49.

Packer L, Tritschler HJ, Wessel K. Neuroprotection by the metabolic antioxidant alpha-lipoic acid. Free Radic Biol Med. 1997;22(1–2): 359–78.

Podda M, Tritschler HJ, Ulrich H, Packer L. Alpha-lipoic acid supplementation prevents symptoms of vitamin E deficiency. Biochem Biophys Res Commun. 1994 Oct 14;204(1):98–104.

Gaetke LM, Chow CK. Copper toxicity, oxidative stress, and antioxidant nutrients. Toxicology. 2003 Jul 15;189(1–2):147–63.

Packer L, Witt EH, Tritschler HJ. Alpha-lipoic acid as a biological antioxidant. Free Radic Biol Med. 1995 Aug;19(2):227–50.

Borek C. Molecular mechanisms in cancer induction and prevention. Environ Health Perspectives. 1993;101:237–45.

Harman D. Free radical involvement in aging. Pathophysiology and clinical implications. Drugs Aging. 1993;3:60–80.

Brunk UT, Terman A. Lipofuscin: mechanisms of age-related accumulation and influence on cell function. Free Radic Biol Med. 2002 Sep 1;33(5): 611–19.

Dei R, Takeda A. Lipid peroxidation and advanced glycation end products in the brain in normal aging and in Alzheimer's disease. Neuropathol (Berl). 2002 Aug;104(2):113–22.

Borek C. Antioxidants and cancer. Sci Med. 1997;4:51–61.

Gey KF. Ten year retrospective on the antioxidant hypothesis of atherosclerosis. J Nut Biochem. 1995;6: 206–236.

Richardson SJ. Free radicals in the genesis of Alzheimer's disease. Ann. NY Acad Sci. 1993;695:73–76.

Russel RM, Suter PM. Vitamin requirements of elderly people: an update. Am J Clin Nut. 1991;1:9–18.

Jama JW, et al. Dietary antioxidants and cognitive functions in a population based sample of older persons. Am J Epidemiol. 1996;144:275–80.

Lykkesfeld J, et al. Age-associated decline in ascorbic acid concentration, recycling, and biosynthesis in rat hepatocytes-reversal with R alpha lipoic acid supplementation. FASEB J. 1998;12:1183–9.

Fleischauer AT, Simonsen N, Arab L. Antioxidant supplements and risk of breast cancer recurrence and breast cancer–related mortality among postmenopausal women. Nutr Cancer. 2003;46(1):15–22.

Jacobs EJ, Henion AK. Vitamin C and vitamin E supplement use and bladder cancer mortality in a large cohort of US men and women. Am J Epidemiol. 2002 Dec 1;156(11):1002–10.

Bonnefoy M, Drai J, Kostka T. [Antioxidants to slow aging, facts and perspectives] Presse Med. 2002 Jul 27;31(25):1174–84 (French).

Fleischauer AT, Olson SH, et al. Dietary antioxidants, supplements, and risk of epithelial ovarian cancer. Nutr Cancer. 2001;40(2):92–98.

Watkins ML, Erickson JD, et al. Multivitamin use and mortality in a large prospective study. Am J Epidemiol. 2000 Jul 15;152(2):149–62.

Blot WJ, et al. Nutrition intervention trials in Linxian, China: supplementation with specific vitamin/mineral combinations, cancer incidence and disease specific mortality in the general population. J Nat Cancer Inst. 1993; 85:1483–92.

Schalch W, Chylack LT. [Antioxidant micronutrients and cataract. Review and comparison of the AREDS and REACT cataract studies] Ophthalmologe. 2003 Mar;100(3):181–89 (German).

Block G, Patterson B, Subar A. Fruit, vegetables and cancer prevention: a review of the epidemiological evidence. Nutr Cancer. 1992;18:1–29.

Gillman M, et al. Protective effects of vegetables on the development of stroke in men. JAMA. 1995;Apr 12;273(14):1113–6.

Hertog MGL, et al. Dietary antioxidants, flavonoids and the risk of coronary heart disease: the Zutphen elderly study. Lancet. 1993;342:1007–11.

Ridker PM, et al. Inflammation, aspirin and the risk of cardiovascular disease in apparently healthy men. NEJM. 1997 Apr 3;336(14):973–79.

McCarty MF. Interleukin 6 as a central mediator of cardiovascular risk associated with chronic inflammation. Med Hypotheses. 1999 May;52(5); 465–77.

Kanta T. C-reactive protein in the cardiovascular system. Rinsho Byori. 2001 Apr;49(4):395–401.

Rader DJ. Inflammatory markers of coronary risk. NEJM. 2000 Oct 19;343 (16):1139–47.

Rifai N, Ridker PM. Inflammatory markers and coronary heart disease. Curr Opin Lipidol. 2002 Aug;13(4):383–89.

Bermudez EA, Ridker PM. C-reactive protein, statins, and primary prevention of atherosclerotic cardiovascular disease. Prev Cardiol. 2002 winter;5(10): 42–46.

CHAPTER 7: COOLING INFLAMMATION: DISEASE PROOFING YOUR BODY

Coussens LM, Werb Z. Inflammation and Cancer. Nature. 2002 Dec 19–26; 420(6917):860–67.

Moran EM. Epidemiological and clinical aspects of nonsteroidal anti-inflammatory drugs and cancer risks. J Environ Pathol Toxicol Oncol. 2002;21(2):193–201.

Cotterchio M, Kreiger N, Sloan M, Steingart A. Nonsteroidal anti-inflammatory drug use and breast cancer risk. Cancer Epidemiol Biomarkers Prev. 2001 Nov;10(11):1213–17.

Corley DA, Kerlikowske K, Verma R, Buffler P. Protective association of aspirin/NSAIDs and esophageal cancer: a systematic review and meta-analysis. Gastroenterology. 2003 Jan;124(1):47–56.

Viner JL, Umar A, Hawk ET. Chemoprevention of colorectal cancer: problems, progress, and prospects. Gastroenterol Clin North Am. 2002 Dec; 31(4):971–99.

Leitzmann MF, Stampfer MJ, et al. Aspirin use in relation to risk of prostate cancer. Cancer Epidemiol Biomarkers Prev. 2002 Oct; 11(10 Pt 1): 1108–11.

Roberts RO, Jacobson DJ. A population based study of NSAID use and prostate cancer. Mayo Clinic Proceedings. 2002 Mar;77:219–25.

Johnson TW, Anderson KE, Lazovich D, Folsom AR. Association of aspirin and nonsteroidal anti-inflammatory drug use with breast cancer. Cancer Epidemiol Biomarkers Prev. 2002. Dec;11(12):1586–91.

Funkhouser EM, Sharp GB. Aspirin and reduced risk of esophageal carcinoma. Cancer. 1995 Oct 1;76(7):1116–9.

Paganini-Hill A. Aspirin and colorectal cancer: the Leisure World cohort revisited. Prev Med. 1995 Mar;24(2):113–15.

Study commissioned by Alzheimer's association, conducted by the Lewin Group, April 3, 2001.

Anthony JC, et al. Reduced prevalence of AD in users of NSAIDs and H2 receptor antagonists. Neurol. 2000;54(11):2066–71.

Breitner JC, et al. Inverse association of anti-inflammatory treatments and AD. Neurol. 1994;44:227–32.

MacKenzie IR, et al. NSAIDs use and Alzheimer-type pathology in aging. Neurol. 1998;50:986–90.

Lim GP, et al. Ibuprofen suppresses plaque pathology and inflammation in a mouse model for Alzheimer's disease. J Neurosci. 2000;20:5709–14.

Mitchell T, Needham A. Over-the-counter drug is treatment for Alzheimer's. Life Extension Magazine. 2000 Nov;51–55.

Mukherjee D. Risk of cardiovascular events associated with selective COX-2 inhibitors. JAMA. 2001 Aug 22–29;286(8):954–59.

Strohmeyer R, Rogers J. Molecular and cellular mediators of Alzheimer's disease inflammation. J Alzheimers Dis. 2001;3(1):131–57.

Tucker ON, Dannenberg AJ, et al. Cyclooxygenase-2 expression is up-regulated in human pancreatic cancer. Cancer Res. 1999 March 1;59(5):987–90.

Jick H, Zornberg GL, et al. Statins and the risk of dementia. Lancet. 2000 Nov 11;356(9242):1627–31.

Wolozin B, Kellman W. Decreased prevalence of Alzheimer's disease associated with statin drugs. Arch Neurol. 2000;57:1439–43.

Horne BD, Muhlestein JB. Statin therapy interacts with cytomegalovirus seropositivity and high C-reactive protein in reducing mortality among patients with angiographically significant coronary disease. Circulation. 2003 Jan 21;107(2):258–63.

Teucher T, Obertreis B, et al. Cytokine secretion in whole blood of healthy subjects following oral administration of *Urtica dioica L.* plant extract. Arzeneimittelforschung. 1996 Sep;46(9):906–10.

Haden ST, Glowacki J, et al. Effects of age on serum DHEA, IGF-1, and IL-6 levels in women. Calcif Tissue Int. 2000 Jun;66(6):41408.

Killer-Galperin M, Galilly R, et al. DHEA selectively inhibits production of TNF-alpha and IL-6 in astrocytes. Int J Dev Neurosci. 1999 Dec;17(8): 765–75.

Reddi K, Henderson B, et al. IL-6 production by lipopolysaccharide-stimulated human fibroblasts is potently inhibited by vitamin K compounds. Cytokine. 1995 Apr;7(3):287–90.

CHAPTER 8: PROTECTING YOUR HEART AND BRAIN BY ENHANCING METHYLATION

McCully KS. Homocysteine and vascular disease. Nat Med. 1996 Apr;2(4): 386–89.

Harpel P, et al. Homocysteine and other sulfhydryl compounds enhance the binding of lipoprotein(a) to fibrin: a potential link between thrombosis, atherogenesis and sulfhydryl compound metabolism. Proc Nat Acad Sci (USA). 1992;89:10193–97.

Langman LJ, et al. Hyperhomocysteinemia and the increased risk of venous thromboembolism. Arch Intern Med. 2000;160:961–64.

Perry IJ, et al. Prospective study of serum total homocysteine concentration and risk of stroke in middle-aged British men. Lancet. 1995;346:1395–98.

Nygard O, et al. Plasma homocysteine levels and mortality in patients with coronary artery disease. NEJM. 1997;337(4):230–36.

Clarke R. Folate, vitamin B_{12}, and serum total homocysteine levels in confirmed Alzheimer disease. Arch Neurol. 1998;55:1449–55.

Duthie SJ, Whalley LJ, et al. Homocysteine, B vitamin status, and cognitive function in the elderly. Am J Clin Nutr. 2002 May;75(5):908–13.

Regland B, Andersson M. Increased concentrations of homocysteine in the cerebrospinal fluid in patients with fibromyalgia and chronic fatigue syndrome. Scand J Rheumatol. 1997;26(4):301–07.

Dhonukshe-Rutten RA. Vitamin B_{12} status is associated with bone mineral content and bone mineral density in frail elderly women but not in men. J Nutr. 2003 Mar;133(3):801–07.

Brattstrom LE. Folic acid responsive postmenopausal homocysteinemia. Metabolism. 1985;34:1073–7.

Hoogeveen EK, Kostense PJ, et al. Hyperhomocysteinemia is associated with the presence of retinopathy in type 2 diabetes mellitus: the Hoorn study. Arch Intern Med. 2000 Oct 23;160(19):2984–90.

Mattson MP, Haberman F. Folate and homocysteine metabolism: therapeutic targets in cardiovascular and neurodegenerative disorders. Curr Med Chem. 2003 Oct;10(19):1923–9.

Bjelland I, et al. Folate, vitamin B_{12}, homocysteine, and the MTHFR 677C->T polymorphism in anxiety and depression: the Hordaland Homocysteine Study. Arch Gen Psychiatry. 2003 Jun;60(6):618–26.

Catargi B. Homocysteine, hypothyroidism, and effect of thyroid hormone replacement. Thyroid. 1999;9:1163–6.

Cattaneo M. High prevalence of hyperhomocysteinemia in patients with inflammatory bowel disease. Thromb Haemost. 1998;80:542–45.

Romagnuolo J. Hyperhomocysteinemia and inflammatory bowel disease: prevalence and predictors in a cross-sectional study. Am J Gastroenterol. 2001 Jul;96(7):2143–9.

Simile MM, Pascale R, et al. Correlation between S-adenosyl-L-methionine content and production of c-myc, c-Ha-ras, and c-Ki-ras mRNA transcripts in the early stages of rat liver carcinogenesis. Cancer Lett. 1994 Apr 29; 79(1):9–16.

Rifai N, Ridker PM. Inflammatory markers and coronary heart disease. Curr Opin Lipidol. 2002 Aug;13(4):383–89.

Ravnskov, U. Cholesterol lowering trials in coronary heart disease: frequency of citation and outcome. Br Med J. 1992;305(6844):15–19.

Olsson AG, Eriksson M, Johnson O. A 52-week, multicenter, randomized, parallel-group, double-blind, double-dummy study to assess the efficacy of atorvastatin and simvastatin in reaching low-density lipoprotein cholesterol and triglyceride targets: the treat-to-target (3T) study. Clin Ther. 2003 Jan;25(1):119–38.

Robinson K, Mayer EL. Hyperhomocysteinemia and low pyridoxal phosphate: common and independent reversible risk factors for coronary artery disease. Circulation. 1995 Nov 15;92(10):2825–30.

Selhub J. Vitamin status and intake as primary determinant of homocysteinemia in an elderly population. JAMA. 1993;270(22):2693–98.

Brattstrom L. Vitamins and homocysteine lowering agents. J Nutr. 1996;126: 1276S–1280S.

Simes RF. Low cholesterol and risk of non-coronary mortality. Aust NZ J Med. 1994;24(10):113–9.

Qureshi AA. Dose-dependent suppression of serum cholesterol by tocotrienol-rich fraction (TRF25) of rice bran in hypercholesterolemic humans. Atherosclerosis. 2002 Mar;161(1):199–207.

CHAPTER 9: PREVENTING GLYCATION:
AGE-PROOFING YOUR ORGANS

Stadtman ER. Protein oxidation and aging. Science. 1992;257(5074):1220–4.

Bierhaus A, et al. AGEs and their interaction with AGE receptors in vascular disease and diabetes mellitus. Cardiovasc Res. 1998;37(3):586–600.

Munch G, et al. Alzheimer's disease—synergistic effects of glucose deficit, oxidative stress and advanced glycation endproducts. J Neural Transm. 1998; 105(4–5):439–61.

Munch G. Influence of advanced glycation end-products and AGE-inhibitors on nucleation-dependent polymerization of beta-amyloid peptide. Biochem Biophys Acta. 1997;1360(1):17–29.

Hipkiss AR. Carnosine protects proteins against methylglyoxal-mediated modifications. Biochem Biophys Res Commun. 1998;248(1):28–32.

Browson C. Carnosine reacts with a glycated protein. Free Radic Biol Med. 2000;28(10):1564–70.

Steurenburg HJ. Concentrations of free carnosine in human muscle biopsies and rat muscle. Arch Gerontol Geratr. 1999;(29):107–13.

Quinn PJ. Carnosine: its properties, functions, and potential therapeutic applications. Mol Aspects Med. 1992;13(5):379–444.

Babizhayev MA. Efficacy of N-acetylcarnosine in the treatment of cataracts. Drugs R D. 2002;3(2):87–103.

Hipkiss AR. Pluripotent protective effects of carnosine, a naturally occurring di-peptide. Ann NY Acad Sci. 1998;854:37–53.

Horning MS. Endogenous mechanisms of neuroprotection: role of zinc, copper, and carnosine. Brain Res. 2000;852(1):56–61.

Ririe DG, Roberts PR, et al. Vasodilatory actions of the dietary peptide carnosine. Nutrition. 2000 Mar;16(3):168–72.

Zaloga GP. Carnosine is a novel peptide modulator of intracellular calcium and contractibility in cardiac cells. Am J Physiol. 1997;272(1Pt2):H462–68.

Roberts PR, Zaloga GP. Cardiovascular effects of carnosine. Biochemistry (Mosc). 2000 Jul;65(7):856–61.

Roberts PR, Black KW, et al. Dietary peptides improve wound healing following surgery. Nutrition. 1998 Mar;14(3):266–69.

McFarland GA. Retardation of the senescence of cultured human diploid fibroblasts by carnosine. Exp Cell Res. 1994;212(2):167–75.

McFarland GA. Further evidence for the rejuvenating effects of the dipeptide L-carnosine on cultured human diploid fibroblasts. Exp Gerontol. 1999;34(1):35–45.

Yuneva MO. Effect of carnosine on age-induced changes in senescence-accelerated mice. J Anti-Aging Med. 1999;2(4):337–42.

CHAPTER 11: DESIGNING YOUR ANTI-AGING SUPPLEMENT PROGRAM

Levine M, Conry-Cantilena C, et al. Vitamin C pharmacokinetics in healthy volunteers: evidence for a recommended dietary allowance. Proc Natl Acad Sci USA. 1996 Apr 16;93(8):3704–9.

Ausman LM. Criteria and recommendations for vitamin C intake. Nutr Rev. 1999 Jul;57(7):222–224.

Carr AC, Frei B. Toward a new recommended dietary allowance for vitamin C based on antioxidant and health effects in humans. Am J Clin Nutr. 1999 Jun;69(6):1086–1107.

Johnston CS. Biomarkers for establishing a tolerable upper intake level for vitamin C. Nutr Rev. 1999 Mar;57(3):71–77.

Wallin R. Arterial calcification: a review of mechanisms, animal models, and the prospects for therapy. Med Res Rev. 2001 Jul;21(4):274–301.

Witteman JC. Aortic calcified plaques and cardiovascular disease (the Framingham Study). Am J Cardiol. 1990;66:1060–4.

Van Noord PA, et al. Mammograms may convey more than breast cancer risk: breast arterial calcification and arteriosclerotic related disease in women of the DOM cohort. Eur J Cancer Prev. 1996 Dec;5(6):483–87.

Jie KSG. Vitamin K status and bone mass in women with and without aerotic athersclorisi: a population based study. Calcif Tissue Int. 1996;59:352–56.

Browner WE. Non-trauma mortality in elderly women with low bone mineral density. Study of Osteoporotic Fractures Research Group. Lancet. 1991;338:355–58.

CHAPTER 12: THE ANTI-AGING LIFESTYLE

Hudgins LC, Hellerstein M, et al. Human fatty acid synthesis is stimulated by a eucaloric low fat, high carbohydrate diet. J Clin Invest. 1996 May 1;97(9):2081–91.

McManus K, Antinoro L, et al. A randomized controlled trial of a moderate-fat, low-energy diet compared with a low-fat, low-energy diet for weight loss in overweight adults. Int J Obes Relat Metab Disord. 2001 Oct;25(10):1503–11.

Tremblay A, Simoneau JA. Impact of exercise intensity on body fatness and skeletal muscle metabolism. Metabolism. 1994 Jul;43(7):814–18.

Sedlock DA, Fissinger JA, Melby CL. Effect of exercise intensity and duration on postexercise energy expenditure. Med Sci Sports Exerc. 1989 Dec;21(6):662–66.

Thornton MK, Potteiger JA. Effects of resistance exercise bouts of different intensities but equal work on EPOC. Med Sci Sports Exerc. 2002 Apr;34(4):715–22.

McCraty R, Barrios-Choplin B, et al. The impact of a new emotional self-management program on stress, emotions, heart rate variability, DHEA and cortisol. Integr Physiol Behav Sci. 1998;33(2):151–70.

Walston KG, Pugh ND, et al. Stress reduction and preventing hypertension. J Altern Complement Med. 1995 Fall;1(3):263–83.

Kamei T, Toriumi Y, et al. Decrease in serum cortisol during yoga exercise. Percept Mot Skills. 2000 Jun;90(3Pt1):1027–32.

Kabat-Zinn J, Lipworth L, Burney R, Sellers W. Four year follow-up of a meditation-based program for the self-regulation of chronic pain: Treatment outcomes and compliance. Clin J Pain. 1986;2:159–73.

Kradin RL, Benson H. Stress, the relaxation response and immunity. Modern Aspects of Immunobiology. 2001;1(3):110–13.

Lehmann JW, Benson H. Nonpharmacologic treatment of hypertension: a review. Gen Hosp Psychiatry. 1982;4:27–32.

Webster A. Mind/body medicine: self-care skills for persons with cancer. Cancer Pract. 1999 Jan/Feb;7:1.

Spiegel K, Leproult R, Van Cauter E. Impact of sleep debt on metabolic and endocrine function. Lancet. 1999 Oct 23;354(9188):1435–39.

Ayas NT, White DP. A prospective study of sleep duration and coronary heart disease in women. Arch Intern Med. 2003 Jan 27;163(2):205–9.

Dawson D, Encel N. Melatonin and sleep in humans. J Pineal Res. 1993;15:1–12.

Brzezinski, A. Melatonin in humans. N Engl J Med. 1997;336:186–94.

CHAPTER 13: EXTENDING HUMAN LIFE SPAN

Ross MH. Length of life and nutrition in the rat. J Nutr. 1961;75;197–210.

Masoro EJ. Caloric restriction and aging: an update. Exp Gerontol. 2000 May; 35(3):299–305.

Stokkan KA, Reiter RJ. Endocrine and metabolic effect of life-long food restriction in rats. Acta Endocrinol (Copenhagen). 1991;125:93–100.

Yu BP, Chung HY. Stress resistance by caloric restriction for longevity. Ann NY Acad Sci. 2001 Apr;928:39–47.

Sohal RS, Weindruch R. Oxidative stress, caloric restriction, and aging. Science. 1996 Jul 5;273(5271):59–63.

Cao, SX, Dhahbi JM. Genomic profiling of short and long term caloric restriction in the liver of aging mice. Proc Natl Acad Sci USA. 2001;98:10630–5.

Weindruch R, Walford RI. Dietary restriction in mice beginning at 1 year of age: effect on lifespan and spontaneous cancer incidence. Science. 1982;215: 1415–18.

Wanagat J, Allison DB, Weindruch R. Caloric intake and aging: mechanisms in rodents and a study in nonhuman primates. Toxicol Sci. 1999 Dec; 52(2 Suppl):35–40.

Walford RL, Mock D, Verdery R, MacCallum T. Calorie restriction in Biosphere 2: alterations in physiologic, hematologic, hormonal, and biochemical parameters in humans restricted for a 2-year period. J Gerontol A Biol Sci Med Sci. 2002 Jun;57(6):B211–24.

Okinawa Centenarian Study data presented at the American Geriatrics Society annual meeting, 2001.

Goodrick CL, Ingram DK. Effects of intermittent feeding upon body weight and lifespan in inbred mice: interaction of genotype and age. Mech Ageing Dev. 1990 Jul;55(1):69–87.

London ED, Waller SB. Effects of intermittent feeding on neurochemical markers in aging rat brain. Neurobiol Aging. 1985 Fall;6(3):199–204.

Goodrick CL, Ingram DK. Effects of intermittent feeding upon growth, activity, and lifespan in rats allowed voluntary exercise. Exp Aging Res. 1983 Fall; 9(3):203–9.

Anson RM, Guo Z. Intermittent fasting dissociates beneficial effects of dietary restriction on glucose metabolism and neuronal resistance to injury from calorie intake. Proc Natl Acad Sci USA. 2003 May 13;100(10):6216–20.

Lee CK, Klopp RG. Gene expression profile of aging and its retardation by caloric restriction. Science. 1999;285:1390–3.

Kirkwood TB. Genes that shape the course of ageing. Trends Endocrinol Metab. 2003 Oct;14(8):345–47.

Barbieri M, Bonafe M, Franceschi C, Paolisso G. Insulin/IGF-I-signaling pathway: an evolutionarily conserved mechanism of longevity from yeast to humans. Am J Physiol Endocrinol Metab. 2003 Nov;285(5):E1064–71.

Dilman VM, Anisimov VN. Effect of treatment with phenformin, diphenylhydantoin or L-dopa on life span and tumour incidence in C3H/Sn mice. Gerontology. 1980;26(5):243–46.

Deutsch, JC. Efficacy of metformin in non-insulin-dependent diabetes mellitus. N Engl J Med. 1996;334(4):269.

Cusi K, DeFronzo RA. Metformin, a review of its metabolic effects. Diabetes Reviews. 1998;6(2):89–131.

Charles MA, Eschwege E. Prevention of type 2 diabetes: role of metformin. Drugs. 1999;58(Suppl 1):71–73.

CHAPTER 14: THE CELLULAR TIME MACHINE

Baur J, Zou Y. Telomere position in human cells. Science. 2001;292:2075–77.

von Zglinicki T, Pilger R, Sitte N. Accumulation of single-strand breaks is the major cause of telomere shortening in human fibroblasts. Free Radic Biol Med. 2000 Jan 1;28(1):64–74.

Epel ES, Blackburn EH, et al. Accelerated telomere shortening in response to life stress. Proc Natl Acad Sci USA. 2004 Dec;101(49):17312–15.

von Zglinicki T. Oxidative stress shortens telomeres. Trends Biochem Sci. 2002 Jul;27(7):339–44.

Xu D, Neville R, Finkel T. Homocysteine accelerates endothelial cell senescence. FEBS Lett. 2000 Mar 17;470(1):20–24.

Serra V, von Zglinicki T, Lorenz M, Saretzki G. Extracellular superoxide dismutase is a major antioxidant in human fibroblasts and slows telomere shortening. J Biol Chem. 2003 Feb 28;278(9):6824–30.

Furumoto K, Inoue E. Age-dependent telomere shortening is slowed down by enrichment of intracellular vitamin C. Life Sci. 1998;63(11):935–48.

Wolf NS, Pendergrass WR. The relationships of animal age and caloric intake to cellular replication in vivo and in vitro: a review. J Gerontol A Biol Sci Med Sci. 1999 Nov;54(11):B502–17.

Kim NW, Piatyszek MA, et al. Specific association of human telomerase activity with immortal cells and cancer. Science. 1994 Dec 23;266(5193):2011–15.

Herbert B. Inhibition of human telomerase in immortal human cells leads to progressive telomere shortening and cell death. Proc Nat Acad Sci. 1999; 96:14276–81.

Bodnar AG. Extension of life span by introduction of telomerase in normal human cells. Science. 1998;279:349–52.

Morales CP, Holt SE. Absence of cancer-associated changes in human fibroblasts immortalized with telomerase. Nat Genet. 1999 Jan;21(1):115–18.

Jiang XR, Jimenez G. Telomerase expression in human somatic cells does not induce changes associated with a transformed phenotype. Nat Genet. 1999 Jan;21(1):111–14.

Cibelli JB, Kiessling AA. Somatic cell nuclear transfer in humans: pronuclear and early embryonic development. E-Biomed: The Journal of Regenerative Medicine. 2001;2:25–31.

Hwang WS, Ryu YJ, et al. Evidence of a pluripotent human embryonic stem cell line derived from a cloned blastocyst. Science. 2004 Mar;303:1669–74.

Thomson JA, et al. Embryonic stem cell lines derived from human blastocysts. Science. 1998 Nov 6;282(5391):1145–47.

Reubinoff BE, Itzykson P. Neural progenitors from human embryonic stem cells. Nat Biotechnol. 2001 Dec;19:12:1134–40.

Schuldiner M, Eiger S. Induced neuronal differentiation of human embryonic stem cells. Brain Research. 2001 Sep 21;913:2:2012–205.

Zhang SC, Wernig M. In vitro differentiation of transplantable neural precursors form human embryonic stem cells. Nat Biotechnol. 2001 Dec;19(12): 1129–33.

Jackson DA, Majka SM, et al. Regeneration of ischemic cardiac muscle and vascular endothelium by adult stem cells. J Clin Invest. 2001 Jun;107:11: 1395–1402.

El Oakley RM, et al. Myocyte transplantation for cardiac repair: a few good cells can mend a broken heart. Ann Thorac Surg. 2001;71:1724–33.

Ostenfeld T, Svendsen CN. Recent advances in stem cell neurobiology. Adv Tech Stand Neurosurg. 2003;28:3–89.

Storch A, Schwarz J. Neural stem cells and Parkinson's disease. J Neurol. 2002 Oct;249 Suppl 3:III/30–32.

Levesque M, Neuman T. Adult stem cells used to repair damage from Parkinson's disease, presented at annual meeting of the American Association of Neurological Surgeons, Chicago, IL, April 2002.

CHAPTER 15: A BRIDGE TO THE FUTURE

Storey KB. Life in a frozen state: adaptive strategies for natural freeze tolerance in amphibians and reptiles. Am J Physiol. 1990;258:R559–R568.

Storey KB. Biochemistry of natural freeze tolerance in animals: molecular adaptations and applications to cryopreservation. Biochem Cell Biol. 1990; 68:687–98.

Storey KB, Storey JM. Frozen and alive. Scientific American. 1990;263:92–97.

Smith A. Studies on golden hamsters during cooling to and rewarming from body temperatures below 0 degrees C. II. Observations during and after resuscitation. Proc R Soc Lond B Biol Sci. 1956 Jul 24;145(920):407–26.

Palmer TD, Schwartz PH. Cell culture: progenitor cells from human brain after death. Nature. 2001 May 3;411(6833):42–43.

Broxmeyer HE, Srour EF. High-efficiency recovery of functional hematopoietic progenitor and stem cells from human cord blood cryopreserved for 15 years. Proc Natl Acad Sci USA. 2003 Jan 21;100(2):645–50.

Wang X, Chen H. Fertility after intact ovary transplantation. Nature. 2002 Jan 24;415(6870):385.

Acknowledgments

Thanks to Saul Kent, Melanie Segala, Amber Needham, Larry Wood, and Michele Morrow, D.O., for their invaluable research assistance and advice. Thanks also to Lynn Sonberg for making the book possible, and to our editor, Toni Burbank, for making it better than it would otherwise have been. And for their unstinting enthusiasm, patience, and support, heartfelt thanks to friends and family, especially Michelle.

M.R.

I want to thank Lynn Sonberg, for her guidance and unflagging support for this project; Monica Reinagel, my writer, for her tenacity and Herculean efforts; and Toni Burbank, my editor at Bantam Books, for her incisive decisions.

A personal note of gratitude is owed, in memoriam, to a very dear friend, Robert Cisowski, who survived and thrived ten years with an "inoperable" lung cancer. His vision, motivation, strength, and zest led me to explore and open my medical approach to a much wider array of possibilities.

On the sixth anniversary of my father's passing, at home, I honor him for showing us through his dignity and strength that the "final passage" is truly part of life's journey.

Thanks to Clifford Grobstein, Ph.D., and Joseph Stokes, III, M.D., both deans of the UC San Diego School of Medicine, who advocated thinking "outside the box" and exemplified the nobility of a life filled with a never-ending pursuit of knowledge.

Among all the colleagues and friends who have encouraged and inspired me over the course of the past decade, special thanks to Ward Dean, M.D., Steven Fowkes, Ph.D., Dharma Singh Khalsa, M.D., Ron Rothenberg, M.D., Eric Braverman, M.D., Elson Haas, M.D., Hyla Cass, M.D., Ron Klatz, M.D., Robert Goldman, M.D., and Robert Superko, M.D.

Very special thanks, with immense gratitude, to Julian Whitaker, M.D., who was instrumental in starting me on a whole new path in medicine.

And, finally, my gratitude to Saul Kent and Bill Faloon of the Life Extension Foundation for their courage, persistence and vision in fighting for the right of all Americans to access a better and more sensible array of nutritional and healthcare products and modalities—the freedom of choice.

Truly the medicine of the future is within reach. It is now up to all of us to grab the brass ring.

Philip Lee Miller, M.D.
Los Gatos, California
February, 2005

Index

About the Authors

Dr. Philip Lee Miller, M.D., founder and medical director of the Los Gatos Longevity Institute, has been in practice for over twenty-seven years.

He graduated from the University of California, Berkeley, in 1968 with a degree in biochemistry and received his medical degree from the University of California, San Diego, School of Medicine in 1972. He then went on to pursue further training in neurology at the University of California, Davis. He has been board-certified in emergency medicine by the American Board of Emergency Medicine.

More recently, Dr. Miller has emerged as a leader in nontraditional medicine after a close one-year association with Dr. Julian Whitaker of the Whitaker Wellness Institute in Newport Beach, California. He is a charter member of the American Academy for Anti-Aging Medicine and is fully board-certified by the American Board on Anti-Aging Medicine.

In addition, Dr. Miller's associations include the European Academy for Quality of Life and Longevity, the American College for the Advancement in Medicine, and the American Academy of Neurology, as well as the Santa Clara Medical Society and the California Medical Association. He serves as a member of the Life Extension Foundation Medical Advisory Board.

Monica Reinagel has authored and edited numerous books, articles, and other publications on nutrition and holistic medicine. She has served as editorial director of the Health Sciences Institute, an alternative medicine information organization with some 100,000 subscribers around the world, as managing editor for the American Academy of Environmental Medicine's weekly *Medical Digest,* and as an editorial consultant to holistic physicians and the natural products industry.

Her work has been published in *Anti-Aging Medical News, Total Health Magazine, The Townsend Letter for Doctors and Patients,* and others. Previous books include *The Secrets of Evening Primrose Oil* (St. Martin's Press, 2000).

About the
Life Extension Foundation

The Life Extension Foundation (LEF) is a nonprofit organization dedicated to the extension of the healthy human life span. Since 1980, LEF has provided its members with cutting-edge articles on the latest scientific breakthroughs in healthcare and longevity in its monthly *Life Extension* magazine and Web site (www.lef.org). The Foundation also enables its members to obtain hundreds of advanced health-building dietary supplements at discount prices and to have free access to expert advisors. LEF currently has 100,000 members.

LEF integrates the findings of thousands of papers from peer-reviewed medical journals and the recommendations of its medical experts in formulating advanced treatment protocols for aging and age-related diseases such as cancer, heart disease, stroke, Alzheimer's disease, and diabetes. These treatments are posted and updated regularly on LEF's Web site and published in its 1,600-page book *Disease Prevention and Treatment,* now in its fourth edition.

LEF has donated tens of millions of dollars for path-breaking life extension research at laboratories throughout the United States. These include BioMarker Pharmaceuticals (www.biomarkerinc.com), which is discovering longevity genes in order to develop therapies to conquer aging in humans; 21st Century Medicine (www.21CM.com), which is developing advanced methods of cryopreservation for transplantation and suspended animation; and Critical Care Research, which is developing technologies to prevent brain damage and revive patients from clinical death.

LEF has also funded pioneering longevity research at the University of Wisconsin in Madison; the University of California at Riverside; the Mayo Clinic in Rochester, Minnesota; Mt. Sinai Medical Center in New York City; the University of Arkansas in Little Rock; the National Institute on Aging in Baltimore; UCLA Medical Center in Los Angeles; the University of Wyoming; and other institutions.

Anyone who wants a longer, healthier life should consider becoming a member of the Foundation. For further information, LEF can be reached at P.O. Box 229190, Hollywood, Florida 33022; by calling toll-free at 1-877-877-9705; or online at www.lef.org

---

The complete text of *Disease Prevention and Treatment* is available as a free CD to anyone who has purchased *The Life Extension Revolution*. If the postage-paid response card is missing from your book, simply call 1-877-877-9705, and request the CD by mentioning code REV.